1904

MECHANICAL
PROPERTIES
OF BONE

Publication Number 881

AMERICAN LECTURE SERIES

A Monograph in

The BANNERSTONE DIVISION *of*
AMERICAN LECTURES IN ANATOMY

Edited by

ALPHONSE R. BURDI, Ph.D.

Associate Professor of Anatomy
Department of Anatomy
Medical School
The University of Michigan
Ann Arbor, Michigan

MECHANICAL PROPERTIES OF BONE

By

F. GAYNOR EVANS, Ph.D.

Professor of Anatomy
The University of Michigan
Medical School
Ann Arbor, Michigan

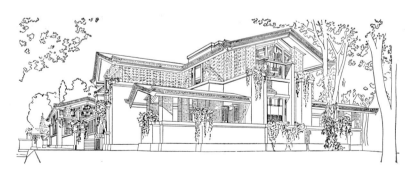

CHARLES C THOMAS · PUBLISHER
Springfield · Illinois · USA

Published and Distributed Throughout the World by

CHARLES C THOMAS • PUBLISHER

Bannerstone House

301-327 East Lawrence Avenue, Springfield, Illinois, U.S.A.

© *1973, by* CHARLES C THOMAS • PUBLISHER

ISBN 0-398-02775-7

Library of Congress Catalog Card Number: 72-93210

*With THOMAS BOOKS careful attention is given to all details of
manufacturing and design. It is the Publisher's desire to present books that are
satisfactory as to their physical qualities and artistic possibilities and
appropriate for their particular use. THOMAS BOOKS will be true to those
laws of quality that assure a good name and good will.*

Printed in the United States of America

C-1

DEDICATION

To the Memory of My Friends

WILFRID T. DEMPSTER AND HERBERT R. LISSNER

PREFACE

During the daily activities of life the bones of the skeleton, individually and collectively, are subjected to a variety of force systems. The response of the bones to these systems is a function, to a large extent, of the mechanical properties of the bones. Of course, the type, magnitude, direction and point of application of the force as well as whether or not it is applied slowly, rapidly, repetitively or for a long duration must also be considered. Additional variables include whether the bone is living or dead, embalmed or fresh, and the age, sex, race and species of animal from which the bone is obtained. The specific bone and part of the bone being studied as well as its microscopic structure influence its mechanical properties as do the amount of moisture in it and the temperature at which the mechanical properties are determined. The effect of all these variables on the mechanical properties of bone, especially that from man, is the subject of this book.

Interest in the mechanical properties of bone is not new but dates at least as far back as 1638 when Galileo Galilei made some comments on the mechanical significance of bone form. After that the subject was more or less forgotten until the latter half of the nineteenth century when the classic studies of Rauber (1876), Messerer (1880), and Hülsen (1896) appeared. The subject was again neglected for some time but within the last few years it has become an active area of research.

Bone is an important tissue component of the human body, constituting 18 percent of the total adult body components compared to 43 percent for muscle, 25 percent for skin and fat, 11 percent for viscera and 3 percent for nervous tissue (Wilmer, 1940). Thus, when studying the mechanical properties of bone one is not dealing with an insignificant component of the body, but one of practical importance to specialists in a variety of fields.

Orthopedic surgeons, neurosurgeons, trauma surgeons, orthodontists, prosthodontists and practitioners of general medicine, surgery, and dentistry are all interested in the influence of forces on the form and structure of bone. Effects of forces exerted on bone by various implants, osteosyntheses, prostheses and arthroplasties are of practical concern to the patient, the surgeon, the dentist, the prosthetist and the physical therapist as well as the designer and manufacturer of the implant device that is used. Pathologists and radiologists are concerned with the effects of various pathological conditions on mechanical properties of bone. Data on the strength characteristics and other mechanical properties of bone might also be useful in the selection of sites for obtaining bone grafts.

A great impetus to research on the mechanical properties of bone, especially its limits of tolerance to various types of impacts, has been created by the recent emphasis on safety in the automobile, aircraft and aerospace industries. Some knowledge of these limits of tolerance is likewise of practical significance to the designers and manufacturers of protective clothing and equipment used in sports such as football, skiing and motor vehicle racing.

The ability of the human body and its components to withstand acceleration and deceleration forces of various magnitudes without severe trauma is of major importance to the safety engineer who must design the automobile, airplane cockpit, or space vehicle to protect the occupant as much as possible from the effects of these forces. In addition to acceleration and deceleration forces encountered in takeoff and landing, the occupant of a space vehicle must also be protected from zero gravitational effects during flight in outer space as well as reduced g forces while on the moon or other celestial bodies.

In all of the aforementioned areas, factual data on the mechanical properties of bone are of considerable practical importance. Such data are also of interest to the anatomist, zoologist, physiologist, anthropologist, physicist, crystallographer and bioengineer. Investigators in these fields are interested in the mechanical properties of bone for a variety of reasons. The biological scientists want to know how the mechanical properties of bone are influenced by age, sex, race, state of health, species and histological structure. The physical scientists are interested in these properties from the viewpoint of the effects of various loading rates, directions, viscoelastic properties, etc., of bone.

Mechanical properties of bone can be studied in whole bones or in bone specimens of a standardized size and shape. In the first method bone is being studied as a structural unit or member while in the second method it is studied as a material. Both methods have advantages and disadvantages. Using intact bones has the advantage of more nearly representing living conditions in which various forces act on whole bones. However, it is very difficult to determine mechanical properties of intact bones because of their irregular shapes, cross-sectional areas and curvatures. The second method has the advantage of eliminating the variables just mentioned. Furthermore, standardized specimens are commonly used for the determination of the mechanical properties of engineering and structural materials.

For the latter reason, this book is restricted, with few exceptions, to a discussion of mechanical property data obtained from experiments made with bone specimens of standardized size and shape. Mechanical properties of whole bones were discussed in my earlier book *Stress and Strain in Bones,* published by Charles C Thomas in 1957.

The preparation of this book involved the assistance of many people and organizations. Those to whom the author especially wishes to express his appreciation and thanks are: his secretaries and editorial assistants, Mrs. Anita Catron and Mrs. Cheryl Hord; Drs. Verne Roberts, James McElhaney and John Melvin of the Highway Safety Research Institute, for their consultation regarding technical questions in mechanics; Miss Esther Schaeffer of the University of Michigan Statistical Research Laboratory, for assistance in the statistical analysis of my data; Mrs. Jean Barnard, University of Michigan Medical Center Library, for aid in obtaining older references; Myron Brownie and David Kikuchi, research assistants, for preparation of some of the tables and illustrations; all the authors and publishers of the various books and journals for their generosity in allowing me to use illustrations from their pubications.

My own research has been supported, in part, by grants from the National Institutes of Health, U.S.P.H.S.

Ann Arbor, Michigan   F. GAYNOR EVANS

CONTENTS

MECHANICAL
PROPERTIES
OF BONE

CHAPTER 1

SOME BASIC CONCEPTS OF MECHANICS

MECHANICS, THE BRANCH of physical science dealing with the effect of forces upon the form or motion of bodies (the state of rest being a special type of motion), consists of two subdivisions: statics and dynamics. *Statics,* the study of bodies at rest or in equilibrium, deals with balanced forces that cause no change in the motion of the body upon which they act. *Dynamics,* the study of moving bodies, is subdivided into kinematics and kinetics. *Kinematics,* the science of motion, describes the relations among displacements, velocities, and accelerations in all kinds of motion without regard to the forces involved. *Kinetics* deals with moving bodies and the forces causing the movement.

One of the basic concepts of mechanics is that of force. A *force* is anything that tends to change the state of a body with respect to motion or the relative position of the molecules composing the body. More simply stated, a force is a push or a pull. The effect of a force upon a body to which it has been applied depends upon (1) the magnitude of the force, (2) the position of the action line of the force within the body, and (3) the direction of the force along the action line. A force is described by these three characteristics.

For every force there is an equal and opposite force (or several forces) whose effect is equivalent to an equal and opposite force (Newton's Third Law of Motion). When a force is balanced by an equal and opposite force or its equivalent, the body is in equilibrium. Such a body remains at rest or continues to move at a uniform rate until some other force obstructs it or changes its rate and direction of motion (Newton's First Law of Motion).

Several different units have been used to measure the magnitude of a force. In the English-speaking countries force is commonly measured in *pounds* (or tons), but in many other countries it is measured in *kilograms.* A *pound of force* is the force necessary to support a one-pound weight (mass) against gravity, or the force that gives a freely falling body a standard acceleration of 32.1740 feet per second per second (32 ft/sec²). A *kilogram of force* is the force necessary to support a one-kilogram weight against gravity, or the force that gives a freely falling body a standard acceleration of 980.665 centimeters per second per second (980 cm/sec²). Many investigators object to the use of pounds and kilograms as units of force because they are also units of mass. In order to avoid ambiguity, the terms *pound force* and *kilogram force* are recommended.

Force is also measured in terms of dynes, poundals, kiloponds, and Newtons. A *dyne* is the force that gives one gram of mass an acceleration of one centimeter per second per second (1 cm/sec²). The force that gives a one-pound mass an acceleration of one foot per second per second (1 ft/sec²) is a *poundal.* A *kilopond* (Kp) is the force required to give a one-kilogram mass an acceleration of 9.80665 meters per second per second (9.8 m/sec²). Consequently, force in kiloponds is equivalent to force in kilograms. A *Newton* is the force required to give one kilogram of mass an acceleration of one meter per second per second (1 m/sec²). Gravitational forces give accelerations varying between 9.78 and 9.83 m/sec².

There are three types of pure force—tension, compression, and shear—each of which is recognized by the effect produced in the body to which the force is applied (Fig. 1). A *tension* (tensile) force tends to lengthen the body to which it is applied, while a *compression* (compressive) force has a tendency to shorten the body. A *shear* force tends to make one part of a body slide in a direction opposite to that of an adjacent part. Except in outer space

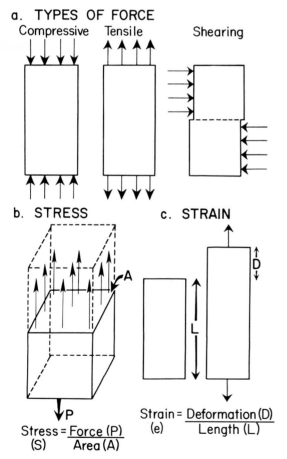

Figure 1. Types of pure force; stress and strain. (Slightly modified from Evans, *Ann NY Acad Sci,* 1955)

a body is also subjected to the force of gravity.

Another basic concept of mechanics is that of stress and strain (Fig. 1), phenomena occurring within a body to which a force has been applied.

Strain is the change in the linear dimensions of a body as the result of the application of a force. Usually strain is invisible but it can be seen if it is sufficiently large, e.g. the stretching of a rubber band. The type of strain in a body is the same as the type of force producing it. Strain is dimensionless but it is frequently recorded as inches per inch, centimeters per centimeter, or percentage.

The tendency of a body to be deformed by the application of a force is resisted by an internal force among the molecules composing the body. The ratio of this internal or restoring force to the area upon which the force is assumed to act is *stress* (Dees, 1945). Since stress is a ratio, i.e. force per unit area (Timoshenko and Young, 1962), it can never be seen, no matter how large, and can only be computed in terms of force (load) per unit area. The kind of force (tensile, compressive, shearing, etc.) applied to a body produces the same kind of stress within the body.

"Stress" is often used synonymously with "strength." However, to speak of the "strength" of a body or of a material has little significance unless the specific type of strength (tensile, compressive, shearing, torsion, or bending) is designated.

The "breaking strength" of a body is often thought to be the same as the "breaking load" but the two phenomena are quite different. For example, suppose a column with a cross section of 1.5 inches by 0.25 inch supported a compressive load of 4,000 lb before it broke. The "breaking load" for the column is 4,000 lb, but its compressive "breaking strength" is 10,700 lb/in² (force or load divided by area). If another column of the same material but a cross section of 2 inches by 4 inches failed under a similar load, its "breaking load" would likewise be 4,000 lb, but its "breaking strength" would be only 500 lb/in². This also illustrates the point that the larger the area over which a force is acting the smaller the stress.

The values for the various strength characteristics and the modulus of elasticity of bone are usually given in pounds per square inch (lb/in² or psi), kilograms per square centimeter (kg/cm²), or kilo-grams per square millimeter (kg/mm²). Some recent investigators have expressed the strength of bone in dynes per square centimeter (dynes/cm²).

When the stresses produced in a body by the application of a force are plotted against the corresponding strains, a *stress-strain curve* or *diagram* is obtained (Fig. 2). The slope of this curve is a general indication of the modulus of elasticity (E) of the body or material. *Modulus of elasticity* is the ratio between unit stress and unit strain and is a measure of the *stiffness* of a material, *not* its elasticity as might be assumed from its name. *Stiffness* is the property of a material enabling it to resist

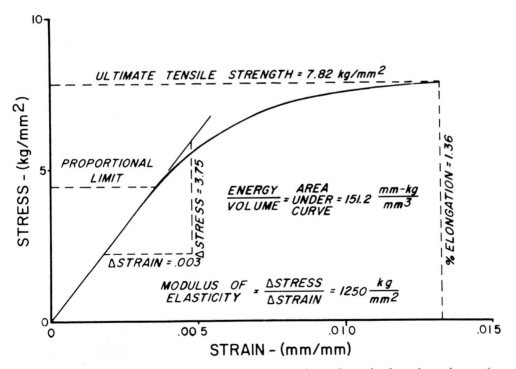

Figure 2. Stress-strain curve for a cortical bone specimen from the lateral quadrant of the distal third of the femur of a 66-year-old white man.

being deformed when a force is applied to it. *Deformation,* the change in the shape of a body, is essentially the same as strain.

The value for the modulus of elasticity, computed in terms of load per unit area (lb/in², kg/cm², or dynes/cm²), is obtained by drawing a tangent to the straightest part of the stress-strain curve (Fig. 2) and dividing the unit stress by the unit strain. The value thus obtained is called the tangent *modulus of elasticity* (Young's modulus) and is the one most commonly used in studies on bone. There is a second type of modulus, the *secant modulus of elasticity,* which is based on a straight line connecting the beginning and the end of a stress-strain curve or two points on the curve.

From the stress-strain curve of a material one can usually determine (1) the *proportional limit* or the limit to which stress and strain are proportional, (2) the *elastic limit* or the limit at which the greatest stress can be applied without leaving a permanent deformation upon removal of the load, (3) the *yield point* or point at which deformation occurs without any increase in load, (4) the *perfect elastic range,* that part of the curve between its beginning and the proportional limit, (5) the *range of plastic deformation,* that part of the curve from the proportional limit to the yield point or failure, (6) the *breaking point,* and (7) the amount of *energy absorbed* by the specimen before it fails. However, all these data cannot always be obtained from the stress-strain curve of every material.

Elasticity, the property that enables a body to return to its original size and shape after removal of a load or force, is another phenomenon encountered in materials testing. There is great variation in the elasticity of different materials and no

material, not even a rubber band, is perfectly elastic.

Hardness, the capacity of one solid to penetrate or scratch another solid or to be penetrated by or scratched by another solid, is an additional concept to be considered. The hardness of a material can be determined with several different kinds of hardness testing machines. The magnitude of the hardness is indicated by an arbitrary (hardness) number which varies with the type of hardness tester used. In general, the larger the hardness number the harder is the material. The hardness of bone and of teeth has usually been determined by penetration or scratch methods.

Ordinarily the harder a material the more brittle it is. A *brittle* material is one that can withstand only a small amount of deformation (strain) before breaking, while a *ductile* material undergoes a large amount of deformation before breaking. Glass and copper are brittle and ductile materials, respectively.

Other concepts involved in a study of the mechanical properties of a material are inertia, mass, weight, and density. *Inertia,* a fundamental characteristic of all matter, is the property that causes a body to remain at rest or in uniform motion in one direction unless acted upon by an external force that changes the body with respect to the state of rest, velocity, or direction.

The *mass* of a body is the quantity of material composing it or "anything which requires a force to cause it to accelerate" (Dees, 1945). Mass is a quantitative measure of the inertia of a body and is involved in Newton's Second Law of Motion which states that the acceleration of a particle (or a body) is proportional to the unbalanced force acting upon it and inversely proportional to the mass of the particle.

Thus, a big push accelerates a small body rapidly while a small push accelerates a big body slowly. Mass is an unchanging property as long as a body retains its original condition.

The *weight* of a body is a measure of the gravitational attraction of the earth on the body and is dependent upon the elevation at which the weight of the body is determined. Thus, a body would weigh more at sea level than it would on top of a mountain but its mass would be the same in both situations. At the surface of the earth the weight of a body is proportional to—but *not equal to*—the mass of the body.

Density, or the concentration of matter, is related to weight, mass, and volume. The *weight density* of a body is its weight per unit volume and is the type usually meant by the term "density." However, there is also a *mass density* or the mass of a body per unit volume (Dees, 1945). The concept of density applies to gases and liquids as well as to solids.

Density is often used interchangeably with specific gravity although the two are not quite the same. *Specific gravity* is the ratio of the mass (or weight) of a body or material to the same mass (or weight) of an equal volume of water at a temperature of $4°$ C. At this temperature the density of water is one, thus making the specific gravity and the density of a material (or body) equal. However, if the density of water is determined at a temperature other than $4°$ C, the values for the specific gravity and density of a material are different.

Momentum, velocity, and acceleration, because of their relation to forces, are also involved in the determination of the mechanical properties of a material. *Momentum* is a function of the mass and of the velocity of a force. *Velocity* is the time rate of change in a given direction while *acceleration* is the time rate of change in velocity.

Another basic concept of mechanics is *time*. This is a factor that is especially significant in the mechanics of fracture because a body, e.g. a bone, can support a greater load before failing if the load is slowly rather than rapidly applied. The importance of the time factor in fracture mechanics was demonstrated by Evans et al. (1958) in their studies on the relation of energy, velocity, and acceleration to skull deformation and fracture. They showed that not only the magnitude of the available kinetic energy (g's) but also the time rate of absorption of the energy are important in the mechanism of skull fracture. Thus, a peak impact acceleration of 686 g's with a total time duration of 0.009 sec produced no skull fracture, while a similar acceleration of only 344 g's and a total time duration of 0.004 sec resulted in a fracture.

There are two kinds of quantities in the world: scalar and vector. A *scalar* quantity has magnitude only, e.g. area, volume, work, money, energy, while a *vector* quantity has both magnitude and direction, e.g. force, velocity, acceleration, momentum. A vector quantity can be represented wholly or in part by a directed, straight line. Thus, the direction of a force can be indicated by an arrow, drawn parallel to the action line of the force, and its magnitude by the length of the arrow according to some arbitrary scale.

One of the most fundamental concepts of mechanics is that of *energy* or the capacity of a body to do work. The magnitude of the energy done by a body can be determined by multiplying the mass (or weight) of a body by the distance through which it operates. For example, if a 100-lb steel ball is dropped through a distance of 20 ft, it does 2,000 ft-lb of work (or energy). The effect of the energy or work done by a body varies with the magnitude of the energy, the time or duration of its action, and the material or object upon which work is done. If the steel ball in the above example were dropped upon soft ground, most of the available energy in the ball would be transferred to the ground and expended in embedding the ball in the ground. However, if the ball were dropped upon a steel stake, there would be relatively little transfer of energy from the ball to the stake and most of the energy in the ball would be expended in driving the stake into the ground.

The energy involved in the falling ball is *kinetic* energy or energy due to motion. The energy due to the position of one body with respect to another body or to the relative parts of the same body is called *potential* energy.

Lissner and Evans (1956) pointed out that all physical injuries of a human body arise from the absorption of energy which can occur in one of three ways: (1) the resting head (or other part of the body) which is free to move can be struck by a moving object, (2) the moving head can strike a resting object, or (3) the moving head can strike or be struck by a moving object. In the first case, the resting head would be accelerated; in the second case, the moving head would be decelerated (what the engineers call negative acceleration); and in the third case, the head can be either accelerated or decelerated depending upon whether the head or the other object is moving faster, and also upon the relative masses and direction of each. Provided the site of the blow and the relative velocity between the head and the striking object are the same, the injury will be identical for the three conditions.

By measuring the area beneath the stress-strain curve with a compensating polar planimeter, one can compute the amount of energy (in-lb or kg-cm) which the body or the material absorbed before it failed (Fig. 2). The energy-absorbing capacity of bone is especially important in fractures, the vast majority of which arises from impacts and, thus, are problems in energy absorption.

Some understanding of the concepts briefly discussed is essential for an appreciation of biomechanical studies of bones and bone. During the daily activity of any vertebrate animal the bones of the skeleton, collectively and separately, are subjected to a variety of force systems arising from body movements, static and dynamic support, gravity, impacts of various sorts, and forces exerted on the skeleton by the contained viscera. Thus, the surrounding bones of the skull are subjected to forces exerted on them by the brain, the eyeballs, and the tongue; the thoracic skeleton to forces arising from the lungs, the heart, and other thoracic viscera; and the bony pelvis to forces produced by the urinary bladder, the uterus, the colon, and the rectum. Blood vessels also apply force to adjacent elements, in some cases producing grooves or even tunnels in the bone against which they lie.

The size, the shape, and the structure (both gross and microscopic) of the bones of the human sekeleton are quite well known but the strength and other mechanical properties of bone have been less thoroughly investigated. This is particularly true with respect to the influence of biological factors, such as species, age, sex, diet, and state of health, on the mechanical properties of bone. Even less information is available on the relation of the microscopic structure of bone to its mechanical properties.

The properties of bone (osseous tissue) with which this book is concerned can be classified into two main categories—mechanical and physical. Although the terms "mechanical and physical properties" are often used interchangeably, they are not the same. According to the American Society for Testing and Materials (ASTM), *mechanical* properties are "those properties of a material that are associated with elastic and inelastic reaction when force is applied, or that involve the relationship between stress and strain" (1966). Examples of the mechanical properties of bone are all kinds of strength (stress) and strain, modulus of elasticity, fatigue life, creep, and hardness. *Physical* properties would include density and specific gravity as well as optical properties and electrical phenomena of bone.

CHAPTER 2

METHODS OF DETERMINING THE MECHANICAL PROPERTIES OF BONE

Bone is a composite, viscoelastic, anisotropic material primarily composed of organic fibers (chiefly collagen), inorganic crystals (hydroxyapatite), cement substance, and water. Although bone is quite different from most engineering materials, the methods and the formulas used for the determination of the mechanical properties of the two classes of materials are the same. However, some of the formulas may not be entirely appropriate for bone because they are based on materials which are usually more homogeneous and isotropic than bone. This is a problem that needs further investigation.

An intact bone in the living body is subjected to a variety of force systems (gravity, muscular activity, static and dynamic support, impacts) which tend to bend and twist it. It would seem logical, therefore, to determine the strength and other mechanical properties of bone from bending and torsion tests. However, for valid reasons which will be discussed, most investigations of the strength and other mechanical properties of bone have been made on standardized specimens tested under a single pure force instead of in bending or in torsion.

When a specimen of any material is tested in bending, its cross-sectional area is subjected to a combination of tensile, compressive, and shearing forces (Fig. 3), none of which is uniformly distributed over the cross-sectional area. The same is true for a part of an intact bone, e.g. the neck of the femur if bent (Fig. 4, Sect. B-B), as pointed out by Zarek (1958).

When a specimen of any material is tested in torsion, the surface of the specimen is subjected to tensile and compressive forces acting at a 45° angle to the long axis of the specimen (Fig. 5), while its cross-sectional area is undergoing torsional shearing stress (Fig. 6). The magnitude of the torsional shearing stress progressively increases from the center to the periphery of the cross section of the specimen. The direction of this stress is the same as that of the force producing the torsion. Thus, in bending and torsion tests it may be difficult to determine the magnitude of the various stresses acting on the specimen, as well as the relative importance of each in causing failure of the specimen.

For the preceding reasons, specialists in the science of materials testing consider bending and torsion to be better tests for evaluating the structure of a material than for determining its mechanical properties.

The preferred method for determining the strength characteristics of a material is to test specimens of a standardized size and shape under a single pure force uniformly distributed over the cross-sectional area of the specimen (Fig. 7). Under these conditions the ultimate breaking stress (strength) of the specimen can easily be computed from the formula

$$S = \frac{P}{A}$$

in which S = stress, P = force, and A = cross-sectional area of the specimen. Subscripts t, c, and s, added to S and A, indicate the type of stress (tensile, compressive, or shearing) involved. The advan-

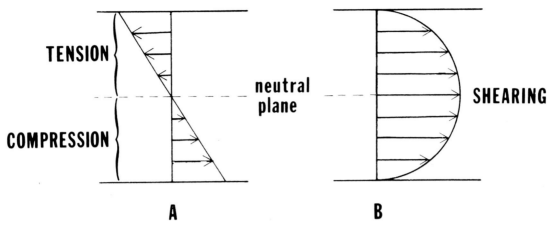

Figure 3. *A*. Tensile and compressive stress distribution over the cross section of a beam type specimen tested in bending. (Modified from Singer: *Strength of Materials.* Courtesy of Harper and Bros.) *B.* Shearing stress distribution over the cross section of a beam type specimen tested in bending. (Modified from Singer: *Strength of Materials.* Courtesy of Harper and Bros.)

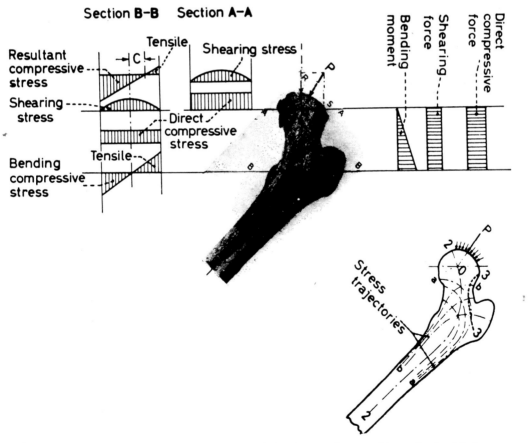

Figure 4. Forces and stresses in the neck of the human femur. (From Zarek: *Modern Trends in Surgical Materials.* Courtesy of Butterworth and Co.)

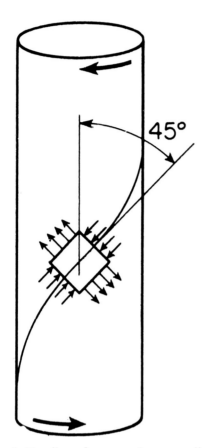

Figure 5. Tensile and compressive stress distribution during torsion in a material, such as bone, which is weaker in tension than in shear. (From Timoshenko and Young: *Elements of Strength of Materials*. Courtesy of D. Van Nostrand Co.)

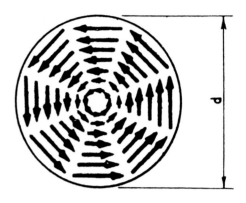

SHEARING STRESS ON CROSS SECTION

Figure 6. Shearing stress on the cross section of a specimen subjected to torsion. The arrows indicate the direction of the shearing stress, which is the same as that of the force producing the torsion. The length of the arrows indicates the magnitude of the shearing stress which progressively increases from the center to the periphery of the specimen. (From Harris: *Strength of Materials*. Courtesy of American Technical Society)

tages of this method, in contrast to testing a specimen in bending or in torsion, are that (1) only one type of force is involved, (2) the cross-sectional area of the specimen is standardized, and (3) the force is uniformly distributed over the cross-sectional area of the specimen.

TENSION, COMPRESSION, AND SHEAR TESTING

All of our determinations on the mechanical properties of bone were based on specimens that had been machined to a standardized size and shape from various parts of the human parietal and major long bones.

The tensile properties of compact (cortical) bone from adult human femurs were determined from elongated flat specimens (Fig. 8A), the middle third of which had a reduced cross-sectional area (Evans and Lebow, 1951, 1952). The tensile strain (percentage elongation) occur-

ring in the reduced region of a specimen during a test was measured over a gauge length of one inch with a Porter-Lipp extensometer calibrated in units of 0.0001 inch. Specially-designed jaws were used to hold the specimen during an experiment (Fig. 9).

The shearing stress of flat bars of cortical bone (Fig. 8C) was also investigated. A special shearing tool to prevent bending held the specimen while a force was applied to the push rod of the tool (Fig. 10).

Elongated flat specimens without a reduced middle region (Fig. 8B) were used in studies on the compressive properties of adult human cortical bone (Evans, 1961a and b). Because of the slenderness of the specimens, a special jig was used to prevent them from buckling during a test (Fig. 11). The jig had a slot on each side so that a Porter-Lipp extensometer, of the same

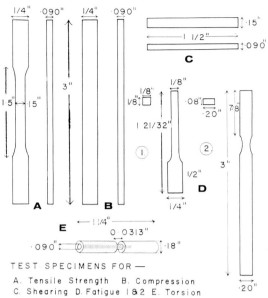

TEST SPECIMENS FOR —

A. Tensile Strength   B. Compression
C. Shearing D. Fatigue 1 & 2 E. Torsion

Figure 8*A-E.* Shape and dimensions of author's test specimens of cortical bone.

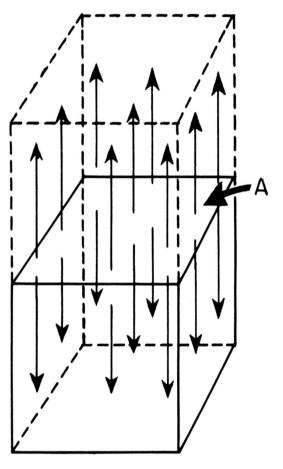

$$\text{Stress} \atop (S) = \text{Force (P)} \atop \text{Area (A)}$$

Figure 7. Uniform stress distribution over the cross section of a specimen tested in pure tension. (From Evans: Instructional Course Lectures, *Am Acad Orthop Surg.* Courtesy of C. V. Mosby)

model as that used in our tension tests, could be attached to each narrow side of the specimen to measure compressive strain.

The ultimate tensile, compressive, and shearing strength of the test specimens was determined by loading them to failure in a 5,000-lb capacity Riehle materials testing machine (Fig. 12) calibrated to an accuracy of ±0.5%. The low-range scale of the machine (0 to 250 lb) was used so that the load was registered in units of 0.5 lb. The specimens were loaded at speeds of 0.035 in/min and 0.045 in/min until failure occurred. Failure was indicated by a sudden decrease in the magnitude of the load registered on the dial of the testing machine. In the tensile and the compressive tests the specimens were loaded in the direction of their long axis, which coincided with that of the shaft of the intact bone, but in the shearing tests the load was applied perpendicular to the long axis of the specimen and to the shaft of the

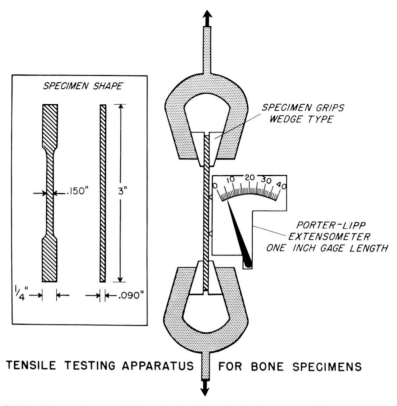

Figure 9. Tensile specimen and jaws for holding it during a test. (From Evans and Lebow: *J Appl Physiol*, 1951)

intact bone. All tests were made at a room temperature of 70° to 75° F and a humidity of 60% to 65%.

During a tensile or compressive test strain readings were taken at regular predetermined load or stress intervals. From the data thus obtained, stress-strain curves were plotted from which the modulus of elasticity of the specimen and the energy it absorbed to failure were calculated.

Directional differences in the tensile stress of human compact bone were investigated by Evans (1964). For this purpose flat tensile specimens, with a reduced middle region, from the major long bones of adults were used. The long axis of some of the specimens coincided with that of the shaft of the intact bone, but in other specimens the long axis was in the radial

or tangential direction with respect to the shaft of the intact bone. The specimens cut in the longitudinal direction had the same dimensions as our regular tensile specimens (Evans and Lebow, 1951, 1952), whereas those cut in the tangential and radial directions were much shorter. All three types of specimens were slowly loaded to failure in the direction of their long axis with the same Riehle testing machine.

Tensile specimens of unembalmed compact bone from the femur of infants and children (Hirsch and Evans, 1965) were flat and of the same general shape as those from adult bones, but much smaller (Fig. 8A). The smallest specimens successfully tested were approximately 25 mm long (with a reduced middle region 5 mm long and 1.3 mm wide), 1 mm thick, and expanded ends 3 mm wide. Special jaws held a specimen while it was loaded to failure, under direct tension, in a Model TT-BM Instron testing machine calibrated to an accuracy of ±1%. The tensile stress was applied to the specimen in the direction of its long axis at a constant speed of 0.1 cm/min. The tests were made at a room temperature of 20° to 22° C and a humidity of 65%.

The tensile strain in the specimens was measured with 3-mm long Budd Metafilm Foil Strain Gauges (Type C12-LXL-M50A), with a gauge factor of 2.01 ± 1% and a resistance of 120 ± 0.5 ohms. A gauge was bonded to a specimen with Eastman 910 cement after the area had been dried with ether. The strain was recorded with a Hottinger Strain Gauge Bridge (Model KWS/T-5) and a Speedomax recorder, using a paper speed of 30 cm/min. Separate stress and strain curves were automatically drawn during a test. From

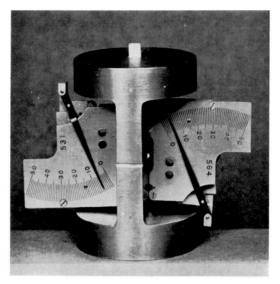

Figure 11. Compression-testing jig with Porter-Lipp extensometers.

these records stress-strain curves were plotted and were used to calculate the tangent modulus of elasticity.

Flat tensile specimens of compact bone of the same general shape as ours but of different sizes were used by Rauber (1876), Hülsen (1896), Carothers et al. (1949), Coolbaugh (1952), Currey (1959, 1962), Dempster and Coleman (1960), McElhaney et al. (1964), Sedlin (1965), Sweeney et al. (1965), and Bonfield and Li (1966). In similar investigations by Yamada (1941), Dempster and Liddicoat (1952), Kimura (1952), Ko (1953), Oda (1955a and b), Uehira (1960), and Mack (1964), the test specimens were round rods of compact bone with a reduced middle region. Wertheim (1847) tested long, thin strips of bone.

The compressive strength of cubes of compact bone was determined by Rauber (1876), Hülsen (1896), and Dempster and Liddicoat (1952). Hülsen also tested rings of bone.

In one respect tensile testing is more difficult than compressive testing because

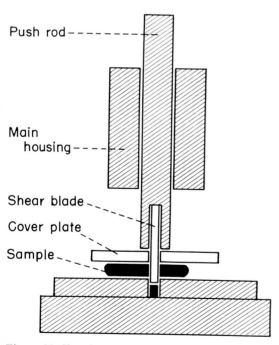

Figure 10. Shearing tool. (From Evans and Lebow: *J Appl Physiol,* 1951)

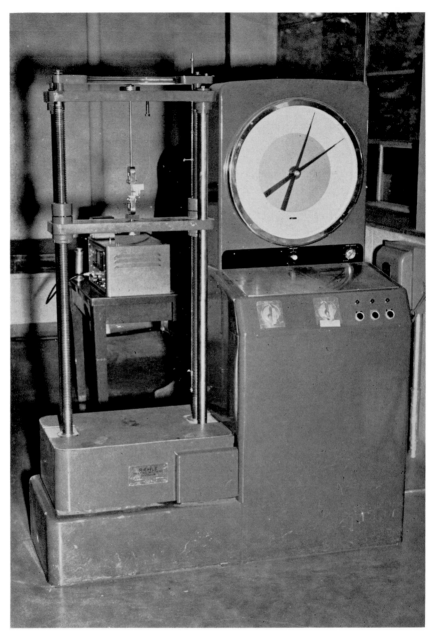

Figure 12. Riehle 5000-lb capacity materials testing machine. (From Evans and Lebow: *Am J Surg*, 1952)

jaws are required to hold a specimen in the testing machine. In order to prevent the specimen from slipping during a test, the jaws usually have two or more chucks with serrated faces so that the grip on the specimen tightens with increasing tension. Sometimes a pin is put through each end of the specimen to hold it.

Tensile specimens must be straight and in alignment with the jaws of the testing machine to ensure that the tensile force is uniformly distributed over the cross-sectional area of the specimen. Reducing the cross-sectional area of the middle part of the specimen concentrates the stress so that failure will occur there. The tensile strain is also measured in the reduced region. In our experiments a test was not considered to be a valid one unless the specimen failed between the gauge marks of the Porter-Lipp extensometer. The fillet, the junction between the reduced and the nonreduced parts of the specimen, should have as large a radius of curvature as possible to decrease stress concentration in that region.

Good compression tests are much more difficult to make than is generally realized. The test specimen must be a cube or, if an elongated specimen is used, straight. Furthermore, the opposite ends of the specimen must be parallel and as smooth as it is possible to make them. If these conditions are not met, the compressive force will not be uniformly distributed over the cross-sectional area of the specimen during a test.

Although it is easier to test cubes in compression than elongated specimens, the cubes tend to be squeezed out from between the heads of the testing machine. In resisting this tendency, quite a high frictional force may develop between the specimen and the heads of the machine. An additional problem is that the upper part of the cube may become impacted into the lower part. When this occurs, abnormally high values for compressive stress and strain may be found. For these reasons we used elongated flat specimens instead of cubes.

When elongated circular or rectangular specimens are used for determining the compressive stress of bone, the effects of column action must be considered. A column is a relatively slender, compression-resisting member, the strength of which,

provided it is composed of homogeneous material and without regard to its size and shape, depends upon (1) the material composing the column, (2) the cross-sectional area of the column, (3) the shape of the cross section of the column, (4) the restraints at the ends of the column, and (5) if the column is circular, the ratio of the smallest diameter of the column to its total length. Although these factors are interdependent to some extent, the cross-sectional shape of the column is the most important one. Thus, a hollow cylinder will support more weight without bending than will a solid column of the same shape and composed of the same kind and the same amount of material.

Because it is impossible to apply a force or load to the exact center of the cross-sectional area of a column, there is always a certain load *(buckling load)* at which buckling or bending of the column will occur. The buckling load for a column is a function of its material, its length, its cross section, and the way it is restrained. The magnitude of the buckling load is directly proportional to the modulus of elasticity of the material composing the column, and inversely proportional to the square of the length of the column. For example, a column twice as long as another of the same material and same cross section has a buckling load only one-fourth as large. A column restrained at both ends will support a load four times greater before buckling than will an unrestrained column of the same length, material, and cross-sectional area. A column restrained at only one end has a buckling load four times less than that of the same column when restrained at both ends (Salvadori and Heller, 1963).

An important characteristic of a column is its *slenderness ratio*, or the ratio of the total length of the column to its least radius of gyration. A slender column, i.e. one with a high slenderness ratio, will buckle at stresses below the yield point of the material and will straighten out after removal of the load provided the elastic limit of the material is not exceeded. The classification of a compression member as a slender column varies with the composition of the column. For instance, a steel column which has a slenderness ratio above 150 and an aluminum- or magnesium-alloy column with a slenderness ratio above 80 are both classified as slender columns.

The load that causes buckling in a simply-supported slender column is called the *critical load*. The column will support the critical load while it is bent but it will fail with any increase in the load. The working load is the load the column will support without buckling failure.

When buckling occurs, the convex side of the bent column or specimen is subjected to tensile stress and strain while the concave side is undergoing compressive stress and strain. Because the stresses are not uniformly distributed over the cross-sectional area of the specimen, it is more difficult to determine the magnitude of each type of stress than if the specimen were tested in pure tension or compression.

In pure shearing tests the magnitude of the shearing stress, provided the shearing force is parallel to the cross section of the specimen, can be computed from the same formula used for pure tension and compression tests. However, the major difficul-

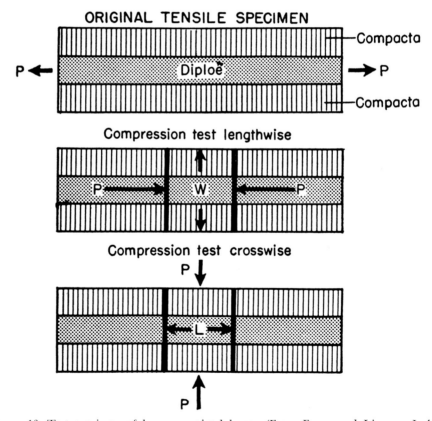

Figure 13. Test specimen of human parietal bone. (From Evans and Lissner: *J Appl Physiol*, 1957)

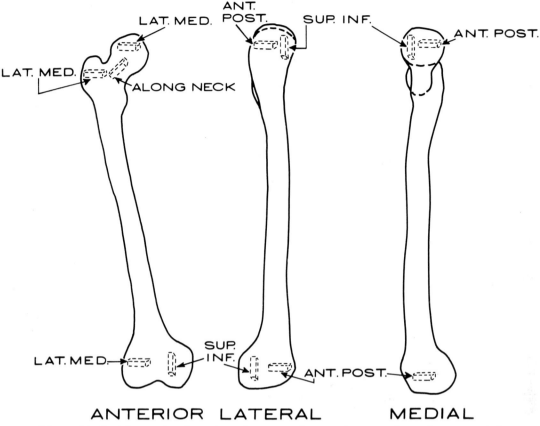

Figure 14. Position and orientation of test specimens of spongy bone from an adult human femur. (From Evans and King: in *Biomechanical Studies of the Musculo-Skeletal System*. Courtesy of Charles C Thomas, Publisher)

ty in computing the shearing stress value is in obtaining an accurate determination of the cross-sectional area upon which the shearing stress is acting.

When a specimen of any material, of uniform cross-sectional area throughout its length, is subjected to a pure tensile or compressive force which is uniformly distributed over the cross-sectional area, the specimen will be either elongated or shortened by the force applied to it. The ratio between the longitudinal deformation (lengthening or shortening) and the lateral deformation (increase or decrease in width or thickness) of the specimen is called *Poisson's ratio*. This is a phenome-

non that has rarely been investigated in bone.

The tensile and compressive strength of standardized specimens of human parietal bone have also been studied (Evans and Lissner, 1957). The test specimens were rectangular bars, composed of the outer and inner skull tables of compact bone separated by diploë (Fig. 13). Since it was necessary to have straight specimens, there was considerable variation in the orientation of the specimens with respect to the intact parietal bone.

Tensile tests were made in a direction parallel to the long axis of the parietal specimens but compression tests were made both lengthwise and crosswise to the long axis of the specimens. All the specimens were stored in a physiological saline solution and tested while wet in the same Riehle testing machine used for the tensile, compressive, and shearing tests of the specimens from the long bones.

Regional and directional differences in the compressive strength and associated mechanical properties of spongy bone from embalmed adult human femurs were likewise investigated (Evans and King, 1961). Ninety-one standardized specimens and sixteen cubic specimens were tested. The standardized specimens were 2.5 cm long and 0.79 cm on each side, with a slenderness ratio of about 11.4. The cubic specimens were 0.79 cm on each side. Data from the latter specimens were not used, however, because of the difficulties already discussed in testing cubes.

Standardized specimens, taken from various parts of the femur (Fig. 14), were loaded in the direction of their long axis.

The specimens were kept in a physiological saline solution and tested wet by slowly loading them to failure in the aforementioned Riehle testing machine. A minimum of twenty load-deformation readings was taken for each specimen during a test. Failure was indicated by a sudden dropping of the load registered on the dial of the testing machine.

The stress-strain characteristics of spongy bone from vertebrae have been investigated by Göcke (1928), Yokoo (1952a), and Sonoda (1962). Similar studies on cubes of spongy bone from different parts of the femur were made by Knese (1958). Hardinge (1949) made one-fourth inch thick cross sections of the head and neck of ninety-four embalmed adult human femurs and then recorded the force required to punch out checker-shaped pieces of spongy bone. Contrary to his belief, Hardinge determined the breaking load instead of the breaking strength, i.e. force per unit area, of his specimens.

TORSION TESTING

When a *twisting* or *torsion* force is applied to a body, tensile and compressive stresses are produced on the surface of the body and torsional shearing stresses on the cross section of the body. The tensile and compressive stresses act at approximately a 45° angle to the long axis of the body (Fig. 5), whereas the shearing stress is perpendicular to the long axis. The direction of the shearing stress on the cross section of the body (Fig. 6) is the same as that of the force producing the torsion. The magnitude of the *twisting moment* (torque) is determined by multiplying the magnitude of the twisting force by the perpendicular distance of the force from the axis about which twisting occurs.

If a straight line is drawn on the surface of a circular bar, parallel to its long axis (Fig. 15), and a twisting force is applied to the right end of the bar while the left end is fixed, the line will be displaced from its original position (A) to a new position (B). The angle between the radius drawn from line A and the radius drawn from line B is the *angle of twist*, i.e. the angle through which the right end of the bar is actually twisted.

If a material is weaker in longitudinal than in transverse shearing, the first cracks arise from axial shearing stresses and appear in a longitudinal direction on the surface of the body. However, if the material is weaker in tension than in shear,

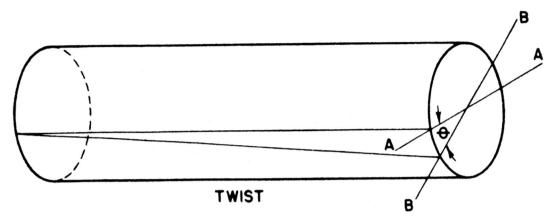

TWIST

Figure 15. Angle of twist in a circular specimen subjected to torsion. (From Harris: *Strength of Materials*. Courtesy of American Technical Society)

it usually cracks along a spiral course inclined at a 45° angle to the long axis of the body. The reason for this is that a state of pure shear is equivalent to a state of tension in one direction and of compression in the opposite direction (Fig. 5). The tension stresses produced the spiral crack in the body.

The torsional properties of compact bone from adult human femurs (Evans, 1964) were determined from cylindrical specimens, which were made with a hole extending three-fourths of their length and a notch encircling their middle (Fig. 8E). In the region of the notch the walls of the specimens had a uniform thickness of 0.150 inch (3.81 mm). The notch concentrated the stress in that area so that the specimens tended to fail from torsional shearing stress instead of tensile stress. The long axis of the specimens coincided with that of the intact bone.

A special torsion jig (Fig. 16) was designed for testing the specimens. The torsion (twisting) force was applied to a specimen by placing weights on a pan which was suspended by a thread wrapped around the rim of a wheel. Two sets of jaws gripped the specimen while being tested. One set of jaws was fixed while the other set rotated with the wheel so that a twisting force was applied to the specimen. The axis about which torsion occurred passed longitudinally through the center of the specimen. Graduated marks on the wheel indicated the angle of twist that occurred in a specimen during a test. The specimens were kept in a physiological saline solution and tested while still wet. The cross-sectional dimensions of the specimens were measured before and after testing to note any effects of swelling.

From the data obtained in the torsion tests a torque vs angle of twist curve (Fig. 17) was plotted for each specimen. From this curve the *shear modulus of elasticity* (G) was calculated and the energy absorbed to failure was determined by measuring the area beneath the curve.

The torsional properties of solid cylinders of compact bone from the middle third of the shaft of beef femurs were determined by Sweeney et al. (1965). The specimens were taken within the cortex between the outer and the inner circumferential lamellae. The long axis of the specimen coincided with that of the intact bone.

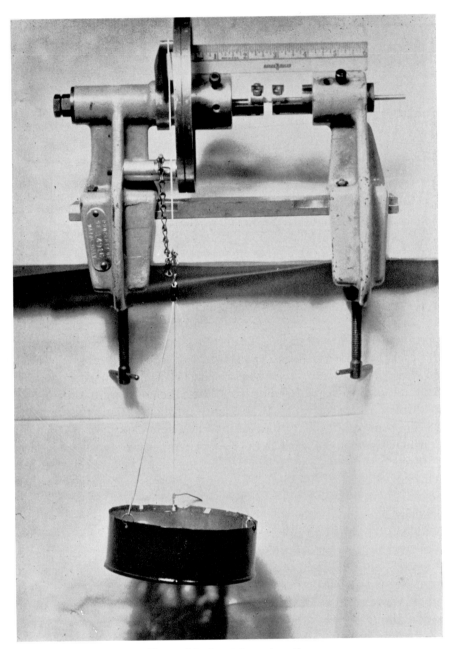

Figure 16. Special torsion jig.

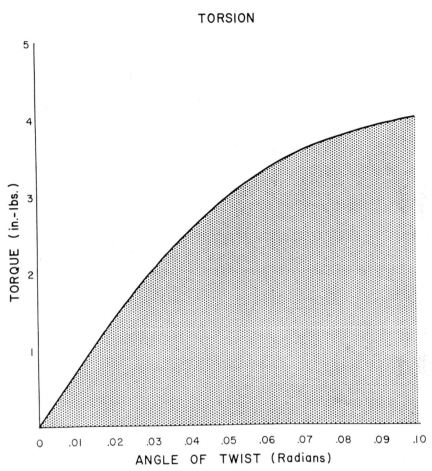

Figure 17. Torque-angle of twist curve for wet specimen of human cortical bone.

FATIGUE TESTING

Fatigue is a well-known phenomenon occurring in engineering structures, most of which are subjected to variations in the applied loads. Such variations cause fluctuations in the stresses of different parts of a structure. If these fluctuating stresses are sufficiently large, failure of a structure may occur provided the stress is repeated often enough. Failure can occur even if the magnitude of the applied stress is considerably less than the static strength of the material. A failure produced by repetitive loading of a material or a structure is called a "fatigue failure," e.g. the breaking of a wire after it has been bent back and forth several times.

Numerous tests have been developed for evaluating the endurance limit of various metals, and certain kinds of machines, specimens, and procedures are in common use. However, the American Society for Testing and Materials (ASTM) has no standardized endurance test for metals. For the classification and description of the different kinds of "repeated" stresses and detailed information on fatigue testing, see Davis et al. (1964).

During the daily activities of life the bones of the skeleton are repeatedly subjected to stress by gravity and muscle action. The response of the bones to this repetitive loading is important in understanding the nature of the so-called "fatigue," "stress," or "march" fracture. Such a fracture usually appears as a hair-line crack in a roentgenogram and often there is no history of trauma in the patient. Fatigue fractures are most commonly seen in the metatarsals, especially the second one, where they are called "march" fractures in the belief that they arise from the repeated loading of the bones during marching.

The fatigue life, i.e. the cycles to failure, of standardized specimens of human compact femoral, tibial, and fibular bone, was determined with a Sonntag Flexure Fatigue Machine (Fig. 18) equipped with an automatic counter which recorded the number of cycles to failure, and a shutoff which stopped the machine when failure occurred. The force was applied to the specimen by a rotating eccentric mass which remained constant at any fixed value for eccentricity. An inertia force compensator spring kept the applied force constant irrespective of the flexibility and the amplitude of the bending of the specimen. During a test the expanded end of the specimen was solidly clamped in place while the other end was bent up and down in a plane perpendicular to the long axis of the specimen and to its greatest dimension in the test area (Fig. 19) until failure occurred.

All the specimens in the first study (Evans and Lebow, 1957) were tested at a stress of 5,000 psi (Fig. 8D ②). If failure had not occurred by ten million cycles, the machine was stopped under the assumption that the specimens would have gone to infinity without failing. Water was allowed to drip on the specimens in order to prevent them from drying and to dissipate any heat generated during the test.

In the second study (King and Evans, 1967) the specimens (Fig. 8D ①) were tested at different stresses. For this purpose twelve test specimens, one from each quadrant of the proximal, the middle, and the distal thirds of thirty-one embalmed adult human femurs were used. The specimens were designed so that the maximum stress occurred at a site 0.82 inch (20.83 mm) from the load.

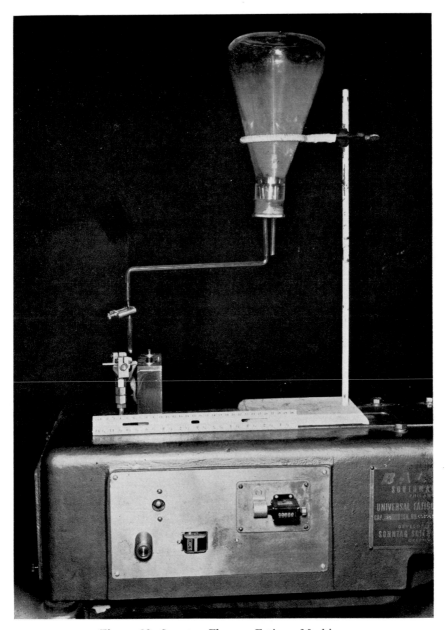

Figure 18. Sonntag Flexure Fatigue Machine.

As the specimens were prepared, they were numbered in sequence from one to twelve. To prevent human judgment from influencing the selection of a specimen for a particular stress level, the twelve specimens from each femur were tested at twelve different stress levels varying from a minimum of 4,375 lbf/in² to a maximum of 11,250 lbf/in² (3.08 kgf/mm² to 7.91 kgf/mm²), with an interval of 625 lbf/in² (0.44 kgf/mm²) between any two stress levels. Thus, specimen number one from the first femur was tested at the maximum stress level, specimen number two at the second highest stress level, etc. Specimen number two from the second femur was tested at the maximum stress level, specimen number three at the second highest stress level, etc., until specimen number one was tested at the minimal stress level. The same procedure was followed with specimens from the other femurs. Consequently, since there were thirty-one femurs, specimens from a specific region (third or quadrant) of a bone were tested at least twice.

While a specimen was being machined, cold air was blown on it to dissipate any heat that might have been generated. Because only a short time was required to machine a specimen, any drying effects produced by the cold air would be insignificant. The limits of accuracy in machining a specimen were well within ±4%. Each specimen was kept in a test tube of physiological saline solution before and after testing. The solution was also used to keep a specimen moist during a test.

The fatigue life of the specimens was determined with three Sonntag Flexure Machines of the same type as that used in the first study. The specimens were tested at a rate of 1,800 cycles/min. However, since the fatigue life of a material is independent of the number of cycles per minute at which it is tested, the specimens would have had the same fatigue life if they had been tested at a rate of only 10 cycles/min. Ten million cycles was selected as the point at which the machine was stopped if failure of the specimen had not yet occurred. A fatigue machine had to run continuously for about four days in order to reach ten million cycles.

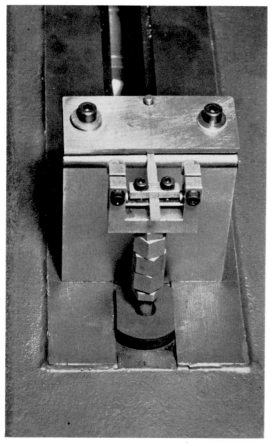

Figure 19. Specimen in Sonntag Flexure Fatigue Machine. (From Evans and Lebow, *J Appl Physiol,* 1957)

The dimensions of each specimen were measured before a test and the machine number, the specimen code, the room temperature, and the relative humidity were noted. The specimens were tested in chronological order. At the end of each test the number of cycles to failure, the specimen number, and the position of the fracture site were recorded.

BENDING TESTS

Bending stress represents a composite of tensile, compressive, and shearing stresses, all of which act on the cross-sectional area of the specimen although none of them is uniformly distributed over the area.

During bending, all the material between the convex surface of the specimen and the neutral plane is subjected to tensile stress while the material between the neutral plane and the concave surface of the specimen is undergoing compressive stress. The magnitude of each type of stress is greatest at the surface of the specimen and decreases to zero at the neutral plane (Fig. 3A). The cross-sectional area of a specimen under bending is also subjected to shearing stress, which has a parabolic distribution over the cross section, being minimal at the surfaces and maximal in the middle of the area (Fig. 3B). Consequently, in bending it is difficult to determine the numerical value for the magnitude of the various kinds of stress and the relative importance of each in the failure mechanism. For these reasons bending is considered to be a rather unsatisfactory test for determining the mechanical properties of a material. In addition to the stresses, a specimen is also subjected to a bending moment.

If a specimen is of uniform dimensions throughout, the bending stress can be calculated from the flexure formula

$$S = \frac{Mc}{I}$$

in which S = maximum stress, M = maximum bending moment on the cross sec-

tion, c = distance from the farthest point in the cross-section to the neutral plane or axis, and I = area moment of inertia of the cross section with respect to the neutral plane through the centroid of the cross section (Harris, 1963).

However, when a specimen is tested under a pure tensile, compressive, or shearing stress, the situation is much simpler because the shearing stress, the neutral plane, the bending moment, and the area moment of inertia are not involved. In this case, the magnitude of the stress is easily calculated from the formula

$$S = \frac{P}{A}$$

in which S = stress, P = force or load, and A = cross-sectional area.

A few investigators have studied the bending properties of bone regardless of its disadvantages. Standardized specimens of cortical bone were tested in bending by Rauber (1876), Maj and Toajari (1937), Olivo et al. (1937), Olivo (1937), Maj (1938a and b), Toajari (1938), Sedlin (1965), and several Japanese investigators (Yamada, 1970).

IMPACT TESTING

Engineering materials are sometimes studied under impact conditions because their behavior when tested under rapidly applied loads is often quite different from that under static, or slowly applied loads. As the velocity of the striking body is changed, there is a transfer of energy from the striker to the test object upon which work is done. The mechanics of impact not only include the induced stresses but also the transfer, the absorption, and the dissipation of energy. As pointed out by Davis et al. (1964), in impact testing a distinction should be made between problems primarily concerned with elastic

energy absorption and those pertaining to energy capacity at failure. The general applicability of the results of ordinary impact tests is limited by this fact. The most commonly used impact tests are the "notch-bar" tests in which only the energy necessary to cause fracture is determined. The energy concentration produced in a specimen by a notch of various sizes and shapes is studied in these tests.

In addition to the conventional methods of studying the bending strength of compact bone, the Japanese have determined its impact bending and snapping strength (Yamada, 1970).

HARDNESS

Although the general concept of hardness, as the quality of matter concerned with solidity and firmness of outline, is easily understood, there is no single method of measuring it that is applicable to all materials. According to Davis et al. (1964), there are five arbitrary "definitions" of hardness that are used as the basis for different hardness tests of engineering and structural materials. These definitions follow:

1. Indentation hardness or the resistance to permanent indentation under static or dynamic loading,
2. Rebound hardness or the energy absorbed under impact loading,
3. Scratch hardness or the resistance to scratching,
4. Wear hardness or the resistance to abrasion,
5. Machinability or the resistance to cutting and drilling.

The indentation hardness of a material can be measured with a Brinell or a Vickers hardness tester. The Brinell hardness number (Bhn) is based on the area of an indentation produced by loading a steel ball of known dimensions. The actual hardness number is computed from the formula

$$Bhn = \frac{P}{\pi Dt}$$

in which P = load, t = depth of indented area (millimeters), and D = diameter of steel ball (millimeters). The depth of the indentation is measured as soon as the load is removed.

The Vickers hardness number (Vhn) is calculated from the ratio P/A in which P = load (kilograms) and A = area of indentation (square millimeters). The indenter is a square-based diamond pyramid with an angle of 136° between the opposite faces. The load can be varied from 5 to 120 kg in 5-kg increments. The diagonal of the square indentation produced in a test is measured to 0.001 mm. The machine can also use 1 mm- and 2 mm-steel balls as indenters. One advantage of the Vickers over the Brinell method is that the diagonal of the square can be measured more accurately than the diameter of a circle where measurements must be made between two tangents to the circle.

The Rockwell hardness tester (Fig. 20) measures the resistance of a material to penetration by a hardened steel ball or by a diamond cone. The machine has two scales of value: a B scale if the indenter is a ball and a C scale if it is a diamond cone. With the Rockwell hardness tester a negative hardness value can be obtained if the penetration of the material is less than a certain depth. The Rockwell test has two distinct advantages over the Brinell test: it uses smaller indenters and smaller loads which makes it useful for testing the hardness of materials beyond the scope of the Brinell test, and it is made more quickly and easily than the Brinell test since the Rockwell hardness number (Rhn) can be read directly from the dial of the machine. For these reasons it is widely used in industry.

Rebound hardness tests are essentially indentation tests in which a load is dynamically applied to a specimen. As in most dynamic testing, the methods of calculating the energy absorbed by the specimen are questionable. Consequently, a standard procedure is used and the values obtained are arbitrary. In order to obtain comparable results when testing similar materials, a standardized testing procedure must be used.

Several types of rebound hardness test-

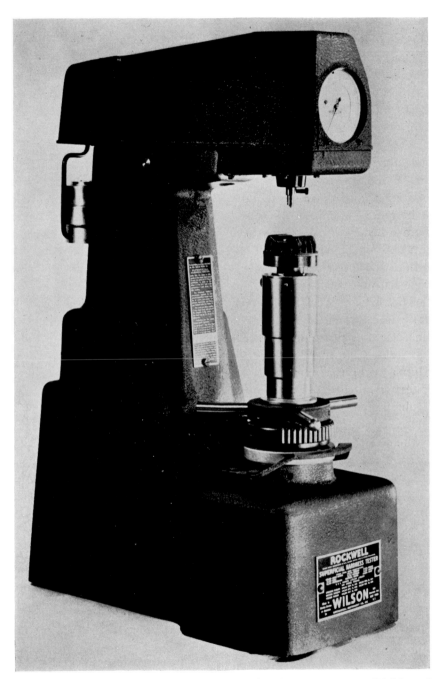

Figure 20. Rockwell hardness tester. (Courtesy of Wilson Instrument Division, American Chain and Cable Co., N.Y.)

ers have been developed by different individuals, but the Shore *scleroscope* is probably the most popular machine at the present time. The scleroscope hardness number (Shn) is equivalent to the height of the rebound of a small hammer within a glass tube, after it has been dropped through a distance of 10 inches onto the surface of the specimen. The standard hammer is about one-fourth inch in diameter, three-fourths inch long, weighs one-twelfth ounce, and has a diamond striking tip with a radius of 0.01 inch. In one type of scleroscope the height of the rebound must be caught by eye but in another type it is recorded on a dial whose hand remains in position until the dial is reset.

The relative hardness of a material can also be determined from scratch hardness tests. Unfortunately, there is no standard scale because there are no materials with an invariable scratch hardness value that can be used for calibration purposes. In scratch hardness tests a quantitative measurement is obtained of (1) the pressure required to make a given scratch in a material or (2) the size of a scratch made by a stylus under a fixed load, as it is drawn across the surface of the material being tested.

The instrument used for making a scratch hardness test is called a *sclerometer*. However, sclerometer tests are not in general use, except for the Bierbaum scratch hardness test for plastics, because they are difficult to standardize and to interpret. In mineralogy the scratch hardness scale most commonly used is the Mohs scale. This is an arbitrary scale in which a mineral that is higher in the scale will scratch a mineral that is lower in the scale.

Wear hardness or abrasion tests have been used for both dry and lubricated metals but have not been adopted except for testing stone and paving bricks. In the Deval abrasion test, the standard one for stone, fifty specimens are "tumbled" in a cylinder to determine the percentage of weight loss. A standard machine and test procedure are utilized. When applicable, the "French coefficient" of wear is calculated by dividing 400 by the wear in grams per kilogram of rock used (see Davis et al., 1964, for further details).

Machinability as a hardness test refers to the ease with which a material can be cut or machined with the usual tools or methods. A material that is easily machined is softer than one that requires specially hardened steel, Carborundum®, or diamond tools to cut it. As far as I am aware, this type of hardness test has not been specifically applied to bone. However, as anyone who has worked with bone knows, it is softer than many engineering materials.

Although cleavage testing was not considered by Davis and his co-workers, it is another method for evaluating the hardness of a material. In this type of test one measures the depth of penetration of a material produced by applying a load to a wedge with a known angle.

In 1951 Evans and Lebow investigated the hardness of human compact bone by means of the *B* scale of the Rockwell Superficial hardness tester. Hardness was measured by applying a 45-kg load for 10 sec to a steel ball one-eighth inch in diameter. All the tests were made on the flat wide surface of the specimen as close to the fracture site as possible. The hardness value was read directly from the dial of the machine—the higher the number, the harder the material. The final hardness value for a single specimen was the average of four tests, two on each side of the specimen.

The hardness (Rockwell or Vickers microhardness) of human and animal compact bone has been determined by Lexer (1928), Carlström (1954), Rosate (1958, 1963), and Amprino (1958, 1961). Rockwell, Vickers, Brinell, scratch, wear (abrasive), and cleavage hardness of compact bone from man and animals was measured by Japanese investigators (Yamada, 1970).

DENSITY AND SPECIFIC GRAVITY

Other factors to be considered in materials testing are the kind, the amount, and the distribution of the material in the specimen being tested. With the same experimental conditions a steel bar behaves differently under a given load than does a wooden bar of the same shape and dimensions because of differences in the mechanical properties of steel and of wood. Similarly a large specimen supports a greater load before breaking than does a small specimen of the same shape and the same kind of material because of the greater amount of material in the large specimen. The distribution of the material is also important. For example, a hollow column is more resistant to bending than a solid column of the same kind and the same amount of material.

The amount of material present in a specimen can be determined from its specific gravity or its density. The *specific gravity* of a specimen can be determined by measuring the amount of water it displaces. *Density,* which can be measured in more than one way, is related to the mass, the weight, and the volume of a material. *Mass density* is the mass of a material per unit volume and *weight density* is the weight of a material per unit volume. The latter is generally meant by the word "density." As discussed in Chapter 1, density and specific gravity are not the same although they are frequently used interchangeably. The specific gravity and the weight density of bone have both been determined by various investigators and methods.

A radioactive Strontium (Sr^{90}) densi-tometer, especially developed for the purpose (Evans et al., 1951a), measured the weight density of our specimens. Strontium^{90}, which is a pure beta ray emitter with a half-life of twenty-five years, was selected because nuclear theory shows that the percentage of beta rays transmitted by any material is proportional to the logarithmic density of the material. Thus, when the log of the intensity (counts per minute) is plotted against the weight per unit area (density × thickness) of the material, a straight line is obtained. Within the maximum and minimum limits of the weight per unit area all materials will fall on this line. Since the concentration of the Sr^{90} was equivalent to approximately 1/100 μc, which is far below the danger thresh-

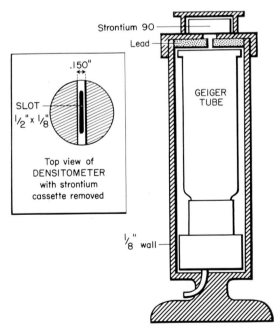

Figure 21. Strontium^{90} densitometer. (From Evans, Coolbaugh, and Lebow: *Science,* 1951)

old for humans, the densitometer could be used without harm to the operator.

The densitometer (Fig. 21) consisted of a TGC2 Geiger tube enclosed in a brass cylinder and a brass cassette for the strontium. The head of the cylinder was lined with lead and had a small groove for the bone specimen which was held in place by clips. At the bottom of the groove there was a slit so that the beta rays, penetrating the part of the specimen overlying the slit, could pass directly to the Geiger tube. The cassette could be adjusted to accommodate specimens of various sizes but when in place it fit tightly on the cylinder head. Reference marks on the cassette and the head of the brass cylinder ensured that the geometry of the strontium and the specimen was always the same. The densitometer was calibrated with four aluminum strips of known density but of varying thicknesses. A Geiger counter connected to an automatic timer (Fig. 22) was used to record the percentage of beta rays transmitted through a bone specimen of known thickness. As a result, a standardized length of time was used for all specimens.

A random (background) counts per minute (cpm), without the strontium or the specimen in place, was taken every day. Then, with the strontium in place the counts per minute was taken for each of the aluminum calibration strips. Three readings were taken for each strip, the final counts per minute being based on the average of all the readings. The background counts per minute was used for all computations. The calibration curve for the aluminum strips was then plotted on semilogarithmic, single-cycle paper (Fig. 23).

With the specimen in place the net

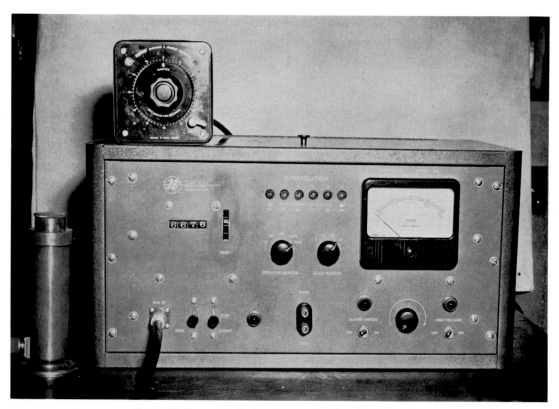

Figure 22. Strontium[90] densitometer with geiger counter.

counts per minute was located on the calibration curve and the weight per unit area (g/cm²) read directly from the curve. Weight per unit area divided by thickness of the specimen gave its density in grams per cubic centimeter. The thickness of the specimen was measured with a micrometer to the nearest 0.0005 inch. A minimum of four thousand counts per specimen was taken. With this method density differences of less than 1% could be detected.

Specimens from adult human femurs, tibias, and fibulas were used for the density measurements of compact bone. All the specimens were air-dried before the measurements were made to avoid the effect of moisture. The same apparatus was used by Evans and King (1961) for evaluating the weight density of standardized specimens of human spongy bone from various regions of the femur. The specimens were dry but this time corrections were not made for air within the spaces of the specimens.

For bone density values obtained by other methods see Garn (1962), Evans (1967), and Blanton and Biggs (1968). Because of its importance in clinical medicine, radiographic density of bones in living subjects has been most extensively studied of all, and has given rise to a vol-

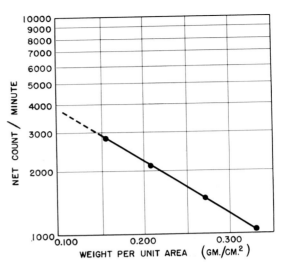

Figure 23. Density calibration curve of aluminum strips. (From Evans, Coolbaugh, and Lebow: *Science,* 1951)

uminous literature with entire books and journals devoted to the subject. Consequently, individual references on radiographic density of bone will not be cited.

Investigations on specific gravity, determined by measuring the amount of water displaced by the bone specimen, have been made by Wertheim (1847), Krause and Fischer (1866), Aeby (1872), Rauber (1876), Hülsen (1896), Gillespie (1954), Woodard (1962), and Blanton and Biggs (1968).

ELECTRICAL PROPERTIES

Bone, like most other biological materials, exhibits electrical phenomena under certain conditions. This is also true of crystals which produce an electric field when they are deformed. The strength of the field, which depends upon the type of crystal being deformed, is proportional to strain. This type of electric field is called *piezoelectricity.*

The electrical potentials produced by deformation of a bone specimen, regardless of whether it is an intact bone or a test piece of a standardized size, are picked up on opposite sides of the specimen by electrodes, which are connected to some type of recording device, e.g. a dynograph, polygraph, oscilloscope, etc.

The "piezoelectric effect" in bone, first reported by Fukada and Yasuda (1957), is dependent upon deformation of the collagen matrix. In 1964 they investigated piezoelectric effects in collagen. Electric phenomena in bone have also been studied by Iida et al. (1956), Iida (1957), Noguchi (1957), Yasuda et al. (1954), Yasuda et al. (1955), Shamos et al. (1963), Shamos and Lavine (1964, 1967), Bassett and Becker (1962), Becker (1963), Basset et al. (1964), Bassett (1965), Becker et al. (1964), Friedenberg and Brighton (1966), McElhaney (1967), Steinberg et al. (1968), and McElhaney et al. (1968). Many of these investigations were made on intact bones.

VISCOUS PROPERTIES

Bone, which is viscoelastic in nature, exhibits the phenomenon of *plastic flow* or *plastic deformation*. Flow is commonly thought to be concerned only with fluids although it also occurs in solids. In fluids the rate of flow is directly proportional to the force and inversely proportional to the viscosity. In solids the problem is not that large forces cause flow but that small forces do not. If a sufficiently large force is applied to a solid, it will be deformed beyond its yield point and the deformation will remain after removal of the load. Such plastic deformation or permanent set has been demonstrated in bone by Roth et al. (1961a). Another example of permanent set is the indentation made in bone during a hardness test.

The laws of rheology, the science dealing with the deformation and flow of matter, are primarily mathematical but are frequently visualized by means of mechanical models (Reiner, 1959). Attempts to explain the mechanical behavior of bone by rheological models have been made by Roth et al. (1961b) and Sedlin (1965).

INTACT BONE TESTING

Determination of the breaking stress (tension, compression, or shear) and associated mechanical properties of an intact long bone is far more difficult than for a standardized specimen because (1) an intact bone is not straight, (2) its cross-sectional shape and area vary continually along the length of the shaft, and (3) it is a very heterogeneous structure consisting of compact and spongy bone, blood, marrow, fat, etc. Therefore, it is difficult to test intact bones under pure tension or compression since the load will not be uniformly distributed over a constant cross-sectional area. The same would be true for shearing stress. When specimens of standardized size and shape are used, one can have straight specimens of uniform cross-sectional shape and area and composed entirely, or primarily, of compact

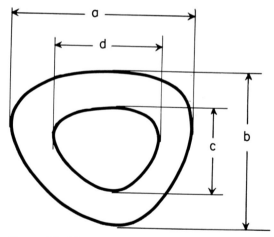

Figure 24. Measurements commonly used for calculating the cross-sectional area of an intact bone for bending tests. The calculation is based on the assumption that the bone is elliptical in its cross-sectional shape. (*a* = maximum external and *d* = maximum internal diameter in major axis of the cross section; *b* = maximum external and *c* = maximum internal diameter in minor axis of the cross section)

or spongy bone. As a result, some of the above-mentioned variables are eliminated.

The breaking stress of intact long bones is generally studied under bending by loading them like a simple beam. In such studies it is usually assumed that the cross-sectional shape of the shaft of the bone is a hollow ellipse with walls of uniform thickness. The outside and inside dimensions, corresponding to the major and the minor axes of the cross section of the bone, are measured (Fig. 24) and the bending stress is calculated from the flexure formula.

The difficulty inherent in such studies is that the cross-sectional shape of most long bones is not a hollow ellipse and the cortex of the bone is not of uniform thickness. Furthermore, because the bones are not straight, bending is apt to be accompanied by some torsion unless the ends of the bone are fixed. If torsion occurs, tensile, compressive, and torsional shearing stresses are also acting on the bone during a test.

SUMMARY

The majority of the methods for determining various mechanical or physical properties discussed in this chapter have been used by the author and his colleagues. A review of extensive studies on the strength of bone made by Japanese investigators can be found in *Strength of Biological Materials* by Yamada (1970).

Readers interested in detailed information on materials testing procedures should consult Davis et al. (1964). A concise but not too technical discussion of some of the principles of mechanics is found in Salvadori and Heller (1963). Useful textbooks on the strength of materials and the formulas for calcuating their mathematical values include Singer (1951), Timoshenko and Young (1962), Harris (1963), and *Marks' Standard Handbook for Mechanical Engineers,* edited by Baumeister (1967).

When calculating the mathematical value for various mechanical properties of bone, it should be remembered that the commonly used formulas are based on engineering materials which are usually isotropic and more homogeneous than bone. Consequently, some of the formulas may have to be modified when applied to bone.

CHAPTER 3

LIVING VERSUS DEAD BONE

PERHAPS THE FIRST and most logical problem to be considered is whether or not there are any significant differences among the mechanical properties of living bone and dead bone. For obvious reasons this problem has not, to my knowledge, been investigated in human bone. However, a comparative study of certain mechanical properties of living and dead rat bone was made by Stevens and Ray (1962).

The material used in the study was obtained from living and dead tibias of ninety-six young, male Long-Evans white rats. The rats were fed on a Rockland Rat Diet and given water *ad libitum* throughout the experiments. At fifteen weeks of age each animal's right hind leg was amputated through the knee joint and the tibia was defleshed, weighed, and put into a sterile test tube. The bone was then frozen for five minutes in a mixture of acetone and carbon dioxide snow, after which it was thawed for five minutes in a water bath at 37° C. This freezing and thawing process was repeated three times for each bone in order to kill the osteocytes. The "killed" tibia was then reweighed and implanted within the sheath of the rectus abdominis muscle of the same animal from which it had been taken.

Groups of six animals were sacrificed at intervals from three hours to 120 days after operation. Immediately after an animal was sacrificed, both tibias were cleanly dissected out as rapidly as possible and studied with respect to (1) whole bone weight, (2) radiographic changes, (3) whole bone strength, (4) specific gravity of the cortical bone, and (5) composition of bone, i.e. ash weights. Items two through four are of special interest at this time.

The breaking load for intact tibias was determined by loading them like a simple beam. The deformation (deflection) occurring during a test was recorded with a kymograph. From the data obtained in the tests, as the authors pointed out, it was impossible to calculate the true stress (strength) and modulus of elasticity values of their specimens, because the cross-sectional area of the bone at the fracture site was not measured. However, they computed an arbitrary value for "strength" of bone from the formula

$$\text{"strength"} = \frac{\text{breaking load}}{\text{bone weight} \times 1,000}$$

On the assumption that no change in bone "strength" occurred in the first twenty-four hours after operation, the mean value for bone "strength" in the first five groups (one to twenty-four hours post operation) was compared with the mean value for "strength" in the other groups. The comparison revealed a decrease in the "strength" of the dead bones in the 10-, 60-, and 120-day groups and an increase in the "strength" of the live bone (Fig. 25). However, no significant differences were found when the data for the dead and live bones in groups one to five were compared with each of the later groups.

Roentgenograms of the paired tibias revealed a continuing growth of the live bones until the animal was sacrificed. No increased radiographic density, as estimat-

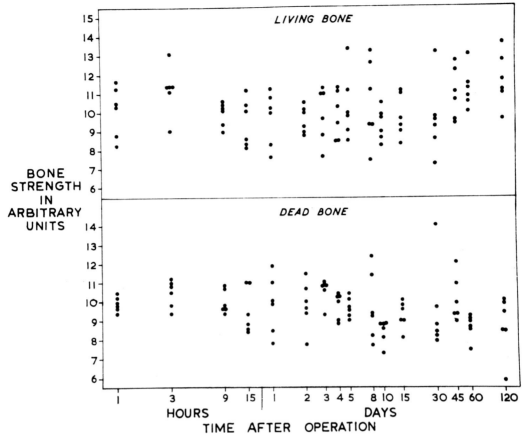

Figure 25. Comparison of the "strength" of living and dead rat tibias. (From Stevens and Ray: *J Bone Joint Surg,* 1962)

ed by the naked eye, occured in the dead tibias.

After the intact tibias were tested, tubular specimens, taken from the "ends" and "shafts" of cortical bone, were prepared by removing the marrow and cancellous bone. The specimens were blotted dry and weighed to determine their "fresh weight." They were then subjected to the following procedure: (1) soaked for eighteen hours at 4° C in distilled water with a wetting agent, (2) weighed again in water at room temperature, (3) carefully dried with blotting paper, and (4) reweighed to obtain their "hydrated weight." The water was then removed from the specimens by heating them in an

oven at 93° to 95° C until a constant "dry-weight" was obtained. The values thus determined represented the weight of the fresh cortex in air, the hydrated cortex in water, the hydrated cortex in air, and the dry cortex in air.

The specific gravity of fresh, of hydrated, and of dry cortex from both living and dead tibias was calculated by application of Archimedes' principle. Fresh living cortex showed a significant increase in specific gravity from 1.92 ± 0.03 at 105 days of age to 2.04 ± 0.02 at 225 days of age. The specific gravity of fresh dead cortex changed from 1.98 ± 0.02 at one hour after operation to 2.02 ± 0.03 at 120 days after operation, a statistically insignificant

difference. Hydrated and dry cortical specimens of the living and the dead tibias
showed no statistically significant variations in their specific gravities.

The composition of the dry specimens
was determined by ashing them in a muffle furnace at 600° C and the final constant
ash weights were recorded. The water, organic, and ash fractions of each sample
were found from the fresh, dry, and ash
weights. The fractions were expressed as
percentages of the original fresh weight.
The only change noted was a very slight
rise in the ash fraction, at the expense of
the water fraction, in the live bone from
the oldest group of animals.

Stevens and Ray's study indicates that
dead bone within the body does not take
up measurable amounts of mineral from
the tissue fluid and retains its original radiographic density, specific gravity, "strength," and composition. The
"strength" of living and dead bone during
the first twenty-four hours after operation
was not significantly different statistically
than that of similar bone in each of the
other groups.

The fact that Stevens and Ray found
no statistically significant differences among
the mechanical properties of living and
dead bone is not surprising when one considers that bone is primarily composed of
nonliving material—collagen fibers, inorganic crystals, cement substance, and water. A much smaller proportion of the total material of bone is represented by the
living constituents which are blood vessels,
blood, nerves, and osteocytes. This is especially true for bone specimens of a standardized size and shape which usually con-
tain no living material. Even if all the
osteocytes in such a specimen were alive,
they would only constitute a small proportion of the total material. This can be de-

duced from the area of the lacunae and
canaliculi, formerly occupied by osteocytes
and their processes, which form less than
3% of the vascular-free volume of cortical
bone of human extremity long bones
(Frost, 1960).

A comparison of the strains produced
in various vertebrae of living anesthetized
and dead embalmed dogs under controlled
acceleration impacts was undertaken by
Lissner and Roberts (1966). Direct strain
measurements were recorded from electric
strain gauges cemented to the anterior aspect of the body of the fifth and the
sixth lumbar vertebrae and to the laminae
and spinous process of the first two thoracic vertebrae. Acceleration was measured
with a Glennite accelerometer mounted on
an aluminum plate, which was screwed to
the spinous process of the first thoracic
vertebra. Consequently, the plate and accelerometer were outside of the dog's
body. Thirty mongrel dogs were used in
the experiments.

A special restraining box held the dog
in an erect sitting position while an acceleration impact was applied to the ischial
tuberosities of the animal. A constant
mean acceleration of 18 g's for a duration
of 170 msec was used in the tests. Jerk or
the time rate of change of the applied acceleration was varied from 250 to 3,000 g's
per second (g/sec) to determine its effect
on skeletal response.

The dogs were first tested in the living
anesthetized condition; then they were sacrificed, embalmed, and left in the restraining box for further testing. Consequently,
the orientation of the dog was the same
in both the living and the dead condition.
The animals were generally embalmed
within twenty-four hours after sacrifice
and tested within seventy-two hours after
embalming. In the interim between sacri-

fice and embalming, the carcass, still in the restraining box, was kept in cold storage. Four dogs were kept in storage for as long as a week prior to testing.

After a dead dog was tested, roentgenograms were taken of it to verify the location of the strain gauges and to determine if any fractures or dislocations had occurred. If malfunction of a gauge was found, the body cavity of the dog was opened to investigate the cause of the malfunction. This procedure also gave an opportunity to evaluate the completeness of the embalming.

The strain gauge and accelerometer data obtained from the tests were presented as dynamic-load factor vs jerk curves. The *dynamic-load factor* is the ratio between strain at a constant acceleration and the initial value obtained with the particular jerk applied in the test. The curves obtained from tests on living anesthetized dogs and on dead embalmed dogs were compared. Direct comparison of data

among individual dogs was difficult to make because of anatomical variations and differences in the exact location of the strain gauges.

The curves based on data from strain gauges on the anterior aspect of the body of the sixth lumbar vertebra of living and of dead dogs (Fig. 26) showed no significant difference in either condition when the dynamic-load factor was less than 1.5. The plateau for the curves based on strain gauge data from the spinous process of the second thoracic vertebra in the two conditions (Fig. 27) was reached at a somewhat higher level than that for the lumbar curves. However, in the thoracic tests the maximum dynamic-load factor for the live animal was 1.7 or greater.

In the lumbar series the maximum variation between the results for the *in vivo* and the dead condition was not more than 20% in the flat part of the curve beyond the transition zone. The dynamic-load factor, as a function of jerk, was always high-

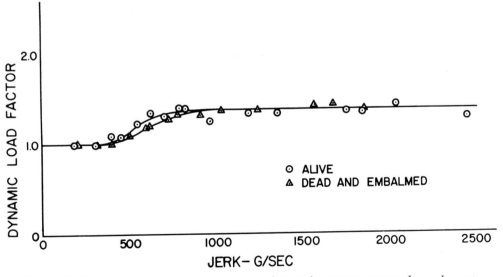

Figure 26. Dynamic-load factor vs jerk curves for strain gauges mounted on the anterior of the body of the sixth lumbar vertebra of living and of dead embalmed dogs. (From Lissner and Roberts: in *Studies on the Anatomy and Function of Bone and Joints.* Courtesy of Springer-Verlag)

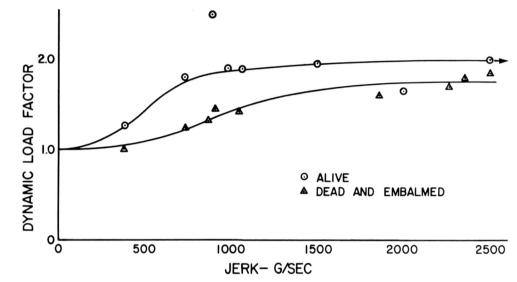

Figure 27. Dynamic-load factor vs jerk curves for strain gauges mounted on the spinous process of the second thoracic vertebra of living and of dead embalmed dogs. (From Lissner and Roberts: in *Studies on the Anatomy and Function of Bone and Joints.* Courtesy of Springer-Verlag)

er in the live than in the dead dog. These results agree closely with those obtained from strain gauges mounted on lumbar vertebrae of embalmed adult human cadavers under similar experimental conditions when the dynamic-load factor was less than 1.5.

The curves for the accelerometer data (Fig. 28) had the same general shape as those for the strain gauge data but the points were more erratic and had a greater scatter. The dynamic-load factor was 2 to 3 in these tests. The location of the accelerometer at the end of a cantilever projection, outside of the dog's body, probably accounts for the scatter in the data. The accelerometer curve for an embalmed dog was lower than that for a live dog but still within the 20% maximum variation found for the strain gauge data. The rise in the curve occurred at a lower acceleration in the living dog than in the dead one.

Lissner and Roberts applied the results

of their study to the prediction of strain response in living human subjects on the basis of cadaver data obtained in acceleration experiments similar to those they used for the dogs. They believed that such predictions could be made with a high degree of confidence. Their experiments also demonstrated that the strain response in the living anesthetized dog was greater than in the dead embalmed one and that the living animal had a decreased sensitivity to jerk at lower levels.

The differences, reported by Lissner and Roberts, between living and dead dogs may be the result of the hardening and stiffening effects of embalming on biological material. These effects, with particular reference to bone, will be discussed in subsequent chapters.

The flexural and the ultimate strength properties of the intact skull and leg bones of adult dogs in the living, the dead, and the embalmed conditions were recently investigated by Greenberg et al.

(1968). The loads were applied by a hydraulic cylinder through a strain gauge type load cell while the deflections in the bones were simultaneously recorded with a linear displacement transducer. Because of individual variation between dogs the experiments were designed so that the results of the various conditions under which each specimen was tested could be compared within a dog.

Loads were applied to the lateral aspect of the skull at a speed of approximately 0.17 in/min to a maximum of 250 lb. The specimen was then permitted to unload itself to zero at approximately the same rate. Afterwards the animal was sacrificed and, without mechanically changing the conditions, retested in the fresh *in situ* condition.

The right tibia was loaded *in vivo* to failure by applying a force in an antero-posterior direction to the center of the bone. The left tibia of the same dog was tested *in vivo* to 50% of the breaking load

for the right tibia and then allowed to unload itself at approximately the same rate at which it was loaded. After sacrificing the animal, the left tibia was retested in the fresh *in situ* condition. The tibia was subsequently removed, put into a 10% formalin solution for one week, and tested again in the embalmed wet condition after which it was placed into water and retested in the wet condition twice at weekly intervals.

Other left tibias were dried over $CaCl_2$ in a vacuum dessicator for about a week to a constant weight. They were then retested in the dry condition to 35% of the original fracture load to determine the hysteresis and flexure changes. The amount of recovery of the strength properties of the wet tibias was measured by retesting the bones after they had been in water for one week. Finally, the bones were loaded to failure and the results were compared with the ultimate strength of the right tibias tested *in vivo*.

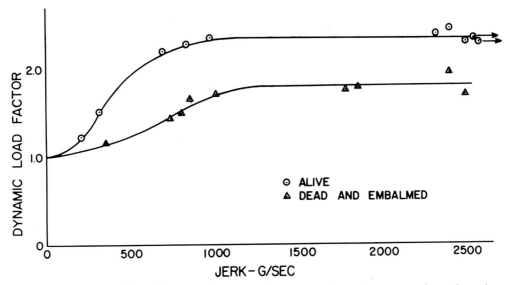

Figure 28. Dynamic-load factor vs jerk curve for an accelerometer mounted on the spinous process of the first thoracic vertebra of living and of dead embalmed dogs. (From Lissner and Roberts: in *Studies on the Anatomy and Function of Bone and Joints*. Courtesy of Springer-Verlag)

The average lateral spring rate load for the intact skull in the fresh *in situ* condition was 5,382 lb/in compared to 5,257 lb/in for the skull *in vivo*. A similar comparison of the average spring rate for the simply supported, center loaded intact tibia-fibula complex showed an average of 2,288 lb/in for the complex in the fresh *in situ* condition and 2,304 lb/in for the *in vivo* condition. The maximum change in the skull was only 5%. The long bones exhibited less change but greater deviation because of less accurate measuring procedures.

The investigations just reviewed indicate that there are relatively few differences between the mechanical properties of standardized specimens of cortical bone or of intact bones in the living and the dead conditions. This conclusion is similar to that of Gurdjian and Lissner (1945) who compared the "stresscoat" pattern, produced under comparable experimental conditions, in the skull of living anesthesized monkeys, the *in situ* skull of the dead monkeys, and the dried skull. The chief difference found between the tensile strain pattern in the skull of the living monkey and that in the same skull when dried, was that the extent of the pattern was somewhat greater in the *in vivo* condition. They, therefore, concluded that interpretations of the mechanical behavior of a bone based on "stresscoat" patterns in dry bone are valid for predicting the behavior of the same bone, under similar experimental conditions, in the living condition.

SUMMARY

Contrary to what may have been expected, the differences between the mechanical properties and biomechanical behavior of living and dead bone, when tested under similar experimental conditions, are few. Consequently, results obtained from experiments with dead bone, especially in the fresh or moist condition, appear to be valid for extrapolation to comparable properties and behavior of bone in the living animal.

CHAPTER 4

EFFECTS OF DRYING

ALTHOUGH THE MECHANICAL properties of bone, especially its strength characteristics and modulus of elasticity, have been studied quite extensively, there is great variation in the values for these properties reported by different investigators. Two important reasons for this variation are (1) the differences in the amount of moisture in the test specimens and (2) the fact that some investigators tested fresh specimens while others used embalmed material.

The amount of moisture in a bone specimen at the time it is tested is a very important factor which must be considered when studying the mechanical properties of bone. In spite of the common expression "as dry as a bone," there is actually a considerable amount of water in cortical bone.

WATER CONTENT OF BONE

Valentin (1847) reported that fresh, air-dried rib bone of horses has a water content of 14.56%. The percentage of water of other tissues is also given by Valentin. Fresh cortical bone from the femur and the tibia of man and of cattle, according to Aeby (1872), has a water content of 12.21% and 9.49%, respectively.

An extensive investigation of the water content of bone, at a temperature of 105° C, was made by Hülsen (1896), who found that fresh specimens of cortical bone from an adult human tibia had 19.78% water while similar specimens from the femur of a newborn infant had 28.06% water. The water content of fresh specimens from an ox was 12.87% for the femoral specimens and 13.24% for the tibial ones. Similar specimens from the femur of a cow and a calf had a water content of 12.47% and 19.65%, respectively. Fresh femoral specimens from a horse had a water content of 13.67%. The percentage of water in fresh specimens from pigs, foxes, wolves, chickens, ducks, and a frog varied from 11.39% in the tibial

specimens of a fox to 31.08% in a frog femur.

Evans and Lebow (1951) reported that standardized specimens of cortical bone from the embalmed femur of a 78-year-old white man lost 12% moisture before attaining a constant weight. The specimens had been dried in a vacuum oven for several days at a temperature of 105° C.

According to Robinson and Elliott (1957), fresh cortical bone from the tibia of puppies had a water content of 73% by volume and 54% by weight, whereas tibial bone of adult dogs had a water content of 21% by volume and 10% by weight.

The water content of bone, according to Neuman and Neuman (1957), varies from 60% in forming bone to 10% in senile cortical bone. Contrary to what was generally assumed, the authors believe that nearly all of the water in bone is bound water.

The dielectric constant and loss of water in standardized flat specimens of fresh human cortical bone from amputated legs were investigated by Marino et al. (1967). The constant and loss were measured at frequencies of 1, 10, 50, and 100 kc and for hydrations (h) from 0 to 65 mg-water/g-bone. The quantity h_c varied from 37 to 48 mg-water/g-bone, depending upon the density of the specimen. It was the author's belief that this quantity represented the bound water in bone at the primary absorption sites.

The percentage of water, organic, and mineral content of human cancellous bone from lumbar vertebral bodies and the iliac crest was determined by Mueller et al. (1966). A total of ninety-seven vertebral specimens, from fifty-four males and forty females, ranging from seven months to 85 years of age was analyzed. Three other specimens were from individuals whose sex was not indicated. The subjects from whom the specimens were obtained were considered to be pathological for various reasons. The iliac material was obtained from selected subjects, most of whom were accident victims who had been hospitalized for less than one day. One hundred specimens, from subjects varying from newborn to 85 years of age and evenly divided as to males and females, were analyzed. There were at least ten specimens from each decade.

The authors reported that the percentage of water per cubic centimeter of hydrated bone decreased for the first twenty-five to thirty years but changed little afterward. No actual values for the water content of their material was given in the text. Their diagrams, in which the percentage of water was plotted against age, revealed the variation in the water content of the unselected specimens to be between 10% and 20% while that of the iliac specimens of trauma victims was approximately 12% to 15%.

EFFECTS OF DRYING

The effects of air drying on tensile strain, in the longitudinal axis, of long strips of cortical femoral and fibular bone from two women, 21 and 60 years of age, and of two men, 30 and 74 years of age, were briefly discussed by Wertheim (1847). He observed that when the bones had been well dried prior to testing, the elongation was practically proportional to the load, i.e. the bones behaved like inorganic bodies, but in fresh bones the coefficient of elasticity did not increase strictly in proportion to load. However, the differences in the two conditions were slight.

The tensile and compressive strength of fresh and dry specimens of cortical bone from the femur of a 28-year-old man was determined by Rauber (1876). The tensile specimens were flat elongated prisms with a reduced middle region and the compressive specimens were cubes. They were loaded parallel to the direction of their fibers. The fresh specimens were put into water which had been briefly heated to 38° C just before testing and were kept at this temperature during a test by wetting them. The dry specimens were tested at an ambient temperature of 15° to 25° C.

The five fresh specimens had an average tensile strength of 10.25 kgf/mm² (14,570 lbf/in²) compared to 11.58 kgf/mm² (16,470 lbf/in²) for the six dry specimens. The average compressive strength was 14.41 kgf/mm² (20,490 lbf/in²) for the seven fresh specimens and 18.63 kgf/mm² (26,490 lbf/in²) for the seven dry specimens.

Seven fresh tensile specimens from the tibia of a cow had an average strength of 11.46 kgf/mm² (16,300 lbf/in²) compared to 12.43 kgf/mm² (17,670 lbf/in²) for six dry specimens.

The deflection and bending modulus of elasticity of three rods of cortical bone, tested in the fresh and the dry condition, from the femur of a 46-year-old man were also investigated by Rauber (Table I). The rods were 80 mm long and were tested under a 100-g load applied intermittently for a brief time at a temperature of 15° to

TABLE I

EFFECTS OF DRYING ON THE MEAN DEFLECTION AND BENDING MODULUS OF ELASTICITY, UNDER A 100-G LOAD AND AT A TEMPERATURE OF 15° TO 25° C, OF FEMORAL CORTICAL BONE OF A 46-YEAR-OLD MAN (Data from Rauber, 1876)

Mean Deflection (mm)		
	Fresh	*Dry*
Specimen 1	11.38	9.5
Specimen 2	12.38	11.15
Specimen 3	15.25	14.00

Modulus of Elasticity			
	Fresh		*Dry*
	kgf/mm²	*lbf/in²*	*kgf/mm²*	*lbf/in²*
Specimen 1	2137	3.04×10^6	2560	3.64×10^6
Specimen 2	2081	2.96×10^6	2311	3.29×10^6
Specimen 3	1891	2.69×10^6	2065	2.94×10^6

25° C. During a test a rod was supported at both ends and loaded in the center.

After specimen number three had been tested in both the fresh and the dry conditions, it was soaked in water for several days and retested. Comparison of the retested results with those in the fresh condition showed that the deflection had increased to 15.25 mm while the modulus of elasticity had decreased to 1,831 kgf/mm² (2.6×10^6 lbf/in²).

Three additional fresh femoral specimens had a modulus of elasticity of 2,339 kgf/mm² (3.3×10^6 lbf/in²), 2,424 kgf/mm² (3.4×10^6 lbf/in²), and 2,213 kgf/mm² (3.1×10^6 lbf/in²). The average modulus of the six fresh specimens was 2,181 kgf/mm² (3.1×10^6 lbf/in²) compared to 2,312 kgf/mm² (3.3×10^6 lbf/in²) for the three dry specimens, an in-

crease of 6% due to drying. Drying reduced the length of the rods from a minimum of 0.25 mm to a maximum of 0.50 mm.

A rod from an ox femur had a mean deflection of 7 mm in the fresh and 6.75 mm in the dry condition. The modulus of elasticity in the fresh and the dry conditions was 2,590 kgf/mm² (3.6×10^6 lbf/in²) and 2,619 kgf/mm² (3.7×10^6 lbf/in²), respectively.

Because the strength values in the bending tests discussed previously were obtained from specimens with different cross-sectional areas, Rauber attempted to correct for this variation by recalculating the strength values on the basis of a common cross-sectional area of 4 mm². The recalculated average bending strength for three fresh specimens from the humerus and the tibia of the 46-year-old man was 1,477 kgf/mm² (21,000 lbf/in²), compared to a strength of 1,709 kgf/mm² (24,300 lbf/in²) for ten dry specimens

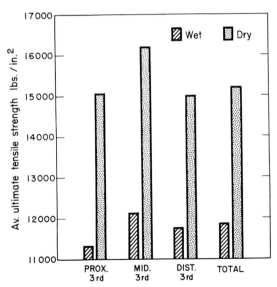

Figure 29. Average ultimate tensile stress for 121 wet-tested and 121 dry-tested standardized specimens of wet cortical bone from various thirds of the shaft of embalmed adult human femurs. (From Evans and Lebow: *Am J Surg*, 1952)

from the humerus of a 30-year-old man and the femur of a 70-year-old man, a 46-year-old man, and a man of unknown age. Thus, the bending strength was increased approximately 16% by drying.

Rauber did not compare the shearing and torsion strength of dry and fresh specimens.

All of Rauber's mechanical property determinations were made on standardized specimens of compact bone from nine femurs of eight men and one woman, three humeri from three men, and three tibias from three men. It is, therefore, difficult to evaluate the effect of drying on the mechanical properties of bone from his data because in only a few instances did he test fresh and dry specimens from the same bone or even from the same individual. In addition, the total number of fresh and dry specimens was too few for statistical analysis.

Hülsen (1896) reported that four fresh flat specimens of cortical bone from the humerus of an adult man had an average ultimate tensile strength of 10.55 kgf/mm² (15,000 lbf/in²) while four similarly-tested dry specimens from the same bone had an average strength of 10.94 kgf/mm² (15,550 lbf/in²). In these specimens drying increased the tensile strength by 3.7%, which is probably not a significant difference. During a test a force or load was applied to a specimen in the di-

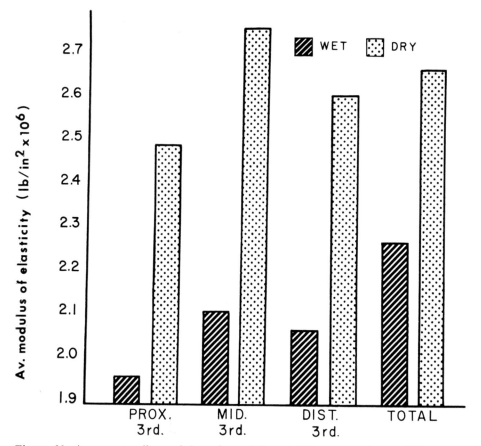

Figure 30. Average tensile modulus of elasticity of 121 wet-tested and 121 dry-tested standardized specimens of wet cortical bone according to shaft third of adult embalmed human femurs.

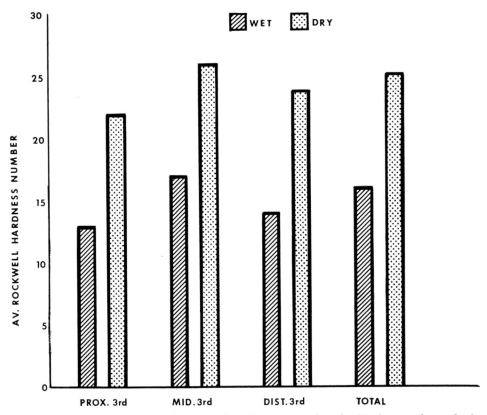

Figure 31. Average Rockwell hardness for 121 wet-tested and 121 dry-tested standardized specimens of wet cortical bone from various thirds of the shaft of embalmed adult human femurs.

rection of its long axis which coincided with that of the intact bone from which it had been taken.

The values given by Hülsen for the compressive strength of fresh and of dry cortical bone were obtained from tests on rings of bone from the humerus and the femur of an adult man. The average compressive strength, in the long axis of the intact bone, of six fresh humeral rings was 20.41 kgf/mm² (29,020 lbf/in²) and of five dry femoral rings 21.08 kgf/mm² (29,970 lbf/in²), a 3% increase due to drying. The age of the individuals from whom Hülsen obtained his material was not given.

The bending modulus of elasticity of two fresh rectangular rods of cortical bone specimens from an ox femur was 2,240 kgf/mm² (3.2 × 10⁶ lbf/in²) and 2,134 kgf/mm² (3.0 × 10⁶ lbf/in²). When the same specimens were tested after drying at a temperature of 105° C, the modulus of the first one had changed to 2,719 kgf/mm² (3.9 × 10⁶ lbf/in²), with an increase of 21%, and that of the second one to 2,667 kgf/mm² (3.8 × 10⁶ lbf/in²), with an increase of 25% due to drying.

In addition, Hülsen found that the specific gravity of small fresh pieces of cortical bone from an adult human humerus was 1.902 compared to 1.936 for similar dry specimens, a specific gravity increase of 1% due to drying. Comparable fresh tibial specimens had a specific gravity of

1.816 while that of dry femoral specimens was 1.933.

The effect of drying on the regional differences of the mechanical properties of embalmed cortical bone was investigated in our laboratory (Evans and Lebow, 1951, 1952). Pairs of specimens from each of the quadrants and thirds of the shaft of both femurs of six adult white men from 47 to 81 years of age were machined

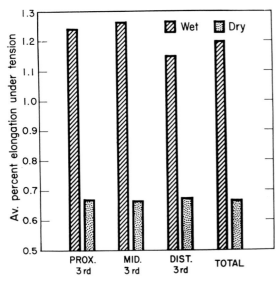

Figure 32. Average percent elongation (tensile strain) for 121 wet-tested and 121 dry-tested standardized specimens of wet cortical bone from various thirds of the shaft of embalmed adult human femurs. (From Evans and Lebow: *Am J Surg,* 1952)

to a standardized size and shape (Fig. 8*A*). A total of 242 specimens was obtained from the twelve femurs of the six men. Generally twenty specimens were made from each femur.

One member of each pair of specimens was put into tap water and tested wet while the other one was air-dried at room temperature and tested dry. A total of 121 specimens was tested wet and the same number dry. The ultimate tensile stress and strain were measured in the direction

of the long axis of the specimen which coincided with that of the intact bone. The shearing stress of the specimens was determined by loading them in a direction perpendicular to the long axis of the specimen and of the bone. Finally, the Rockwell superficial hardness of the specimens was measured.

The results of our experiments showed that air drying the specimens increased their average ultimate tensile strength (Fig. 29), their modulus of elasticity (Fig. 30), and their hardness (Fig. 31), but reduced their tensile strain or percentage elongation (Fig. 32) and their single shearing strength (Fig. 33).

The average values for the mechanical properties of specimens from the various individuals are given in Table II and similar data for all the specimens, regardless of the individual from whom they were obtained, in Table III. When the percentage change due to drying was computed from the data in Table III, it was found that drying increased the average tensile strength by 28%, the modulus of elasticity by 18%, and the hardness by 56%. However, the average single shearing strength, perpendicular to the long axis of the specimen, was reduced 18% and the tensile strain 45% by drying.

An additional effect of drying was a change in the shape of the tensile stress-strain curve. The dry-tested specimens tended to have a linear stress-strain curve while that of wet-tested specimens deviated from a straight line at the proportional limit (Fig. 34). This conforms with Wertheim's (1847) observation that dry bone behaves more like an inorganic material than does wet bone.

Perhaps the most important result of our investigation was the demonstration that drying reduces the energy-absorbing capacity of bone. This can be readily seen

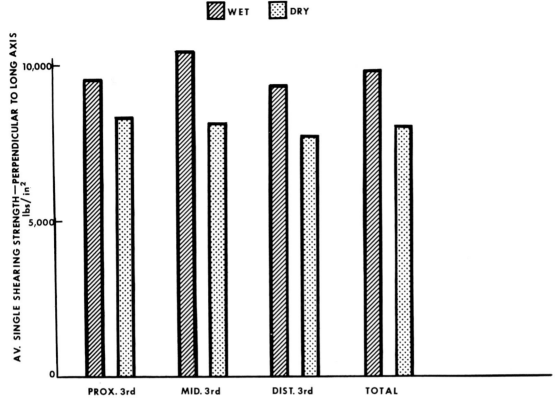

Figure 33. Average single shearing stress for 121 wet-tested and 121 dry-tested standardized specimens of wet cortical bone from various thirds of the shaft of embalmed adult human femurs.

by comparing the area below the stress-strain curve of a dry specimen with that of a similarly tested specimen of comparable tensile strength (Fig. 34). The amount of energy absorbed by a specimen can be calculated by measuring the area below its stress-strain curve with a compensating polar planimeter. When this was done for each of nineteen dry-tested and twenty-one wet-tested specimens from the femur of a 78-year-old white man, it was found that the wet specimens absorbed an average of 83.6 in.lb/in^3 of energy before failing compared to an average of only 60.0 in.lb/in^3 for the dry specimens. We also discovered that the energy-absorbing capacity of the specimens, both in the wet and the dry conditions, was directly related

to its percentage elongation or tensile strain (Fig. 35).

The capacity of bone to absorb considerable amounts of energy without breaking is an important safety factor in the ability of an animal to resist various stresses and strains to which it is subjected in daily life. The energy-absorbing capacity of bone is also a factor to be considered in fracture mechanisms because most fractures are caused by impacts and thus involve problems of energy absorption. To our knowledge, the energy-absorbing capacity of bone had not been previously investigated.

An analysis of variance was made between the means for the mechanical properties of wet- and of dry-tested specimens

TABLE II

Effect of Drying on the Mechanical Properties of Cortical Bone from
Embalmed Femurs of Six Adult White Males (Data from Evans and Lebow, 1951)

Age	Cause of Death	Test	Shearing Strength		Tensile Strength		Modulus of Elasticity		Hardness (Rockwell)	Tensile Strain (% Elongation)
			lbf/in²	kgf/mm²	lbf/in²	kgf/mm²	×10⁶ lbf/in²	kgf/mm²		
47	Tuberculosis	W	9,140	6.43	10,650	7.49	1.71	1,202	2	1.16
		D	7,620	5.36	14,510	10.20	2.16	1,518	11	0.61
58	Infectious hepatitis	W	10,640	7.48	11,690	8.22	1.92	1,350	75	1.24
		D	7,950	5.59	16,040	11.28	2.45	1,722	33	0.73
63	Pneumonia	W	8,290	5.83	10,500	7.38	2.15	1,500	3	1.37
		D	9,840	6.92	16,540	11.63	2.39	1,680	23	0.79
70	Tuberculosis	W	10,680	7.51	12,590	8.79	2.39	1,680	27	0.98
		D	7,140	5.02	12,980	9.12	2.89	2,032	34	0.46
78	Coronary occlusion	W	—	—	11,490	8.08	2.09	1,469	16	1.10
		D	—	—	15,410	10.83	2.49	1,750	25	0.72
81	Arteriosclerosis	W	10,650	7.49	12,910	9.08	2.08	1,462	15	1.63
		D	8,850	6.22	17,600	12.37	2.86	2,011	24	0.85

W = wet
D = dry

TABLE III

Effect of Drying on the Mechanical Properties of Cortical Bone from Embalmed Femurs of Adult White Males (Data from Evans and Lebow, 1951)

	Wet	*Dry*
Number of specimens	121	121
Tensile stress* (lbf/in²)	11,840	15,530
Tensile stress* (kgf/mm²)	8.32	10.92
Shearing stress† (lbf/in²)	9,800	8,000
Shearing stress† (kgf/mm²)	6.89	5.62
Modulus of elasticity (× 10⁶ lbf/in²)	2.27	2.67
Modulus of elasticity (kgf/mm²)	1,596	1,877
Tensile strain (% elongation)	1.20	0.66
Hardness (Rockwell)	16	25

* Parallel to long axis of specimen and bone.
† Perpendicular to long axis of specimen and bone.

of unembalmed bone from the distal third of the femur from above-knee amputations. This analysis (Table IV) revealed that the tensile strength, the modulus of elasticity, and the hardness of the dry specimens were each greater, at the 0.01 significance level, than were the same properties of the wet specimens. However, the latter specimens had a greater tensile strain, at the 0.01 significance level, than that of the dry specimens.

The ultimate tensile strength has been compared (Evans, 1964) in standardized wet- and dry-tested specimens from embalmed and unembalmed adult human tibias (Fig. 36). A statistical analysis of the results of the comparison showed that the mean ultimate tensile strength of the dry specimens from both embalmed and

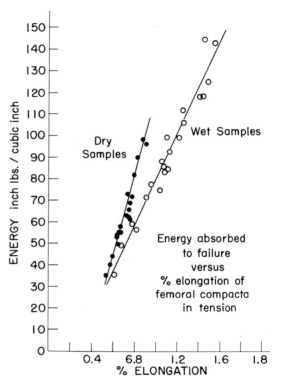

Figure 35. Energy absorbed to failure vs percent elongation curves for wet-tested and dry-tested specimens of embalmed cortical bone from the femur of a 78-year-old white male. The average energy absorbed to failure for all the dry-tested specimens was 69.0 in-lb/in³ compared to an average of 83.6 in-lb/in³ for all the wet specimens. (From Evans and Lebow: *J Appl Physiol*, 1951)

unembalmed bones was significantly greater at the 0.01 level than that of the wet specimens.

Another investigation of the influence of drying on the tensile and compressive strength and the modulus of elasticity of human cortical bone was made by Dempster and Liddicoat (1952). The material

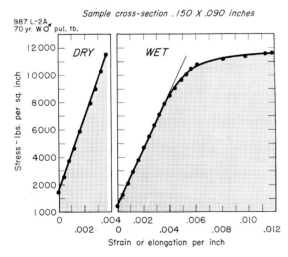

Figure 34. Stress-strain diagram for a wet-tested and dry-tested standardized specimen of cortical bone from embalmed adult human femurs. (From Evans and Lebow: *J Appl Physiol*, 1951)

TABLE IV

VARIATION BETWEEN THE MECHANICAL PROPERTIES OF UNEMBALMED WET AND DRY CORTICAL BONE OF HUMAN FEMURS

Variable	N (1)	N (2)	F-Ratio	Mean (1)	Sigma (1)	Mean (2)	Sigma (2)
$E \times 10^6$ lbf/in²	20	8	45.115*	1.74	.44495	2.86625	.24366
UTS (lbf/in²)	20	8	24.787*	9,433.00	2,491.69	14,800.00	2,795.15
Percent elongation	20	8	16.145*	1.4895	.71736	.455	.10071
Hardness (Rockwell)	17	8	87.087*	.588	9.014	36.375	8.782

　* 0.01 or better significance level.
　(1) = unembalmed wet, (2) = unembalmed dry, E = modulus of elasticity, UTS = ultimate tensile strength.

used in their study was obtained from thirty-one femurs, ten fibulas, and five humeri selected at random from a university osteological collection. No obviously pathological bones were used. The age, the sex,

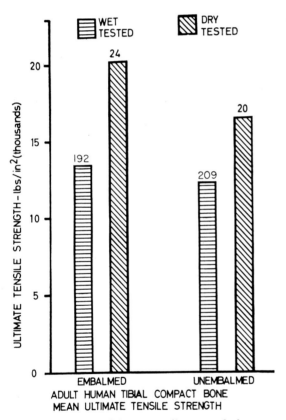

Figure 36. Mean ultimate tensile strength for embalmed wet and dry and unembalmed wet and dry standardized specimens of cortical bone from adult human tibias. (From Evans: in *Proceedings of the First European Bone and Tooth Symposium.* Courtesy of Pergamon Press)

the race, and the method of preservation of the bones were unknown.

Tensile specimens, with a reduced middle region, of two general types—round rods and rectangular prisms—were used. The compression specimens were columns with a rectangular or circular cross section and a length-thickness ratio of approximately 7:1. All test specimens were taken from the middle third of the bone, usually the anterior aspect, and were tested dry or wet. The condition of the latter was obtained by soaking them in water overnight or for twenty-four hours. The only "fresh" specimens were those from the femur of a middle-aged man. The strain occurring in a specimen during a test was measured with one or two Porter-Lipp, Huggenberger, or Tuckermann extensometers. The average values and standard deviations Dempster and Liddicoat found for the modulus of elasticity (Table V) and for tensile and compressive stress (Table VI) were higher in the dry specimens than in the wet ones.

The percentage change calculated from Dempster and Liddicoat's data revealed that the average modulus of elasticity in compression (Table V) increased 26% (two gauges used) and 24% (one gauge used) in drying. Drying had an even greater effect on the modulus of elasticity in tension which increased 55% (two gauges) and 61% (one gauge).

TABLE V

AVERAGE VALUES AND STANDARD DEVIATIONS OF THE MODULUS OF ELASTICITY OF ADULT HUMAN COMPACT BONE
(Data from Dempster and Liddicoat, 1952)

	No. of Specimens	Two Gauges		One Gauge	
		$\times 10^6$ lbf/in²	$\times 10^3$ kgf/mm²	$\times 10^6$ lbf/in²	$\times 10^3$ kgf/mm²
In Compression					
Dry bone	5	2.60 ± .167	1.83 ± .117	—	—
	6	—	—	2.53 ± .301	1.78 ± .211
Wet bone	5	2.06 ± .117	1.45 ± .82	2.04 ± .290	1.43 ± .203
In Tension					
Dry bone	10	2.69 ± .420	1.89 ± .295	—	—
	12	—	—	2.86 ± .612	2.01 ± .430
Wet bone	7	1.73 ± .128	1.22 ± .899	—.	—
	3	—	—	1.77 ± .232	1.24 ± .163

A similar calculation of the differences between the average compressive and tensile strength of their specimens (Table VI) showed that drying increased the compressive strength 62.7% and the tensile strength 49.5%. These are probably significant differences although Dempster and Liddicoat did not analyze their data statistically.

It is preferable to use two strain gauges on a test specimen because it is possible to determine more readily if bending is occurring in the specimen during a test. If bending does occur, it means that the load has not been uniformly applied over the cross-sectional area of the specimen during the test and that both tensile and compressive stresses and strains are acting on the specimen.

Dempster and Liddicoat (1952) found that the stress-strain curve for dry bone in tension is approximately a straight line to failure in contrast to that for wet bone, which, in both tension and compression, deviates from a straight line beyond the proportional limit (Fig. 37).

A comparison of the bending properties of twenty-four wet- and air-dried standardized specimens of cortical bone from adult human femurs made by Sedlin (1965) showed that the average ultimate fiber stress (Table VII) progressively increased with the length of time the specimens were air dried. The bending modulus of elasticity tended to decrease while the energy absorbed to failure tended to increase with the length of time the specimens were air dried. However, these tend-

TABLE VI

ULTIMATE LONGITUDINAL COMPRESSIVE AND TENSILE STRENGTH OF ADULT HUMAN COMPACT BONE
(Data from Dempster and Liddicoat, 1952)

	No. of Specimens	lbf/in²	kgf/mm²
In Compression			
Dry bone	38	25,680 ± 4740	18.05 ± 3.33
Wet bone	29	15,775 ± 3880	11.09 ± 2.73
In Tension			
Dry bone	11	17,090 ± 3940	12.01 ± 2.77
Wet bone	14	11,428 ± 1540	8.03 ± 1.08

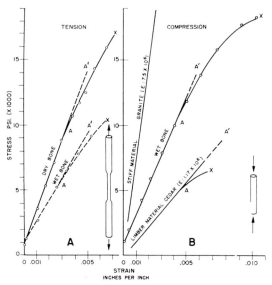

Figure 37. Stress-strain curves in tension and compression of wet vs dry adult human compact bone. (From Dempster and Liddicoat: *Am J Anat,* 1952)

encies were not consistent. An analysis of variance showed that the mean ultimate fiber stress was the only mechanical property that exhibited significant changes

(greater than 0.01) in relation to the length of time of air drying of the specimens. Statistically significant differences were found between subjects but not between various states of hydration. Five to ten minutes of air drying produced no changes in the bending properties of the specimens.

Microhardness is another mechanical factor of cortical bone that is affected by drying. Amprino (1958) reported that drying produced a highly significant increase in the Vickers microhardness value of primary and secondary cortical bone from the limbs of man and several other mammals. Vickers microhardness values (kilograms per square millimeter) for strictly comparable areas of fresh and dried specimens of primary and secondary cortical bone from cattle (Table VIII) showed that the value increased with the temperature at which drying occurred. Each value in Table VIII is the mean of ten measurements.

TABLE VII

EFFECTS OF AIR DRYING ON BENDING PROPERTIES OF HUMAN CORTICAL BONE (Data from Sedlin, 1965)

Subject, Age, and Cause of Death	Wet	Time in Air (Min.)				Average
		15	30	45	60	
Mean Ultimate Fiber Stress (Kp/mm²)						
Female, 41, breast carcinoma	21.3	24.6	19.1	22.2	26.0	22.6
Female, 46, uremia	21.2	19.2	22.8	23.3	26.2	22.5
Male, 55, bronchopneumonia	19.2	17.5	20.5	20.9	19.4	19.5
Male, 56, cerebral hemorrhage	19.2	20.5	22.1	22.7	24.0	21.8
Male, 91, myocardial infarct	13.4	17.1	19.2	19.3	19.5	17.7
Average	18.9	19.9	20.7	21.7	23.0	20.8
Modulus of Elasticity (× 10³ Kp/mm²)						
Female, 41, breast carcinoma	1.85	1.90	1.60	1.58	1.56	1.70
Female, 46, uremia	1.97	1.44	1.65	1.73	1.72	1.70
Male, 55, bronchopneumonia	1.57	1.30	1.38	1.31	1.28	1.37
Male, 56, cerebral hemorrhage	1.76	1.66	1.64	1.62	1.70	1.68
Male, 91, myocardial infarct	1.28	1.38	1.47	1.42	1.37	1.38
Average	1.69	1.54	1.55	1.53	1.52	1.57
Energy (× 10⁻² Kpcm/mm²) Absorbed to Failure						
Female, 41, breast carcinoma	12.7	16.3	11.5	11.1	13.2	13.0
Female, 46, uremia	11.3	9.43	10.9	9.85	14.7	11.2
Male, 55, bronchopneumonia	7.45	6.90	7.89	8.27	6.82	7.47
Male, 56, cerebral hemorrhage	8.28	9.39	9.01	10.6	11.4	9.47
Male, 91, myocardial infarct	6.11	8.40	7.66	12.4	13.2	9.55
Average	9.17	10.1	9.39	10.4	11.9	10.2

TABLE VIII

DRYING AND TEMPERATURE EFFECTS ON THE VICKERS
MICROHARDNESS OF PRIMARY COMPACT BONE FROM
CATTLE* (Data from Amprino, 1958)

	50g Load[†]	50g Load[†]	100g Load[‡]
Fresh bone	49.7	55.7	53.1
Bone dried at 38° C	63.0	69.1	67.7
Bone dried at 60° C	73.0	76.0	77.4
Bone dried at 120° C	97.0	99.7	94.0

* Each value is the mean of ten measurements.
† 6-month bovine bone.
‡ 8-month bovine bone.

By alternately oven drying specimens at 38°, 60°, or 120° C and soaking them in saline solution for six to forty-eight hours, an increase in microhardness was produced after drying and a decrease after rehydration. However, a gradual decrease in microhardness was found in consecutive sets of measurements.

Amprino's investigations indicated an inverse relation between moisture content and microhardness of bone. Thus, decreasing the amount of moisture in bone by heating it at various temperatures resulted in a progressive and consistent increase in its microhardness.

Greenberg et al. (1968) reported that the average spring rate for a simply supported, center loaded intact dry tibia-fibula complex of adult dogs was 2,988 lb/in and 2,304 lb/in for the same complex in the *in vivo* condition. When the dry specimens were remoistened and then retested, the average spring rate was found to have decreased.

Japanese investigators, cited by Yamada (1970), who have studied the effects of drying on the mechanical properties of compact bone from man and other animals reported that drying increased the ultimate tensile and compressive stress and modulus of elasticity, the bending strength and modulus, the modulus of rigidity, the compressive strain, and the Rockwell and Brinell hardness values. Tensile strain and ultimate specific deflection in bending were reduced by drying.

SUMMARY

The research briefly reviewed in this chapter clearly demonstrates the importance of moisture in bone. All investigators who have studied the problem have found that the tensile and compressive strength characteristics, the modulus of elasticity, and the hardness of bone are increased by drying. The shearing strength of bone, in a direction perpendicular to its long axis, and its energy-absorbing capacity are both decreased by drying.

CHAPTER 5

PRESERVATION EFFECTS

A PROBLEM OF GREAT practical importance in studies on the mechanical
properties of bone is the preservation of a
specimen during the time between preparation and testing. Ideally, only fresh bone
should be used and the tests on it should be
made as soon as possible after a specimen is
prepared. However, this is often difficult to
accomplish and a considerable length of time
may elapse between preparation and testing
of specimens. The chief concern, as discussed in Chapter 4, is to prevent a specimen
from drying. This can be done by keeping
it in water, physiological saline solution, embalming fluid, alcohol, or by freezing it or
wrapping it in moist skin, moist cloth, or
flesh. The possible effects on the mechanical
properties of bone vary with the method
and with the length of time a specimen is
preserved before it is tested.

EFFECTS OF ALCOHOL FIXATION

The deformation produced in specimens
of human cortical bone after alcohol fixation was investigated by Sedlin (1965). For
this purpose femoral specimens with a cross-
sectional area of 3.5 mm^2 and a moment of
inertia of 1 mm^4 were loaded like a cantilever beam. All of the specimens were frozen prior to the experiment as most of them
had previously been used in the determination of other mechanical properties. Two
series of experiments were conducted.

In the first series thirty specimens were
thawed at room temperature and then
stored in 40% alcohol for ten days before
they were tested. Later, the specimens were
put in Ringer's solution for three hours and
then retested.

In the second series twenty-five specimens
were thawed and tested at room temperature
in Ringer's solution. They were then put in
40% alcohol for five days, tested again, replaced in Ringer's solution for twenty-four
hours, and tested a third time.

The specimens were deformed at a rate
of 1 cm/min up to a 100-g load. This load
produced an average maximum bending moment of 3 Kpmm and a resultant average
maximum stress of 3 Kp/mm^3. The deflection produced by a 100-g load was measured
in each test.

The mean deflection of twenty-four of
the specimens in the first series was 4% less
in alcohol than in Ringer's solution, a difference significant at better than the 1%
level. In the twenty-five specimens of the
second series the mean deflection was 2.5%
less after five days in alcohol, a decrease also
significant at better than the 1% level.
These specimens did not show an increased
deflection after being replaced in Ringer's
solution. Because the effect of alcohol fixation was not reversible, Sedlin did not use
it as a means of preservation in his study.

EFFECTS OF FREEZING

Freezing is another method of preservation whose effects on the mechanical properties of bone were investigated by Sedlin
(1965). Forty-three specimens, 2 × 1 mm or
2 × 2 mm in cross section, were tested three
hours after removal from the body while

TABLE IX

EFFECTS OF FREEZING UPON THE MEAN VALUES FOR SOME MECHANICAL PROPERTIES IN BENDING OF CORTICAL BONE FROM ADULT HUMAN FEMURS (Data from Sedlin, 1965)

	Fresh	*Frozen*	*Probability*
Number of specimens	43	31	—
Ultimate fiber stress (Kp/mm²)	16.7 ± 3.0	17.6 ± 3.2	$> .05$
Modulus of elasticity ($\times 10^3$ Kp/mm²)	1.41 ± 0.24	$1.39 \pm 0.23*$	$> .05$
Energy absorbed to failure ($\times 10^{-2}$ Kpcm/mm³)	9.16 ± 2.72	$9.67 \pm 3.05*$	$> .05$
Total deflection to failure (mm)	1.81 ± 0.64	$1.60 \pm 0.53*$	$> .05$

* Only 23 specimens. Valid maximum stress values could be obtained but not for the other mechanical properties.

thirty-one other specimens were frozen at $-20°$ C for three to four weeks. The latter specimens were thawed and then heated to $37°$ C before being tested. Both groups of specimens had representatives from all quadrants of three adult human femurs but it was impossible to obtain an equal number of specimens from each quadrant.

Sedlin reported that freezing and subsequent heating produced no statistically significant differences in the mechanical properties of his specimens (Table IX). The same was true with respect to the mechanical properties of fresh and fresh-frozen specimens from each individual. Consequently, he concluded that freezing at $-20°$ C did not significantly change the mechanical properties of human cortical bone.

In evaluating Sedlin's work on the mechanical properties of bone, it should be remembered that the data were obtained from bending tests, which are considered to be better tests for analyzing the structure of a material or an object than for determining its mechanical properties. During bending, a specimen is subjected to longitudinal (horizontal) tensile, compressive, and shearing stresses, none of which is uniformly distributed over the cross section of the specimen. Consequently, a value for the extreme fiber stress does not provide a great deal of information unless the particular kind of stress (tensile, compressive, or shearing) is stated. For example, the convex side of the specimen, when it is bent, undergoes tensile stress and strain while the concave side undergoes compressive stress and strain. However, the location of the stresses is reversed as soon as the specimen is bent in the opposite direction. If the neutral plane is not midway between the two external surfaces, the magnitude of the stresses (tensile or compressive) will be unequal.

EFFECTS OF EMBALMING

One of the most common methods of preserving biological material is to inject some kind of embalming fluid into the blood vessels of the cadaver. Consequently, one must consider the effects of embalming on the mechanical properties of bone. This is especially important with respect to studies on human bone because of the great difficulties in obtaining adequate amounts of fresh unembalmed material.

Differences in the compressive strength between fresh and embalmed human cortical bone from the middle third of the shaft of seven femurs and tibias were investigated by Calabrisi and Smith (1951). Two types of test specimens were used. One type consisted of hollow tubes with walls machined to a uniform thickness; the second type, of miniature cylinders three-eighths inch long and an approximate diameter of one-eighth inch. The miniature specimens were used to determine the effect of specimen size on the compressive strength of bone.

Two nearly identical tubular test specimens were machined from each bone. One specimen of each pair was tested in the fresh condition and the other specimen after forty-three to fifty-six days in an embalming fluid consisting of equal volumes of 95% alcohol, 10% formalin, and chemically pure glycerin.

The results obtained from the tubular specimens, loaded in the direction of their long axis (Table X), showed that the compressive strength of all the embalmed specimens, except the one from the tibia of the 53-year-old man, was less than that of the fresh specimens. The average ultimate compressive strength of the seven fresh specimens was 27,171 lbf/in² (19.1 kgf/mm²) compared to an average of 23,289 lbf/in² (16.4 kgf/mm²) for the seven embalmed ones, a 17% decrease in the compressive strength due to embalming.

The average compressive strength, in the long axis, of the seven fresh miniature specimens from the middle third of the tibial shaft from a 69-year-old woman was

25,200 lbf/in² (17.7 kgf/mm²). The two tubular specimens from the same bone had an average compressive strength of 26,400 lbf/in² (18.6 kgf/mm²), only 4.8% greater than the average strength of the miniature specimens. This was not considered to be a significant difference. Consequently, Calabrisi and Smith concluded that miniature specimens were satisfactory for studying the compressive strength of bone.

Evans (1964), who compared the ultimate tensile strength of embalmed and unembalmed wet- and dry-tested specimens of cortical bone from tibias of adult white men, found that embalmed specimens, both wet and dry, were stronger than similarly tested unembalmed specimens (Fig. 36). An analysis of variance showed that the tensile strength of the embalmed dry-tested specimens was greater, at the 0.01 significance level, than that of the unembalmed dry specimens. A similar comparison revealed that the strength of the embalmed wet specimens was significantly greater, at the 0.05 to 0.01 level, than the strength of the unembalmed wet specimens.

A more recent study conducted in this laboratory on mechanical properties of em-

TABLE X

EFFECTS OF EMBALMING ON THE COMPRESSIVE STRENGTH OF TUBULAR SPECIMENS OF HUMAN CORTICAL BONE
(Data from Calabrisi and Smith, 1951)

Bone	Sex	Age (Years)	Days Embalmed	(lbf/in²) Fresh Specimens	Embalmed Specimens	(kgf/mm²) Fresh Specimens	Embalmed Specimens
Femur	M	50	0	31,000	—	21.8	—
			50	—	25,600	—	18.0
Femur	M	53	0	29,300	—	20.6	—
			43	—	23,000	—	16.2
Femur	F	23	0	31,000	—	21.8	—
			50	—	23,500	—	16.6
Tibia	M	59	0	23,100	—	16.2	—
			50	—	20,200	—	14.2
Tibia	M	53	0	21,100	—	14.9	—
			43	—	26,700	—	18.8
Tibia	F	65	0	31,400	—	22.1	—
			56	—	27,000	—	19.0
Tibia	F	52	0	23,300	—	16.4	—
			43	—	17,020	—	12.0

TABLE XI

Variation Between Embalmed and Unembalmed Wet-tested Cortical Bone from Human Tibias

Variable	N (1)	N (2)	F-Ratio	Mean (1)	Sigma (1)	Mean (2)	Sigma (2)
$E \times 10^6$ lbf/in^2	251	149	34.860*	2.4904	.60373	2.14134	.51292
UTS (lbf/in^2)	252	150	17.124*	13513.77	2754.50	12289.93	3049.15
Percent elongation	228	141	22.897*	1.55439	.79242	1.95872	.78265
SSS (lbf/in^2)	115	127	2.261	11458.78	1280.58	11115.75	2120.92
Hardness (Rockwell)	114	134	115.400*	11.377	10.184	−3.075	10.866
SSS/UTS × 100	114	127	3.236	88.0518	18.4586	92.526	19.984

* 0.01 or better significance level.
(1) = embalmed, (2) = unembalmed, E = modulus of elasticity, UTS = ultimate tensile strength, SSS = single shearing strength.

balmed and unembalmed wet specimens of cortical bone from tibias of adult men showed that the mean ultimate tensile and single shearing strength, tensile strain, modulus of elasticity, and Rockwell superficial hardness of the embalmed specimens were greater than those of the unembalmed ones (Table XI). An analysis of variance in the data revealed that all the differences, except for single shearing strength, were significant at the 0.01 or better level. The difference in single shearing strength of the embalmed and unembalmed specimens was not significant. Thus, embalming significantly affects mechanical properties of human cortical bone but, according to McElhaney et al. (1964), has little influence on those of beef bone except for compressive strength (Table XII).

The effects of embalming on the bending modulus of elasticity of specimens of cortical bone from the femur of an 83-year-old man were investigated by Sedlin (1965). Ten fresh tensile specimens, without prior warming, were loaded at a rate of 2 mm/min until a load of 8 to 9 kg (approximately 2 to 2.3 kg/mm²) had been applied. The load was then removed and the specimens were retested after being in a 10% formalin solution for three weeks. The average modulus of elasticity was 400 ± 54 Kp/mm² for the fresh specimens in comparison with 417 ± 41 Kp/mm² for the embalmed ones,

a 4.3% increase in modulus of elasticity due to embalming was not significant.

The spring rates for a simply supported, center loaded intact tibia-fibula complex in the *in vivo* and wet embalmed conditions of adult dogs were determined by Greenberg et al. (1968). The average spring rate was 2,399 lb/in for twelve wet embalmed specimens compared to 2,304 lb/in for seven *in vivo* specimens. They also found that the ultimate bending strength of the complex was increased by embalming.

An extensive investigation of the effects of embalming on the mechanical properties of beef cortical bone was made by McElhaney et al. (1964). Small tension and compression specimens were machined to a standardized size and shape from eight femurs of cattle from 2½ to 3 years of age. During the machining, the specimens were kept in contact with water at all times in order to maintain the water content of the specimens as close to that of the living bone as possible. Specimens were alternately tested in the fresh condition and after being in embalming fluid for a minimum of fifteen hours, which was considered to be long enough to embalm the specimens. Four embalming fluids of different chemical composition were used. The fresh specimens were tested within forty-eight hours after the death of the animal.

The results of the experiments (Table

TABLE XII

EFFECTS OF EMBALMING ON THE AVERAGE MECHANICAL PROPERTIES OF BEEF CORTICAL BONE
(Data from McElhaney et al., 1964)

	Fresh	Embalmed	Percentage Change
In Tension			
Ultimate strength (lbf/in²)	13,300	12,850	−3.4
Ultimate strength (kgf/mm²)	9.349	9.033	−3.4
Maximum strain (× 10⁻⁶ in/in)	5,030	4,800	−4.6
Maximum strain (× 10⁻⁶ cm/cm)	5,030	4,800	−4.6
Modulus of elasticity (× 10⁶ lbf/in²)	2.98	2.94	−1.3
Modulus of elasticity (kgf/mm²)	2,094	2,066	−1.3
In Compression			
Ultimate strength (lbf/in²)	19,360	16,990	−12.2
Ultimate strength (kgf/mm²)	13.61	11.94	−12.2
Maximum strain (× 10⁻⁶ in/in)	4,820	4,610	−4.4
Maximum strain (× 10⁻⁶ cm/cm)	4,820	4,610	−4.4
Modulus of elasticity (× 10⁶ lbf/in²)	4.18	3.92	−6.2
Modulus of elasticity (kgf/mm²)	2,938	2,755	−6.2
Hardness			
Rockwell H	97.4	98.2	+0.8

XII) showed that the tensile and compressive property values of beef cortical bone were reduced by embalming while the hardness value was increased. The reductions (12%) in the values for the compressive properties were significantly greater than those for the tensile properties.

SUMMARY

Investigations of the effects of different methods of preservation on the mechanical properties of cortical bone reveal that alcohol fixation causes a significant and irreversible decrease in the deflection of human tibial bone when tested in bending. However, no statistically significant changes occurred in the bending properties of human cortical bone that had been frozen at −20° C for three to four weeks and subsequently heated before testing.

Embalming increases, at the 0.01 or better significance level, the mean ultimate tensile strength and strain, modulus of elasticity (in tension), and Rockwell superficial hardness of wet cortical bone from adult male tibias. Single shearing strength is also increased but not in a statistically significant amount.

The compressive strength of beef cortical bone is significantly reduced (12%) by embalming but tensile strength, maximum strain, and modulus of elasticity, are only slightly decreased. Hardness was insignificantly increased by embalming.

The spring rate of the simply supported, center loaded tibia-fibula complex of adult dogs and usually its ultimate bending strength are increased by embalming.

CHAPTER 6

TEMPERATURE EFFECTS

BENDING PROPERTIES

THE FIRST INVESTIGATION of the effects of different temperatures on the mechanical properties of fresh and dry rods of cortical bone was made by Rauber (1876) who determined the bending modulus of elasticity of one humeral specimen from a 30-year-old man, one femoral and two tibial specimens from a 46-year-old man, and one femoral specimen from an ox. The test specimen had rectangular, or occasionally, quadratic cross sections.

The humeral specimen from the 30-year-old man was dry-tested whereas the other specimens were tested in the fresh condition. All specimens were tested at 10° C (50° F), which was obtained by artificially lowering the room temperature. Then separate tests were made on the dry and moist rods. The dry one was exposed to sunlight for a sufficient period of time and tested at 40° C (104° F), while the fresh specimens were continuously wetted during the test with water which had been heated to 38° C (100.4° F) before testing.

During a test the total flexure, the elastic flexure, the elastic flexure increase, and the elastic aftereffect were measured. Loads from 100 g to 300 or 400 g were applied to each specimen. The mean flexure and the mean modulus of elasticity for a 100-g load were calculated at 10° C and 40° C for the dry specimen and at 10° C and 38° C for the fresh ones.

Rauber found that heating fresh moist or dry human cortical bone at slightly above the normal body temperature reduced its bending modulus of elasticity (Table XIII). The highest temperatures at which the specimens were tested, i.e. 38° C for the fresh and 40° C for the dry, would be a slight and a high fever, respectively, for a normal human adult. How the results of the test were affected by the age of the subject, the bone from which the specimens were taken, and the moisture content of the specimens, are additional factors to be considered.

Smith and Walmsley (1959) investigated the influence of temperature variation on the elastic properties of cortical bone by measuring the deformations produced in standardized specimens by bending stress and by axial tensile and compressive stress. The test specimens, obtained from a human tibia, a horse radius, a dog femur, and the

TABLE XIII

EFFECTS OF TEMPERATURE ON THE MEAN BENDING MODULUS OF ELASTICITY OF HUMAN CORTICAL BONE
(Data from Rauber, 1876)

Bone	Test Condition	Modulus of Elasticity (kgf/mm^2)				Modulus of Elasticity ($\times 10^6\ lbf/in^2$)			
		10° C	40° C	10° C	38° C	10° C	40° C	10° C	38° C
Humerus	Dry	2,315	2,091	—	—	3.3	3.0	—	—
Tibia	Fresh moist	—	—	2,337	2,041	—	—	3.3	2.9
Tibia	Fresh moist	—	—	1,983	1,871	—	—	2.8	2.7
Femur	Fresh moist	—	—	2,213	1,982	—	—	3.1	2.8

metacarpus of an ox and a sheep, were rods about 3 inches long with an average cross section of 0.02 in².

A special apparatus was developed for measuring the bending modulus of elasticity under cantilever loading and the tensile and compressive modulus under axial loading. The specimen was surrounded by a closely fitting metal collar to prevent buckling during a compression test. The collar, which was about one-sixteenth inch shorter than the specimen, had windows for the attachment of a Lyndley extensometer by which compressive strain was measured to an accuracy of 1/20,000 inch. The bending and axial tension tests were made with the specimen immersed in a fluid of known temperature. Since it was impossible to do this with the compression tests, they were made in air.

The purpose of the axial tension and compression tests was to determine if the modulus for bone is the same under both conditions, as is true for most other materials. This comparison was necessary because the value for the modulus, assumed to be the same in tension and compression, was used in calculations of the modulus of elasticity in the cantilever bending tests. The compressive modulus of elasticity was 3% greater than the tensile modulus, a difference which the authors attributed to friction between the specimen and the collar enclosing it. The difference between the tensile and compressive modulus was not considered to be a significant one.

The specimens were immersed in saline solution for one hour to overcome any evaporation effects during preparation. After the fluid bath had come to the desired

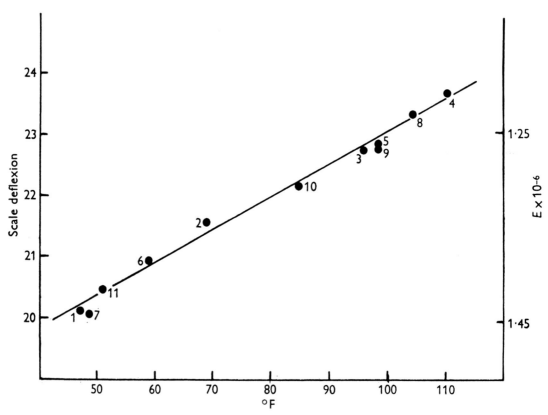

Figure 38. Relation between temperature and bending modulus of elasticity of cortical bone. (From Smith and Walmsley: *J Anat,* 1959)

temperature, the specimen was placed in it for thirty minutes, during which time heating was assumed to be uniform. The bending test of the immersed specimen was then performed under a known load and its deflection recorded. The fluid bath was then raised to a higher temperature and after thirty minutes the test was repeated with the same load. With this procedure the deformations produced by a constant load at temperatures of 40° F to 110° F (4.4° C to 43.3° C) were measured.

An approximately linear but inverse relationship was shown to exist between temperature and bending modulus of elasticity of cortical bone as a result of these experiments (Fig. 38). The value for the modulus of elasticity decreased from 1.45×10^6 lbf/in^2 (1,019 kgf/mm^2) at 40° F (4.4° C) to 1.25×10^6 lbf/in^2 (878 kgf/mm^2) at 99° F (37.2° C). Temperature effects on the modulus of elasticity of bone were completely reversible.

EFFECTS OF WET AND DRY HEAT

A thorough investigation of the effects of wet and dry heat, used in different experimental conditions, on the mechanical properties of standardized specimens of human cortical bone was made by Sedlin (1965). The majority of the tests were done in bending.

Experiment 1

The relation between heat and bending was determined for ten standardized femoral specimens, $2 \times 2 \times 50$ mm, from a 66-year-old woman who died from bronchopneumonia. After being tested in Ringer's solution at room temperature, the fresh specimens were dried in a glass "sandwich" for four days at 105° C (221° F). They were retested dry, returned to Ringer's solution for twenty-four hours, and tested a third time.

The specimens were tested like 30-mm cantilever beams with loads up to 250 g applied at a rate of 0.5 cm/min. From the deformation measurements obtained in each of the three tests, the tangent modulus of elasticity of each specimen was calculated. Because shrinkage after dry heating caused a 13% change in the average moment of inertia, the modulus rather than the deformation (deflection) was evaluated.

Sedlin reported that the mean modulus of elasticity was $1.34 \pm 0.14 \times 10^3$ kp/mm^2

in the first test, $1.56 \pm 0.24 \times 10^3$ kp/mm^2 after drying at 105° C for four days, and $0.91 \pm 0.15 \times 10^3$ kp/mm^2 after rewetting. The differences in the values for the modulus of the individual specimens were statistically significant.

Experiment 2

In another study, test specimens previously subjected to a 100-g load after immersion in Ringer's solution at room temperature were boiled in Ringer's solution for one hour and returned to Ringer's solution at room temperature for thirty minutes before testing. The specimens were then refrigerated for one day and tested again in Ringer's solution at room temperature.

The deflections occurring in each test were measured and compared for each specimen. For example, before the boiling and cooling test the specimens had an average deflection of 0.66 mm while afterwards the deflection decreased to 0.63 mm. One day in Ringer's solution increased the mean deflection to 0.70 mm, a change of only borderline significance.

Experiment 3

A third group of specimens was heated at a temperature of 105° C for one hour before testing. Otherwise, the experiment was the same as the preceding one. The re-

TABLE XIV

Changes in the Bending Properties of Human Cortical Bone After Four Days of Dry Heat (105°C) (Data from Sedlin, 1965)

	Wet	Oven-Dried	Probability
Number of specimens	23	12	—
Ultimate fiber stress (Kp/mm²)	18.2 ± 4.3	17.2 ± 3.1	> .05
Modulus of elasticity (× 10³ Kp/mm²)	1.64 ± .37	2.58 ± .37	> .001
Energy absorbed to failure (× 10⁻² Kpcm/mm³)	9.14 ± 3.51	0.157 ± .044	> .001
Total deflection to failure (mm)	2.03 ± .45	0.54 ± .06	> .0005

sults of this study were similar to those of the boiling experiment but more pronounced and consistent. The average deflection was 0.69 mm in the control test, 0.65 mm after heating and immediate rewetting, and 0.75 mm one day later. These were significant differences.

Experiment 4

Sedlin also investigated the effect of four days of dry heat at a temperature of 105° C on some other physical properties of corti-

cal bone (Table XIV). Twelve specimens were obtained from a 41-year-old woman who died from carcinoma of the breast, a 56-year-old man who died from a cerebral hemorrhage, and a 91-year-old man who died from a myocardial infarction. After heating the specimens, they were loaded like a simple beam to failure at a deformation rate of 1.0 cm/min.

Comparison of the mechanical properties of the specimens oven-dried for four days at 105° C with those of wet specimens re-

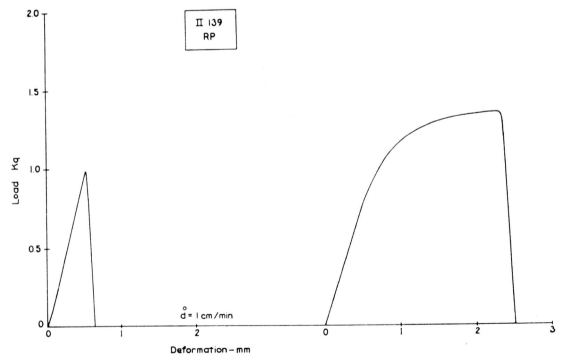

Figure 39. Bending load vs deformation diagram showing effects of 4 days of heat drying. (From Sedlin: *Acta Orthop Scand,* 1965)

vealed that oven-drying produced a statistically significant decrease in the energy absorbed to failure and the total deflection of the specimens, but an increase in the modulus of elasticity. Oven-drying produced a decrease in the ultimate fiber stress, athough it was not a statistically significant one (Table XIV). The load-deflection curves for the dry specimens were almost linear to failure but the curves for the wet specimens had a major change at 40% to 50% of the breaking load (Fig. 39).

Although Sedlin does not mention it, age, especially in the specimens obtained from the 91-year-old man, may have had some influence on the results of the experiments.

As Sedlin points out, the combined effect of heating and dehydration on the mechanical properties of bone is greater than that produced by either heating or drying alone. Four days of dry heat and subsequent rewetting decreased the modulus of elasticity by 32%, whereas drying at room temperature for the same length of time and rewetting the specimen only produced a 5% decrease in the modulus of elasticity. The concept of the relative effects of heating and dehydration vs drying alone was substantiated by the one-hour tests in which boiled specimens showed a deflection increase of 6.1% one day later compared to an 8.7% increase in oven-heated specimens.

Experiment 5

Tests to determine the effect of four days of dry heat on stress relaxation and on hysteresis were also made. Ten specimens from a 66-year-old woman who died from bronchopneumonia were tested by cantilever loading after the following treatments: (1) wet-testing in Ringer's solution at room temperature, (2) dry-testing after four days of incubation at a temperature of 105° C and, (3) wet-testing in Ringer's solution twenty-four hours later.

The specimens were tested for hysteresis by loading them to 250 g and then unloading them at a rate of 0.5 cm/min. After two minutes a stress-relaxation test was made without changing the orientation of the specimen. After loading the specimen, the heads of the testing machine were stopped and the recorder was permitted to run for one minute. Thus, the deformation of the specimen was constant while the change in resistance of the specimen during that time was recorded. Each specimen was tested for the three conditions. By this method it was possible to measure the decrease in stress in every specimen after one minute in addition to the residual deformation in the testing cycle when the specimen registered no resistance.

The hysteresis tests showed that the average residual deformations at zero stress were 0.05 mm in the control group, 0.01 mm for the group dried by heating, and 0.21 mm for the rehydrated group. In the stress relaxation tests the average decrease in stress after one minute was 4.3% in the control group, 2.1% in the heated group, and 13.4% in the rehydrated group. All the hysteresis and stress relaxation changes were highly significant.

Experiment 6

The ultimate fiber stress, the modulus of elasticity, the energy absorbed to failure, and the total deflection in seventy-seven standardized specimens were likewise investigated by Sedlin. He obtained the specimens from a 34-year-old man who died from suffocation, a 67-year-old man who died from massive trauma, and a 75-year-old woman who died from a pulmonary embolism. These specimens were divided into two groups with site-matched specimens in each. One group was tested in Ringer's solution at a temperature of 21° C (69.8° F) and the second one at a temperature of

37° C (98.6° F). The specimens were loaded to failure in bending at a deformation rate of 1.0 cm/min. An increase ($0.05 > p > 0.01$) in the total deflection of the specimens at the higher temperature was the only significant difference between the mechanical properties of the specimens tested.

Experiment 7

Experiments were also made on the effect of two different temperatures on the deformation of specimens loaded like a cantilever beam. For this purpose specimens were tested in Ringer's solution at 27° C (80.6° F) and then warmed in the solution for one hour at 37° C before being retested. Loads up to 100 g were applied to the specimens at a rate of 1.0 cm/min.

An average deformation of 0.77 mm was found when the specimens were tested at a temperature of 21° C and of 0.82 mm when tested at 37° C. The modulus of elasticity at the two temperatures was 1,250 Kp/mm² and 1,190 Kp/mm², respectively, a statistically significant change. The values for the modulus of elasticity confirmed the results of the study by Smith and Walmsley (1959) that the modulus decreases with an increase in temperature.

Experiment 8

A problem of considerable practical importance, especially to dentists, is the heat produced in bone by dental drills. Thompson (1958) reported that the temperature of bone varied from 38° C to 67° C (152.6° F) as the speed of drilling increased. However, Rafel (1962) found that the maximum temperature at a distance of 3 mm from a dental bur was only 24° C (75.2° F).

Sedlin investigated this problem in five compression blocks of bone from a 50-year-old man who died from uremia and a 53-year-old man who died from cardiac failure. Three Honeywell thermocouples, 0.1 mm in diameter, were placed in holes at various distances from the grinding surface. The thermocouples were connected to an amplifier which was joined to a four-channel recorder. The specimens, in a vise, were put into a pan of water at room temperature (23° C or 73.4° F). With this apparatus temperature changes in the specimen and the surrounding fluid could be read at three different points simultaneously. A Carborundum wheel, which was lowered to the specimen at a constant rate, was used for the grinding. The apparatus was calibrated at temperatures of 40° C and 100° C (212° F).

Four different tests were conducted: (1) Intermittent grinding for approximately 10 sec in increments of 0.1 mm at 2,800 revolutions per minute (rpm) of the grinding wheel. The specimen was ground, parallel to the long axis of the osteons, until the thermocouples were destroyed. (2) Constant grinding at a rate of 0.02 mm/sec and the same revolutions per minute, parallel to the long axis of the osteons, until the thermocouples were destroyed. (3) Constant grinding, perpendicular to the long axis of the osteons, was used in two other specimens; the wheel and grinding rates were the same as in (2). Finally, (4) constant grinding at a rate of 0.02 mm/sec, parallel to the long axis of the osteons, but at a speed of 1,000 rpm of the grinding wheel.

When a surface temperature of 100° C was used, Sedlin found that the temperature of the specimen was 83° C (181.4° F) at a distance of 4 mm from the surface, 65° C (149° F) at a distance of 1.3 mm from the surface, and 55° C (131° F) at a distance of 2.7 mm from the surface. With a surface temperature of 40° C the corresponding temperature values were 36° C (98.6° F), 32.5° C (90.5° F), and 29° C (84.2° F). At no time was the specimen temperature higher than 40° C. The results of the study showed that the maximum temperature reached by the element within the specimen was a direct function of its distance from the heat source.

The results of Sedlin's tests suggest that not enough heat was generated to alter the mechanical properties of bone with the methods used by different investigators in the preparation of their specimens.

TENSILE PROPERTIES

Elastic and Plastic Strain

Elastic and plastic strain (deformation) produced by tensile loading and unloading of cortical bone at room temperature (25° C) as well as variations in ultimate tensile stress at temperatures ranging from −196° to 200° C have been investigated by Bonfield and Li (1966). Flat tensile specimens with a gauge length of one inch and a cross section of 0.18×0.60 inch machined from beef femurs and tibias were used. Presumably the specimens were unembalmed although it was not so stated by the authors. The specimens were loaded in the direction of their long axis which coincided with that of the intact bone.

Prior to testing, the specimens were refrigerated under identical conditions and tested as nearly at the same time as possible. Comparative tests were made on specimens from the same section of the bone. Again, the specimens were probably unembalmed and tested in the moist condition although this information was not given by the authors.

The specimens were subjected to direct tensile stresses, at increasingly higher levels, in the direction of their long axis. A load-unload technique was used. A constant strain rate of $3.3 \times 10^{-4} sec^{-1}$ was applied with an Instron testing machine while the strain over a gauge length of one inch was measured with a Tuckerman strain gauge having a sensitivity of 2×10^{-6} in/in. The total strain (elastic and plastic) at stress and the residual plastic strain after unloading were measured for each stress level. From these data the authors determined the microscopic yield stress (i.e. the stress required to produce the first detectable plastic strain of 2×10^{-6} in/in) and the subsequent strain rate of hardening to failure. The load-unload procedure was performed in a continuous way at stresses below the microscopic yield stress in order to determine whether or not closed hysteresis loops, indicating anelastic behavior, were found.

The results of the tests at room temperature (Fig. 40) showed that plastic yielding (microscopic yield stress) began at about 600 lbf/in² (.4218 kgf/mm²). This was accompanied by elastic deformation without closed hysteresis loops. An elastic modulus of 3.8×10^6 lbf/in² (2671.4 kgf/mm²) was computed from the stress-total strain diagram (Inset, Fig. 40). Microscopic yield stress, determined from ten similar tests on other specimens, varied from 190 to 780 lbf/in² (.1336 to .5483 kgf/mm²) with an average of approximately 400 lbf/in² (.2812 kgf/mm²). The values for microscopic yield stress were not significantly different for specimens from various regions of the same bone nor for those from different bones.

Above the microscopic yield point plastic strain increased progressively with applied stress (Fig. 40) and amounted to 160×10^{-6} in/in just before failure. Generally within two minutes after unloading a large anelastic contraction occurred, followed within five to ten minutes, by a smaller relaxation until equilibrium was attained. The amount of relaxation was a function of an increase in the level of previously applied stress. Thus, permanent contractions at zero stress of 44%, 63%, and 67% of the initial plastic

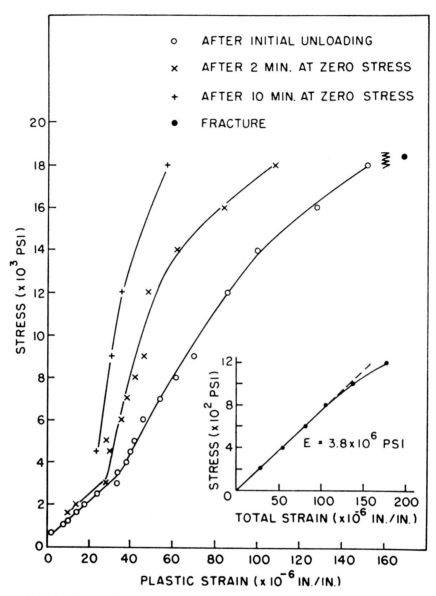

Figure 40. Variation of plastic strain with stress in the longitudinal direction in cortical beef bone. (From Bonfield and Li: *J. Appl Physics,* 1966)

strain were found in specimens after unloading them from stresses of 4,500, 9,000, and 12,000 lbf/in² (3.164, 6.327, 8.436 kgf/mm²), respectively. The percentage of contraction in each load-unload cycle tended to increase if the tests were repeated to the same stress level. In one specimen (Table XV) the initial plastic strain produced by a second, third, and fourth load-unload cycle was almost completely recovered. However, recovery of the residual plastic (permanent) strain found for the first load-unload cycle was not improved with additional cycles.

TABLE XV

EFFECTS OF TENSILE LOAD-UNLOAD CYCLES AT 25° C ON RELAXATION IN BEEF CORTICAL BONE
(Data from Bonfield and Li, 1966)

Applied Stress lbf/in²	Load-Unload Cycle	Plastic Strain After Unloading (× 10⁻⁶ in/in)	Residual Plastic Strain After Relaxation (× 10⁻⁶ in/in) In Each Cycle	Total	Percentage Contraction In Each Cycle
7,000	1	60	22	22	63
	2	44	0	22	100
	3	50	4	26	92
	4	52	0	26	100

Ultimate Tensile Stress

In a similar series of experiments longitudinal tensile specimens were loaded to failure at the same strain rate used in the previous studies but at temperatures varying from −196° to 200° C. Temperatures of −196°, −70°, 0°, and 100° C were obtained by putting the specimens, contained in glass tubes, into baths of liquid nitrogen, dry ice and acetone, ice and water, and boiling water, respectively. To obtain temperatures of 200° to 900° C, specimens under a helium atmosphere were heated in a furnace for ten minutes. During a test the temperature change was < 5° C.

The results of these tests (Fig. 41) showed that ultimate tensile stress is temperature dependent with maximum failure stress occurring at 0° C. Reducing or raising the temperature caused a decrease in the magnitude of the failure stress although the decrease occurred at a more rapid rate as the temperature was increased to 200° C.

Temperature differences in the fracture profile were also observed. Thus, at −196°, −70°, and 100° C the profile was more serrated while at 200° C a ninety degree brittle fracture occurred.

In a more recent publication Bonfield and Li (1968) report the results of their continued studies on the relation of temperature to tensile deformation in cortical bone from beef femurs. However, instead of testing all their specimens at room temperature (25° C), as was done in their earlier investigation, specimens were tested at temperatures varying from −58° to 90° C. The methods of preparing and testing the specimens were the same as those employed in their previous study.

All specimens were tested in the direction of their long axis at various temperatures but a constant strain rate of $3.3 \times 10^{-4} \text{sec}^{-1}$ to a given stress at which the total strain was measured. The specimens were then unloaded at the same strain rate and the amount of residual nonelastic strain was determined. The stress producing the first measurable departure from elastic behavior, i.e. a residual nonelastic strain of 2×10^{-6} in/in, was called the microscopic yield stress. As the specimens always exhibited some recovery after unloading, the anelastic strain (decrease in residual strain with time) and the plastic strain (equilibrium residual strain) were likewise measured. The values for the slopes of the stress/total strain and stress/residual nonelastic strain were obtained by repeating the tests for an increasing series of stress up to a maximum of 4,700 lbf/in² (3.304 kgf/mm²).

Precise comparisons between different temperatures and specimens were made by following an identical loading sequence and series of stress levels in each test. Between each stress cycle the specimens remained at

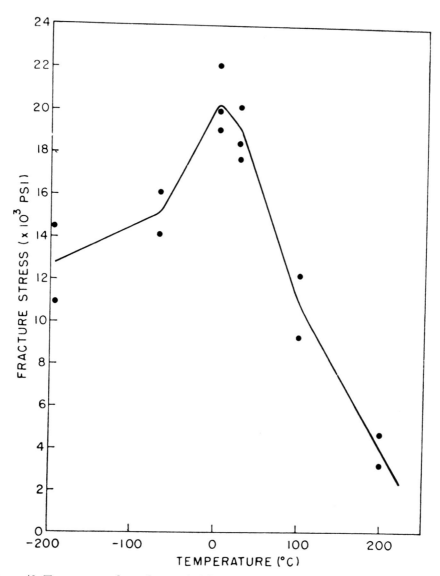

Figure 41. Temperature dependence of ultimate tensile stress in beef cortical bone tested at a constant strain rate. (From Bonfield and Li: *J Appl Physics*, 1966)

zero stress for four minutes during which all or most (depending on the applied stress) of the anelastic strain was recovered.

Tests at −58° to 25° C

Results of tests conducted at temperatures varying from −58° to 25° C show that the stress/total strain curves are nonlinear and that the slope of the curve at any given stress decreases with increasing temperature (Fig. 42). Three successive stress/total strain determinations for a given specimen at each temperature revealed a reproducibility within 2%. This was also true if the curve was first determined at a given temperature, then at a second temperature, and again at the first temperature. The absolute value of variation between different specimens at a given temperature was about 12%.

The amount of total strain at each stress

level is a summation of its elastic, anelastic, and plastic components. These components were differentiated by measuring the residual nonelastic strain (anelastic and plastic strain) after unloading. Typical values for nonelastic strain measured immediately after unloading as a function of previously applied stress can be obtained from the curve in Figure 43 which exhibit only small variations in slope. The microscopic yield stress, indicated by the first point on each curve, was similar at all temperatures between −58° and 25° C with a range of variation from 180 to 570 lbf/in² (.1265 to .4007 kgf/mm²) and an average of 420 lbf/in² (.2953 kgf/mm²).

By allowing the specimens to remain at zero stress after unloading, the anelastic and plastic components of nonelastic strain were separated. The amount of contraction in length of the specimen with time represents recovery of the anelastic strain. When equilibrium in length has been attained, any residual strain indicates the plastic component of the total strain.

Relaxation curves (Fig. 44) for specimens tested at temperatures of −58° and 25° C showed a decrease in nonelastic strain with time after unloading from a maximum stress of 4,700 lbf/in² (3.304 kgf/mm²). An equilibrium length was reached after fifteen minutes. In both cases a significant residual plastic strain was found after recovery.

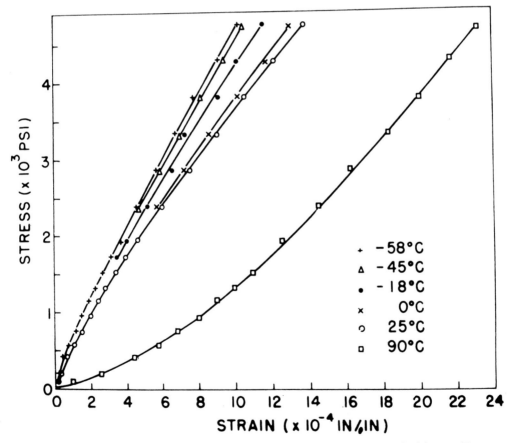

Figure 42. Temperature effects of stress-total strain relations in beef cortical bone. (From Bonfield and Li: *J Biomech,* 1968)

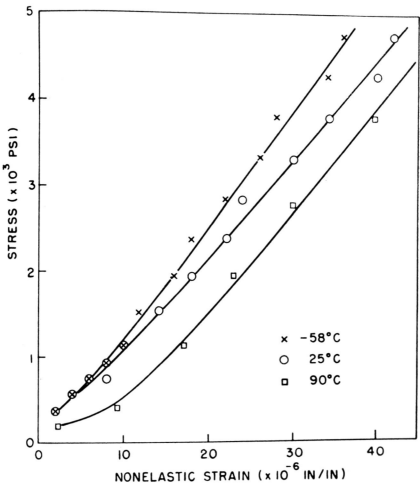

Figure 43. Temperature effects of stress-nonelastic strain relations in beef cortical bone. (From Bonfield and Li: *J Biomech,* 1968)

Tests at 50° to 90° C

At temperatures of 50°, 70°, and 90° C determination of stress/total strain relations after unloading was complicated by rapid contraction of the specimen to less than its original length (Fig. 44). In some cases, equilibrium was not attained until seventy-two hours after unloading. Consequently, the absolute value for stress/total strain is a function of the time between loadings. At temperatures less than 25° C the four minute time between loadings corresponded with the contraction of the specimen to its original length. These were the conditions under which the stress/total strain values were computed. At 90° C the slope of this curve was less than those at lower temperatures (Fig. 42). However, the slope tends to decrease as the stress level is raised.

Reproducible values for stress/total strain were obtained for tests repeated at 50°C, but at 70° and 90° C the total strain at a given stress was a function of the time the specimen was maintained at the particular temperature (Table XVI). At temperatures between −58° and 25° C the slope of the stress/total strain curve was considerably reduced from that seen after exposures to higher temperatures. Thus, total strains, measured at a stress of 4,700 lbf/in² (3.304 kgf/mm²), of 1,372, 2,380, and 2,214 × 10⁻⁶ in/in were found for three successive tests at temperatures of 25°, 90°, and 25°, respectively.

In the 50° to 90° C temperature range the yield stress (average 240 lbf/in²; .1687 kgf/mm²) and the stress/residual nonelastic strain were generally smaller than at lower temperatures. However, because of the rapid recovery of the specimen after unloading at these temperatures, the scatter of the data was greater.

In discussing the results of their experiments Bonfield and Li note that there are

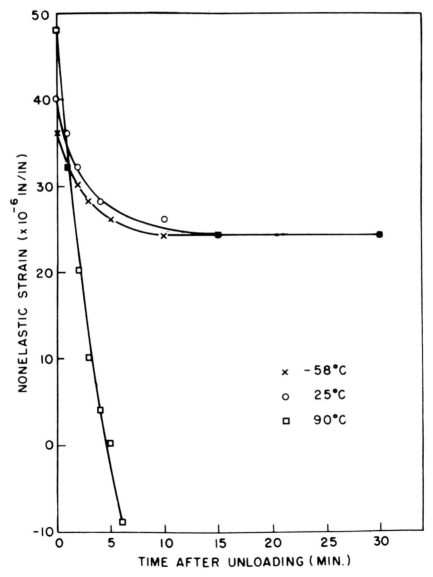

Figure 44. Temperature effects on contraction of beef cortical bone after unloading. (From Bonfield and Li: *J Biomech,* 1968)

TABLE XVI

Increase in Total Strain with Time at Temperature
(Data from Bonfield and Li, 1968)

| Temperature (° C) | Total Strain (× 10⁻⁶ in/in) at 4,700 psi | |
	1st Loading	2nd Loading After 24 hr at Temperature
50	1,574	1,566
70	1,616	1,648
90	2,334	2,468

two stages in the dependence of bone deformation on temperature. At temperatures ranging from −58° to 25° C there is a small elastic deformation to the microscopic yield stress (Stage I) followed by elastic and nonelastic flow (Stage II). With increasing tem-

perature the slope of the stress/residual nonelastic strain curve decreased while the anelastic and permanent strain remained approximately constant. Since the variation in the nonelastic strain was not large enough to account for the temperature change in stress/residual nonelastic strain, the authors concluded it was due to differences in elastic strain and modulus of bone.

They computed the modulus directly from the slope of the stress/residual nonelastic strain curves in Stage I or obtained it by subtracting the nonelastic strain, after unloading, from the total strain in Stage II. These procedures were based on the assump-

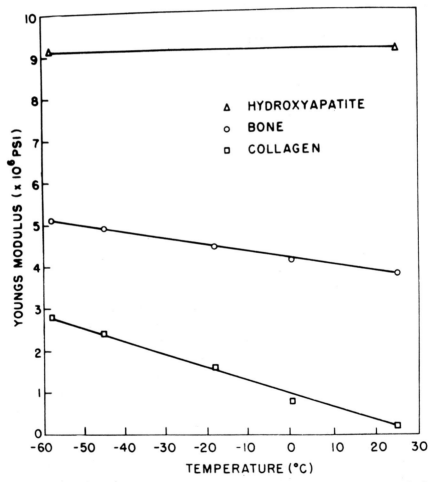

Figure 45. Temperature effects on modulus of elasticity in beef cortical bone, hydroxyapatite, collagen. (From Bonfield and Li: *J Biomech*, 1968)

tion that the continued nonelastic flow and recovery during unloading were small. Reasonably good results were obtained by both methods, the modulus exhibiting an approximately linear dependence on temperature in the −58° to 25° C range (Fig. 45). A similar linear dependence of modulus of elasticity of bone on temperature was previously noted by Smith and Walmsley (1959), who found a modulus increase of about 0.51 percent per degree at temperatures between 9° and 43° C, and by Currey (1965) who reported an increase of about 0.4 percent per degree in the range from 3° to 37° C.

Bonfield and Li's studies showed that at temperatures between −58° and 25° C and at stress levels greater than 400 lbf/in², bone deformation consists of elastic, anelastic, and plastic strain. The modulus of elasticity increases as temperatures are reduced from 25° to −58° C while the microscopic yield stress and the stress/residual nonelastic strain remain approximately constant.

The authors account for the variation in the modulus of elasticity at temperatures from 25° to −58° C on the basis of a composite model of bone in which the modulus of collagen is temperature dependent while that of hydroxyapatite is not. Thus, the decrease in the ratio of the modulus of hydroxyapatite to that of collagen with reduction in temperature produces an increase in the proportion of the load supported by the collagen. They also noted that deformation of bone at temperatures between 50° and 90° C is compounded by non-equilibrium recovery and an irreversible change in bone structure.

COMPRESSIVE PROPERTIES

Effects of variations in temperature on compressive properties of cortical bone from beef femurs was recently investigated by Armstrong et al. (1971). Ten cylindrical compression specimens, 0.186 inch (4.72 mm) × 0.500 inch (12.70 mm) machined from bones dried by aging for two years, and ten tetragonal specimens, 0.400 inch (10.16 mm) in height with a cross section of 0.200 inch (5.08 mm) per side made from wet bones within two weeks after death were used. Five of the specimens were annealed in a vacuum of 10^{-5} mm Hg at 100° C for 170 hours and tested a short time later.

A specially designed cylindrical compression chamber immersed in liquid baths of different temperatures held the specimens while they were tested in an Instron testing machine. Thus, specimens were tested while the compression chamber was immersed in liquid nitrogen (−196° C), in a mixture of dry ice and acetone (−80° C), in methyl alcohol kept at 0° C by a surrounding dewar of ice and water, and in stirred silicone oil maintained at 100° C and at 190° C by immersed heating elements.

Usually the specimens were loaded to failure at a constant strain rate of about 10^{-3} sec⁻¹ while a load-time curve was automatically recorded. The direction of loading was not stated but presumably it was in the long axis of the specimen and the bone.

The anelasticity of bone was confirmed by successively loading and unloading one specimen at room temperature from a specific stress on the original loading curve. A closed hysteresis loop was found for each unloading cycle until fracture during the final loading occurred at about the same stress as found in other specimens loaded directly to failure.

By means of resistance strain gauges mounted on the specimens, stress-strain curves to failure were obtained from a tetragonal and an annealed specimen tested

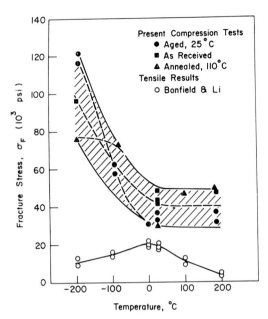

Figure 46. Comparison of temperature effects on ultimate compressive and tensile stress in beef cortical bone. (From Armstrong, Arkayin, and Haddad: *Nature,* 1971)

ing to the Griffith energy release hypothesis, on the basis of a single critical flow governing fracture strength of a material. They also believe that the lower limit of the ratio may be significant because the initiation of a brittle fracture in a normally ductile polycrystalline material can sometimes be described by equating the ductile yield stress of the material to the brittle fracture stress, in compression or in tension. Thus, bone might, at room temperature, exhibit significant plastic yielding at a stress of about 20,000 lbf/in² (14.06 kgf/mm²) but continued deformation at higher stresses is necessary for a brittle compression fracture to occur.

Armstrong et al. then compared their compressive data, obtained at room temperature (25° C) from a non-annealed and an annealed specimen, with tensile data from Bonfield and Li (1966). At lower stresses it was found that the compressive strains were relatively larger than the tensile ones, but at higher strains the specimen exhibited a linear elastic behavior essentially identical to the extended stress-strain behavior for the tensile specimen (Fig. 47). Both types of specimens had an elastic modulus of 3.8 × 10⁶ lbf/in² (2,671 kgf/mm²). The compression specimen had a yield point drop with an accompanying elastic strain de-

at room temperature. The direction in which strain was measured was not given but very probably it was longitudinal to coincide with the direction of loading.

Specimens tested at room temperature had a compressive stress varying from 29,000 lbf/in² (20.387 kgf/mm²) to 48,000 lbf/in² (33.744 kgf/mm²), compared to an average compressive strength, based on data from Currey (1964) and Calabrisi and Smith (1951), of 25,000 lbf/in² (17.575 kgf/mm²). The maximum tensile strength, about 20,000 lbf/in² (14.06 kgf/mm²) is much lower than the comparable compressive strength.

The ratio of ultimate compressive and tensile stress varied between 8.0 and 12.0 at −200° C, between 1.5 and 2.5 at room temperature, and again between 8.0 and 12.0 at 200° C (Fig. 46). The authors believe that the upper limiting value of the ratio may be significant because a theoretical fracture stress ratio on 8.0 can be predicted, accord-

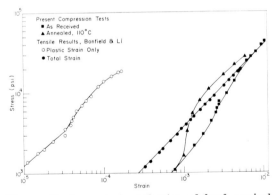

Figure 47. Stress-strain behavior of beef cortical bone in compression or tension at 25° C. (From Armstrong, Arkayin, and Haddad: *Nature,* 1971)

crease at 7,600 lbf/in² (5.343 kgf/mm²). The authors account for this on the basis of imperfections in the geometry of the test specimens. This idea was confirmed by the stress-strain behavior of the annealed specimens which apparently was better fab- ricated and aligned than the other speci- mens. Thus, the annealed specimen showed the expected linear stress-strain behavior af- ter lower strains with an expected increased elastic modulus of 5.0 × 10⁶ lbf/in² (3,515 kgf/mm²).

ENERGY ABSORBING CAPACITY

Bonfield and Li (1966) also demonstrated that the energy absorbing capacity of stan- dardized specimens of beef cortical bone is influenced by temperature. Notched and un- notched impact specimens, cut longitudinal- ly and transversely with respect to the shaft of the femur and the tibia, were tested in a modified Charpy impact tester with which an energy of 5.1 in-lb was applied to the midpoint of the specimen. At the moment of impact the surface of the specimen was subjected to an estimated strain rate of 60 sec⁻¹. The energy absorbed to failure by the longitudinal and transverse specimens, in the notched and unnotched conditions, was determined at temperatures varying from −196° to 900° C. These temperatures were obtained by the methods previously de- scribed for their tensile tests. The fracture surface of the specimen was studied by means of chromium shadowed carbon rep- licas.

The results of the experiments showed that the energy absorbed to failure by the longitudinal unnotched specimens (Fig. 48) was maximum at about 0° C but was mark- edly reduced by lowering the temperature to −70° C and showed little change between −70° and −196° C. Raising the temperature above 0° C also caused a progressive reduc- tion in the magnitude of the energy ab- sorbed to failure which became approxi- mately zero at 200° C and remained there between 300° and 900° C, the highest tem- perature used in the experiments. The color of the specimens did not change at temper- atures below 100° C but at about 200° C

they became light brown, at about 500° C they were black, and at 700° to 900° C they were white in color.

At all temperatures the energy absorbed to failure by the unnotched transverse speci- mens (Fig. 48) was significantly less than that absorbed for the longitudinal speci- mens. Only a small maximum in the energy- absorbed versus temperature curve was noted for the transverse specimens when the measurement was made at room tempera- ture (25° C). Both longitudinal and trans- verse specimens absorbed zero energy at tem- peratures greater than 200° C. Notching re- duced the amount of energy absorbed at temperatures between −196° and 100° C in both types of specimens (Fig. 49). How- ever, the notched specimens resembled the unnotched ones by having the maximum energy absorbed at temperatures from 0° to 25°C.

At temperatures from −196° to 100° C the unnotched longitudinal specimens had an irregular serrated fracture, while at 200° C and at all temperatures from 500° to 900° C there was a more continuous fracture. The fracture surface was more even and had more tear marks at temperatures between −196° and 100° C than it did at tempera- tures above 200° C.

The authors attributed the differences they found to the annular growth structure of bone which, macroscopically, exhibits "growth rings of slightly different color." The meaning of this statement is not clear from the text. Probably they are referring to osteons because they state "It may be reasoned that these rings are of varying composition and structure and separated by interfacial regions in which the bonding is less developed than within any given ring." Presumably the "interfacial regions" are cement lines between osteons.

Bonfield and Li qualitatively correlate the fracture behavior of bone with these interfacial regions, and suggest the probability that fractures will be initiated by the interfaces. In transverse specimens the fracture is quite easily propagated through the interfacial region in a unidirectional continuous way. However, in longitudinal specimens, fractures cannot propagate along the interface because it is perpendicular to the direc-

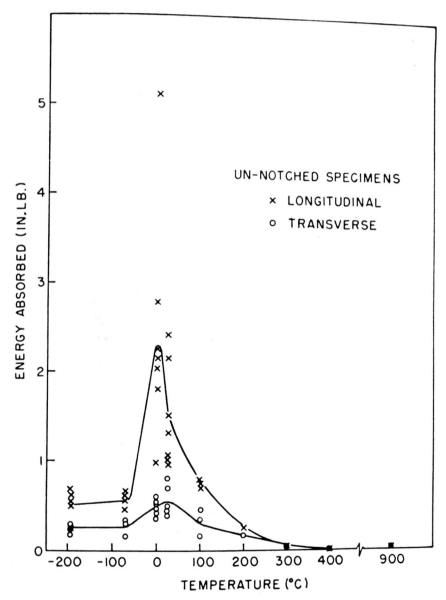

Figure 48. Temperature effects on energy absorbed to failure by unnotched longitudinal and transverse specimens of beef cortical bone. (From Bonfield and Li: *J Appl Physics,* 1966)

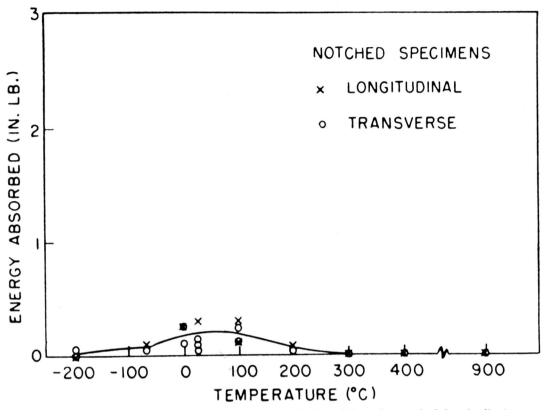

Figure 49. Temperature effects on energy absorbed to failure by notched longitudinal and transverse specimens of beef cortical bone. (From Bonfield and Li: *J Appl Physics*, 1966)

tion of applied stress. Consequently, in order to continue, the fracture must shear across the adjacent ring to the next facial region or area of weakness. Under these conditions the fracture occurs at a 45° angle to the stress axis to conform with the maximum resolved shear stress on the specimen. Continuation of the crack in the same manner results in an irregular, serrated fracture.

They also noted that from −196° to 100° C the temperature dependence of fracture behavior of bone was not due to a permanent structural change but more probably resulted from a reversible structural change or mode of deformation. The smaller temperature dependence of unnotched transverse specimens in contrast with that of similar longitudinal ones was interpreted as

a result of less significant changes, as a function of temperature, in the interfacial region than within a growth ring.

The much smaller energy absorbing capacity of the notched specimens was taken as an indication of the susceptibility of bone to surface defects. It was concluded, therefore, that most of the energy absorbed in fracture is expended in the initiation of a crack of a critical size while little energy is required for continued propagation of the crack. The zero energy absorbed during fracture at temperatures from 200° to 900° C for all specimens tested was attributed to permanent changes in bone structure caused by its progressive decomposition. This was an irreversible change as indicated by annealing specimens at temperatures higher than 200° C and impacting them at 0° C. The energy absorbed by all specimens was at or near zero in contrast to the behavior of specimens tested at temperatures from −196° to 100° C.

If Bonfield and Li's "rings" represent osteons and their "interfacial regions" are cement lines then their idea that the latter are "areas of relative weakness" supports a similar interpretation of cement lines made by Maj and Toajari (1937), Evans (1958), Dempster and Coleman (1960), and Evans and Bang (1966) who also noted a relation between fracture cracks and cement lines.

In the experiments of Bonfield and Li

and of Armstrong et al., bone was treated strictly as an engineering material with no regard to its biological functions. Therefore, their data have relatively little relevance to bone biology because living bone would never be subjected to the extreme range of temperatures employed in their experiments. This would be particularly true for mammalian and avian bone because of the constant body temperature in these animals. Even bones of cold-blooded vertebrates would not be subjected to the extremely high and low temperatures employed in their studies.

MICROHARDNESS

The effects of heat on the microhardness of cortical bone from the long bones of man, cattle, horses, a giraffe, and an elephant were studied by Amprino (1958, 1961). Longitudinal and cross sections, at least 150μ thick, were cut from the cortex of the bones. One of the surfaces of the specimens was highly polished. Loads of 15 to 300 g were applied to the polished surface of the bone specimen with a Leitz-Durimet hardness tester equipped with a square-based Vickers pyramid diamond indenter with angles of 136°. The hardness of the specimens was based on the Vickers pyramid hardness number.

The microhardness, in strictly comparable areas of the same specimen, was first determined in fresh wet specimens, and then after heating them for a few hours at temperatures of 38°, 60°, 120°, 200°, and 300° to 800° C (1,472° F). The effects on microhardness of dehydration, dehydration followed by rehydration, carbonization, ashing, calcification, and directional differences, with respect to the orientation of the collagen fibers, were also investigated.

Amprino found that removal of moisture

from bone by oven-drying at temperatures of 38°, 60° (140° F), and 120° C (248° F) produced a progressive and consistent increase in its microhardness (Table XVII). The amount of moisture absorbed by dry bone after rehydration is approximately equal to that lost in drying. A marked decrease in microhardness occurs after carbonization and more so after ashing at temperatures of 300° to 500° C (572° to 932° F) but at higher temperatures the microhardness increases (Fig. 50). The microhardness of glycol-ashed bone was considerably less than that of bone dried at 38°C.

The microhardness of human bone specimens, mineralized at a temperature of 400° C (752° F) was slightly increased by

TABLE XVII

MICROHARDNESS VALUES FOR GLYCOL-ASHED COMPACT BONE FROM THE METACARPUS OF AN EIGHT-MONTH-OLD CALF* (Data from Amprino, 1958)

	25g Load	50g Load	100g Load
Bone dried at 38° C	—	50.5	51.9
Glycol-ashed bone	10.5	10.4	9.8

* Each value is the mean of ten measurements in structurally identical areas.

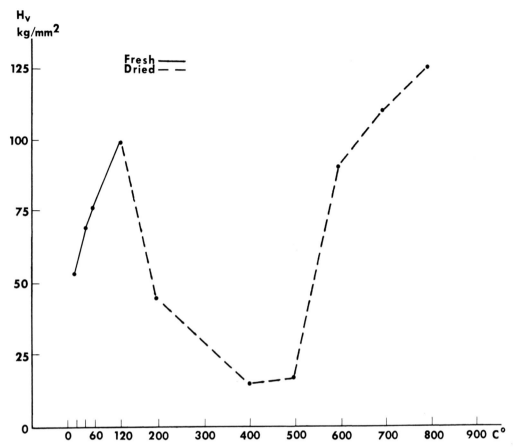

Figure 50. Micohardness of primary periosteal calf bone tested fresh and after drying and incineration at various temperatures. Each point is a mean for 10 determinations. (From Amprino: *Acta Anat,* 1958)

heating them at 500° C. Heating the specimens at 600° C (1,112° F) increased their microhardness to twice that of wet specimens. Additional increases in microhardness were found when the specimens were heated at temperatures of 700° and 800° C (1,292° and 1,472° F). A sudden increase in microhardness apparently occurred at approximately 500° C but the exact point at which this change took place could not be accurately determined because the temperature of the muffle-furnace arose in 100° C increments. Experiments with specimens from different species showed a microhardness increase from eight to fifteen times after heating the specimens at 400° C.

SUMMARY

The bending modulus of elasticity of cortical bone has an approximately linear but inverse relationship with temperatures within the normal body range. These temperature effects are completely reversible. Heating and dehydration affect the flexure properties of human cortical bone more than heating or drying alone. The ultimate fiber stress in bending of human cortical bone is significantly increased by heating to normal body temperature. Studies of the temperature produced in bone by drilling show that bone is a poor conductor of heat.

Longitudinal impact specimens and similar tensile specimens of cortical bone from beef femurs and tibias exhibit plastic yielding at an average stress of about 400 lbf/in² (.2812 kgf/mm²) when tested at room temperature (25° C). With increasing stress, plastic strain progressively increases to an average total plastic strain of approximately 160×10^{-6} in/in just before failure. After unloading to zero stress, plastically strained bone has a large anelastic contraction.

Energy absorbed to failure by longitudinal impact and similar tensile specimens of beef cortical bone, when tested at temperatures from $-196°$ to 100° C is maximum at 0° C. Raising or lowering the temperature reduces the amount of energy absorbed to failure with the greater reduction at temperatures above 0° C. Within the same temperature range unnotched longitudinal impact specimens absorbed more energy to failure than similar transverse specimens. Notching greatly reduced the energy absorbing capacity of both types of specimens. At temperatures above 200° C the energy absorbed to failure by both types of specimens decreased to zero. Temperature dependence of unnotched transverse specimens is less than for longitudinal specimens.

Deformation of beef cortical bone at temperatures between $-58°$ and 25° C and at tensile stresses greater than 400 lbf/in² (.2812 kgf/mm²) has three components—elastic, anelastic, and plastic strain. The tensile modulus of elasticity of the bone was increased as the temperature was lowered from 25° to $-58°$ C but the stress/residual nonelastic strain remains almost constant. Between 50° to 90° C the tensile deformation of beef cortical bone is complicated by non-equilibrium and an irreversible structural change.

The ultimate compressive strength of cortical beef bone, determined at several temperatures between $-200°$ and 200° C, is reasonably constant above 0° C but increases rapidly below 0° C. The ratio of compressive strength to tensile strength is a variable function of temperature with a minimum value near 0° C. The stress-strain behavior of bone at room temperature is very similar for compression and tension except that the ultimate tensile strength is lower than the ultimate compressive strength.

The microhardness of cortical bone is consistently and progressively increased by oven-drying at temperatures of 38°, 60°, and 120° C. Carbonization, ashing, and mineralization by high temperatures (300° to 600° C) markedly increase the microhardness of cortical bone.

CHAPTER 7

DIRECTIONAL DIFFERENCES

BECAUSE BONE is an anisotropic material, the values obtained for its mechanical properties depend upon the direction, with respect to the various axes of the intact bone, in which the test specimen is loaded. The axes of the specimen itself also influence the values obtained for its mechanical properties.

COMPACT BONE

Long Bones

TENSILE PROPERTIES

A survey of the literature shows that Hülsen (1896) was the first to investigate directional differences in the tensile strength of standardized specimens of compact bone. He found that fresh specimens from the tibia of an ox had a greater tensile strength parallel to the long axis of the bone than perpendicular to it (Table XVIII). The difference between the average values in the two directions was 23%. This is probably a significant difference although the number of specimens tested by Hülsen is too few for proper statistical analysis.

The tensile strength of wet and dry standardized specimens of cortical bone from adult human tibias, according to Dempster and Coleman (1960), is greater in a direction parallel to the grain, or predominant direction of the haversian systems, than it is across the grain of the bone (Fig. 51; Table XVIII). The dry-tested specimens were stronger than the wet ones. The specimens were obtained from museum material which had probably been embalmed.

Evans (1964) reported that the ultimate tensile strength of wet-tested specimens of cortical bone from embalmed adult human femurs and tibias was about eight times greater in the longitudinal direction than in the radial or tangential direction with respect to the axes of the intact bone (Fig. 52; Table XVIII). An analysis of variance revealed that the mean tensile strength in the longitudinal direction was greater, at better than the 0.01 significance level, than that in the tangential or radial direction. The difference between the strength in the latter two directions was not statistically significant.

Directional differences in the mechanical properties of standardized test specimens of compact bone from cattle femurs were investigated by Sweeney et al. (1965). The specimens, consisting of haversian bone without outer or inner circumferential lamellae, were taken from the middle third of the femoral shaft of presumably healthy animals, approximately one year old, that had been fed an identical diet. These specimens were cut and loaded in the longitudinal and the transverse directions with respect to the long axis of the intact bone. After being made, the specimens were stored in a solution of equal parts of alcohol and water for one to three weeks before testing. The surface of a specimen was hand-dried and the test performed within an hour. Preliminary tests on human bone were also made to evaluate their technique.

Tensile and compression tests were made with an Instron Type TT-C-L testing ma-

TABLE XVIII

DIRECTIONAL DIFFERENCES IN THE TENSILE STRENGTH OF COMPACT BONE

Author	Source	Bone	No. Spec.	Spec. Type	Spec. Condition	Loading Direction	kgf/mm^2	lbf/in^2
Hülsen, 1896	ox	tibia	4	flat	fresh	parallel to long axis	11.80	16,780
	ox	tibia	5	flat	fresh	perpend. to long axis	9.12	12,970
Dempster and Coleman, 1960	adult human	tibia	20	flat	embalmed (?) dry	parallel to grain	14.02 ± 2.19	19,939 ± 3,120
	adult human	tibia	6	circular	embalmed (?) dry	parallel to grain	13.45 ± 2.25	19,138 ± 3,200
	adult human	tibia	10	flat	embalmed (?) wet	parallel to grain	9.71 ± 2.75	13,818 ± 3,910
	adult human	tibia	1	circular	embalmed (?) wet	parallel to grain	9.19	13,068
	adult human	tibia	20	flat square	embalmed (?) dry	across grain	1.16 ± 0.33	1,648 ± 472
	adult human	tibia	9	flat square	embalmed (?) wet	across grain	1.01 ± 0.30	1,432 ± 420
Evans, 1964	adult human	femur	70	flat	embalmed wet	parallel to long axis	8.50	12,090
	adult human	tibia	62	flat	embalmed wet	parallel to long axis	8.92	12,688
	adult human	femur	112	flat	embalmed wet	tangent. to long axis	1.64	2,326
	adult human	tibia	103	flat	embalmed wet	tangent. to long axis	1.34	1,910
	adult human	femur	46	flat	embalmed wet	radial to long axis	1.62	2,298
	adult human	tibia	11	flat	embalmed wet	radial to long axis	1.54	2,193
Sweeney, Byers, and Kroon, 1965	bovine	femur	(?)	flat	unembal. (?) moist	parallel to long axis	13.12	18,660
	bovine	femur	(?)	flat	unembal. (?) moist	perpend. to long axis	5.72	8,135

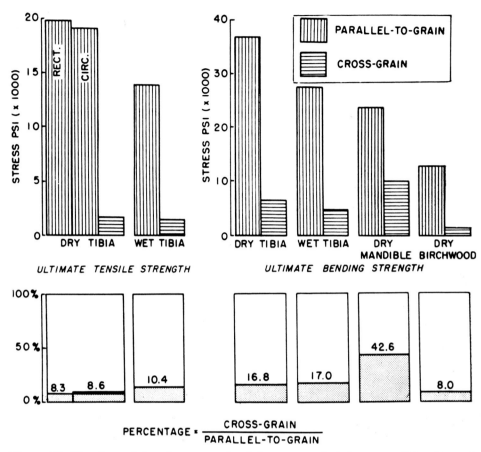

Figure 51. Tensile and bending strength of human cortical bone parallel with and across the grain. (From Dempster and Coleman: *J Appl Physiol,* 1960)

chine. The load measuring equipment consisted of a load cell attached to the stationary crosshead of the testing machine for the tension tests or to the base of the machine below the crosshead for the compression tests. Load-displacement curves, which could be converted into stress-strain curves, were automatically plotted during a test.

It was found that the longitudinal specimens had a higher ultimate tensile stress and strain than the transverse specimens (Table XVIII; Fig. 53).

Directional differences in tensile and impact properties of standardized specimens of beef cortical bone, tested at various temperatures, were reported by Bonfield and Li (1966). The specimens were prepared so that their long axis was longitudinal or transverse with respect to the shaft of the intact bone. Some of the impact specimens had a notch at their midpoint.

Two marked directional differences were found for the impact data: (1) transverse specimens absorbed significantly less energy at all test temperatures than longitudinal specimens; and (2) only a small maximum was measured in the energy absorbed vs temperature curve.

The energy absorbed by notched specimens appeared to be independent of specimen orientation and, as for unnotched longitudinal and transverse specimens, was maximum at temperatures between 0° C and 25° C.

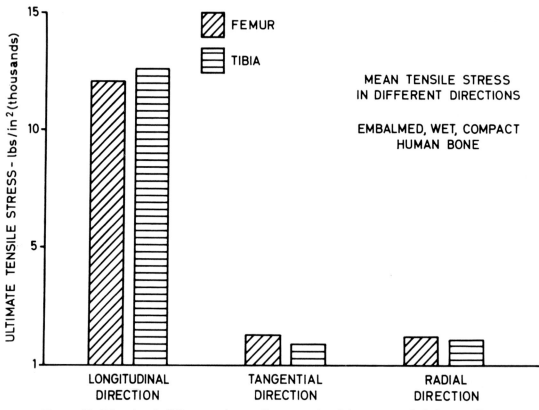

Figure 52. Directional differences in tensile strength of human cortical bone. (From Evans: in *Proceedings of the First European Bone and Tooth Symposium.* Courtesy of Pergamon Press)

COMPRESSIVE PROPERTIES

Compressive strength, with respect to directional differences of bone, has been studied more extensively than tensile strength. Rauber (1876) reported that the ultimate compressive strength of dry cubes of bone from the femur, tibia, and humerus of a 40-year-old man was greater in a direction parallel than perpendicular to the long axis of the bone (Table XIX).

Similar directional differences in the compressive strength of cortical bone from an adult human tibia and humerus were found by Hülsen (1896). Fresh fibular specimens from an ox also had a higher compressive strength parallel than perpendicular to the long axis of the bone (Table XIX). In both directions the compressive strength of ox bone was greater than that of human bone.

Hülsen's values for the compressive strength of fresh specimens were generally higher than those of dry specimens tested by Rauber. This presents a rather puzzling problem since, according to most investigators, drying tends to increase the compressive strength of bone. The explanation may be that Hülsen's data were obtained from a younger man.

Carothers et al. (1949) likewise demonstrated directional differences in the compressive properties of specimens of compact bone from the shaft of adult human femurs and tibias. All specimens were from

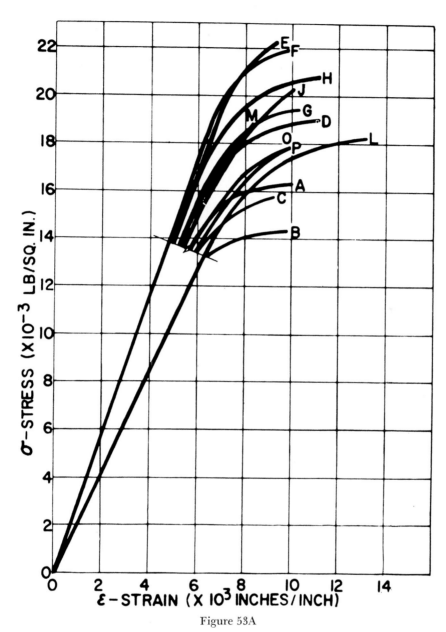

Figure 53A

Figure 53. Tensile stress-strain curves for cortical beef bone tested in the longitudinal (*A*) and the transverse (*B*) directions. (From Sweeney, Byers, and Kroon: Courtesy of Amer Soc of Mech Eng publication, 1965)

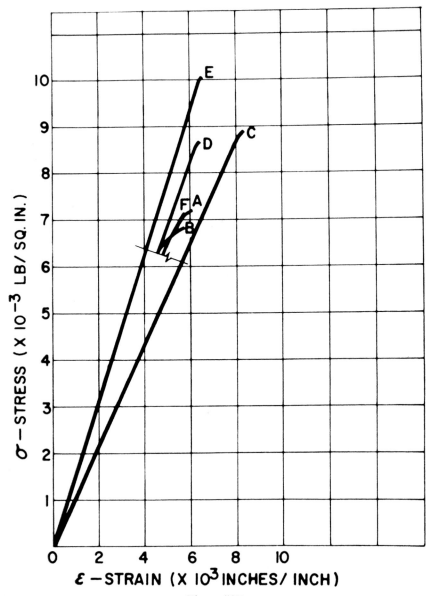

Figure 53B

embalmed, dissecting-room cadavers. Of the total number of specimens, eight femurs had been air-dried for several years. Prior to dissection the cadavers were refrigerated at 38° F. The specimens were not put into a fluid before testing.

Three types of specimens were used: (1) whole sections, with smooth parallel ends but a varying cross-sectional shape, area, and wall thickness, taken from the middle third of the shaft of the bone; (2) hollow cylinders, machined to a standardized size with walls of uniform thickness; and (3) solid cylinders of standardized size. In addition, a 0.615-in block from a femur was tested.

The results of their experiments showed that the hollow cylindrical specimens from the femur had a greater compressive strength parallel than perpendicular to the direction of the fibers. Unfortunately, the first and third types of specimens from the same bone were tested only in one direction. The block specimen was tested perpendicular to the direction of its fibers. For all the specimens loaded parallel to the direction of the fibers, the average compressive strength was 5,656 lbf/in² (3.98 kgf/mm²) compared to an average of 13,085 lbf/in² (9.20 kgf/mm²) when loaded perpendicular to the direction of the fibers (Table XIX).

Dempster and Liddicoat (1952) compared the compressive strength of wet and dry cubes of compact bone from four adult human femurs and three humeri. The cubes were compressed in the longitudinal, the radial, and the tangential directions with respect to the long axis of the intact bone. It was found that the compressive strength of dry bone in the radial and tangential directions was only 65% and 63%, respectively, of that in the longitudinal direction (Fig. 54; Table XIX). The compressive strength of wet bone in the radial and tangential directions was 89% and 82%, respectively, of that in the longitudinal direction.

Sweeney et al. (1965) found that longitudinal specimens of cortical bone from beef femurs had a greater ultimate compressive strength than transverse specimens (Fig. 55). Similar behavior was noted in a few specimens from human femurs tested to evaluate the technique. However, transverse specimens, judging from their stress-strain curves, had a higher average compressive strain than longitudinal specimens.

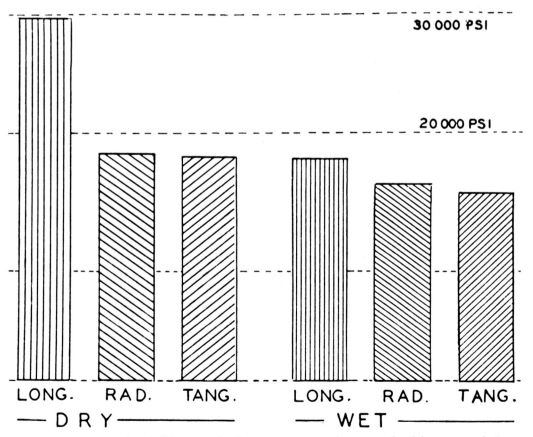

Figure 54. Directional differences in the mean compressive strength of human cortical bone. (From Dempster and Liddicoat: *Am J Anat,* 1952)

TABLE XIX

DIRECTIONAL DIFFERENCES IN THE COMPRESSIVE STRENGTH OF COMPACT BONE

Author	Source	Bone	No. Spec	Spec. Type	Spec. Condition	Loading Direction	kgf/mm^2	lbf/in^2
Rauber, 1876	40-yr.-old man	femur	5	cube	dry	parallel to long axis	19.48	27,700
	40-yr.-old man	femur	6	cube	dry	perpend. to long axis	17.80	25,310
	40-yr.-old man	tibia	5	cube	dry	parallel to long axis	17.24	24,515
	40-yr.-old man	tibia	5	cube	dry	perpend. to long axis	12.60	17,920
	40-yr.-old man	humerus	5	cube	dry	parallel to long axis	13.65	19,410
	40-yr.-old man	humerus	6	cube	dry	perpend. to long axis	11.30	16,070
Hülsen, 1896	adult human	tibia	4	cube	fresh	parallel to long axis	20.93	29,760
	adult human	tibia	3	cube	fresh	perpend. to long axis	14.48	20,590
	adult human	humerus	2	cube	fresh	parallel to long axis	20.42	29,040
	adult human	humerus	2	cube	fresh	perpend. to long axis	16.50	23,460
	ox	fibula	5	cube	fresh	parallel to long axis	21.12	30,030
	ox	fibula	4	cube	fresh	perpend. to long axis	18.20	25,880
Carothers, Smith, and Calabrisi, 1949	adult human	femur	8	hollow cylinder	embalmed dry	parallel to fibers	17.82	25,350
	adult human	tibia	1	section of shaft	embalmed dry	parallel to fibers	14.34	20,400
	adult human	tibia	4	hollow cylinder	embalmed dry	parallel to fibers	19.53	27,775
	adult human	femur	1	section of shaft	embalmed dry	perpend. to fibers	19.75	28,100
	adult human	femur	3	hollow cylinder	embalmed dry	perpend. to fibers	17.01	24,200
Dempster and Liddicoat, 1952	adult human	femur & humerus	21	cube	embalmed (?) dry	longitud.	20.79 ± 1.81	29,575 ± 2,580
	adult human	femur & humerus	21	cube	embalmed (?) dry	radial	13.50 ± 2.21	19,203 ± 3,139
	adult human	femur & humerus	21	cube	embalmed (?) dry	tangent.	13.11 ± 2.15	18,653 ± 3,064
	adult human	femur & humerus	7	cube	embalmed (?) wet	longitud.	13.36 ± 2.18	19,007 ± 3,100
	adult human	femur & humerus	7	cube	embalmed (?) wet	radial	11.94 ± 3.23	16,988 ± 4,600
	adult human	femur & humerus	7	cube	embalmed (?) wet	tangent.	10.78 ± 1.97	15,336 ± 2,800

Author	Source	Bone	No. Spec.	Spec. Type	Spec. Condition	Loading Direction	kgf/mm²	lbf/in²
Sweeney, Byers, and Kroon, 1965	adult human	femur	(?)	flat	unembal. (?) moist	longitud.	20.39	29,000
	adult human	femur	(?)	flat	unembal. (?) moist	transverse	15.33	21,800
	bovine	femur	(?)	flat	unembal. (?) moist	longitud.	22.34	31,781
	bovine	femur	(?)	flat	unembal. (?) moist	transverse	15.60	22,184

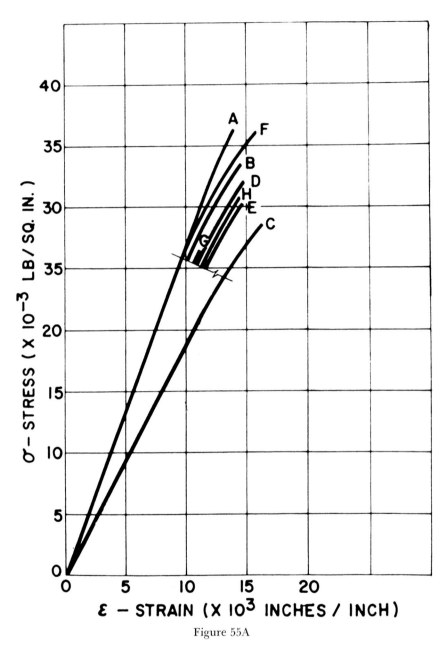

Figure 55A

Figure 55. Stress-strain curves of cortical beef bone compressed in the longitudinal (*A*) and the transverse (*B*) directions. (From Sweeney, Byers, and Kroon: Courtesy of Amer Soc Mech Eng publication, 1965)

Beef cortical bone has a greater compressive strength in both directions than does human bone (Table XIX).

Directional variations in the compressive properties of short cylinders of cortical bone from fresh beef femurs, tested at different stress rates, have been reported by Bird et al. (1968). Test specimens whose long axis varied with respect to the shaft of the bone (Fig. 56) were tested in an ARA universal testing machine at low (1×10^2 lbf/in²/sec; 0.073 kgf/mm²/sec) and high (5×10^5 lbf/in²/sec; 351.5 kgf/mm²/sec) stress rates of loading. After preparation all specimens were refrigerated in physiological saline until tested. The specimens were tested wet and within twenty-four hours after their preparation.

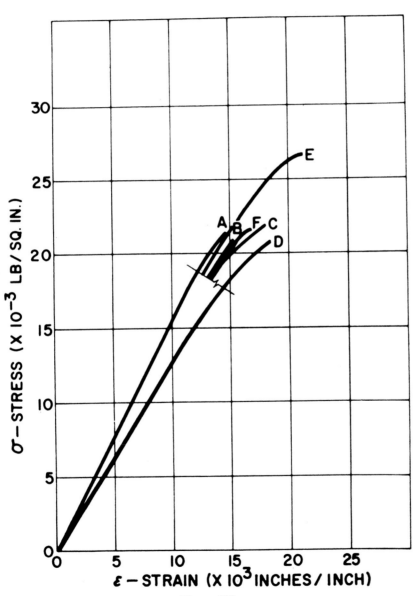

Figure 55B

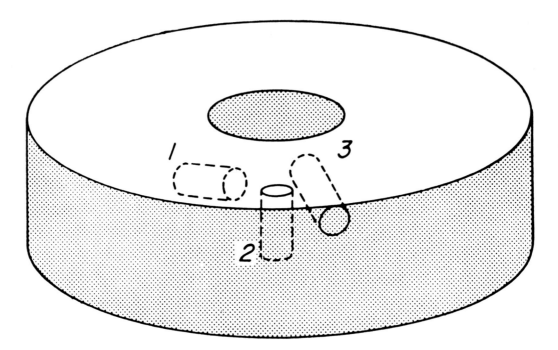

1. Circumferential Sample
2. Longitudinal Sample
3. Radial Sample

Figure 56. Orientation of compression specimens of fresh cortical bone from beef femurs. (From Bird, Becker, Healer, and Messer: *Aerosp Med,* 1968)

At low stress rates of loading the longitudinal specimens had the highest compressive strength and modulus but the lowest strain to failure while the radial specimens had the lowest strength and highest strain (Fig. 57). Mechanical property values varied the most in the radial specimens and the least in the circumferential ones.

At high stress rates of loading the stress-strain curve envelopes had similar characteristics but significant differences were seen in the magnitudes of failure stress and strain and in the elastic and secant moduli of the different types of specimens (Fig. 58).

SHEARING PROPERTIES

Directional differences in the shearing strength of fresh rods, with a square cross section 2 mm on each side, of compact bone from the femur of a 30-year-old man were determined by Rauber (1876). Some of the rods were cut in the longitudinal direction and others in the transverse direction with respect to the long axis of the intact bone. Rauber's results demonstrated that specimens cut parallel to the long axis of the bone and loaded perpendicular to it had an average shearing strength more than twice that of specimens cut transverse to the long axis of the bone and loaded parallel to that axis (Table XX).

Frost et al. (1961) investigated directional differences in the punching shear strength of cortical bone from the femur and tibia of two people, 18 and 63 years of age. The determinations were based on the force required to punch out pieces from longitudinal and cross sections of fresh undecalcified bone. The sections were 70μ thick and unembedded. The direction of the shearing force was perpendicular to the plane of the sections; thus, the cross sections were loaded in the longitudinal direction and the longitudinal sections in the transverse direction.

The average shearing strength in the longitudinal direction for the thirteen valid cross section tests was 7.5 kgf/mm² (10,665 lbf/in²) with a range of variation from 6.94 kgf/mm² to 8.15 kgf/mm² (9,867 to 11,589 lbf/in²). The six valid tests of the longitudinal sections had an average shearing strength in the transverse direction of 8.4 kgf/mm² (11,945 lbf/in²) and a variation from 8.0 kgf/mm² to 8.8 kgf/mm² (11,376 to 12,514 lbf/in²).

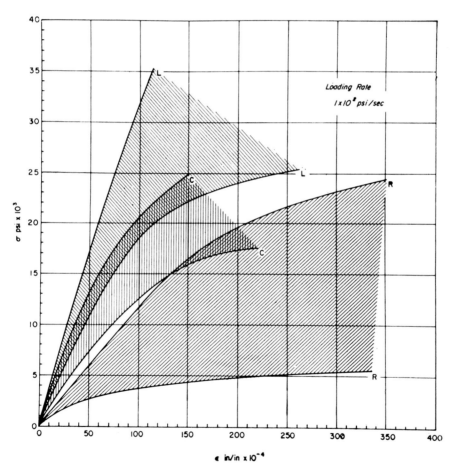

Figure 57. Compression stress-strain curve envelopes for fresh cortical bone from beef femurs tested at low stress rate (1 × 10² psi/sec) of loading. L = longitudinal specimens; C = circumferential specimens; R = radial specimens. (From Bird, Becker, Healer, and Messer: *Aerosp Med,* 1968)

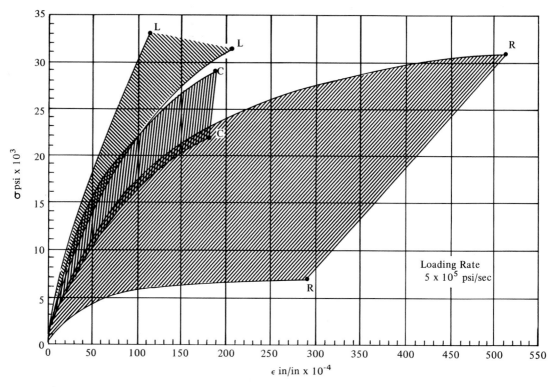

Figure 58. Compression stress-strain curve envelopes of fresh cortical bone from beef femurs tested at high stress rate (5×10^5 psi/sec) of loading. L = longitudinal specimens; C = circumferential specimens; R = radial specimens. (From Bird, Becker, Healer, and Messer: *Aerosp Med,* 1968)

BENDING PROPERTIES

The breaking load in bending of twelve small rectangular bars of compact bone from ox tibias was determined by Maj and Toajari (1937). The bars were cut parallel, radially, and tangentially to the long axis of the bone and had different orientations within the bone. Each bar was described in terms of the orientation of its length first and then its width with respect to the long axis of the bone, e.g. longitudinal radial, tangential radial, etc. In order to test the specimens, they designed an apparatus called a clasimeter consisting of two knife blades, 7 mm apart, which supported the bar while a load was applied to it midway between the supports.

Maj and Toajari found that the breaking load for bars cut longitudinally with respect to the long axis of the bone was three times greater than that for bars cut tangentially to the axis and six times greater than that for bars cut radially to the axis (Table XXI). The breaking load of the tangentially cut bars was about twice as great as that for the radially cut ones.

In another series of tests Olivo et al. (1937) investigated the breaking load and the deflection, in load units of 0.01 mm/5 kgf, of several bars of compact bone from the same cross sections of the metacarpals and metatarsals of a 6-year-old ox, a mule, and femurs of two women, 42 and 90 years of age. The specimens were tested with the clasimeter.

The results of the study showed a definite tendency toward an increase in the antero-

TABLE XX

DIRECTIONAL DIFFERENCES IN THE SHEARING AND BENDING STRENGTH OF HUMAN COMPACT BONE

Author	Source	Bone	No. Spec.	Spec. Type	Spec. Condition	Loading Direction	kgf/mm^2	lbf/in^2
SHEARING STRENGTH								
Rauber, 1876	30-yr.-old man	femur	5	rectang. rod	fresh	perpend. to fibers	23.70	33,700
	30-yr.-old man	femur	6	rectang. rod	fresh	parallel to fibers	10.06	14,305
BENDING STRENGTH								
Dempster and Coleman, 1960	adult human	tibia	15	flat square	embalmed (?) dry	parallel to grain	25.83 ± 2.80	$36,743 \pm 3,980$
	adult human	mandible	10	flat square	embalmed (?) dry	parallel to grain	16.48 ± 4.78	$23,438 \pm 6,800$
	adult human	tibia	3	flat square	embalmed (?) wet	parallel to grain	19.14 ± 1.19	$27,224 \pm 1,690$
	adult human	tibia	15	flat square	embalmed (?) dry	across grain	4.33 ± 1.31	$6,161 \pm 1,860$
	adult human	mandible	10	flat square	embalmed (?) dry	across grain	7.01 ± 2.39	$9,978 \pm 3,400$
	adult human	tibia	3	flat square	embalmed (?) wet	across grain	3.26 ± 0.66	$4,639 \pm 940$

TABLE XXI

DIRECTIONAL DIFFERENCES IN THE BREAKING LOAD UNDER BENDING OF BARS, 2.65 MM WIDE AND 1.2 MM THICK, OF COMPACT BONE OF OX TIBIAS (Data from Maj and Toajari, 1937)

Orientation of Specimen	Breaking Load (kgf)			
	Exp. 9	Exp. 10	Exp. 11	Mean
Longitudinal radial*	14.25	15.50	14.50 ⎱	
Longitudinal tangential	16.00	15.00	15.25 ⎰	15.00
Tangential longitudinal	4.50	5.25	4.50 ⎱	
Tangential radial	5.25	4.50	5.25 ⎰	5.00
Radial longitudinal	2.50	3.00	2.75 ⎱	
Radial tangential	2.50	2.00	2.50 ⎰	2.50

* The first word refers to the length and the second to the width of the specimen with respect to the long axis of the bone.

posterior direction in the magnitude of the breaking load and a decrease in the deflection (Fig. 59). No such tendencies were observed in the lateromedial direction.

Dempster and Coleman (1960) reported

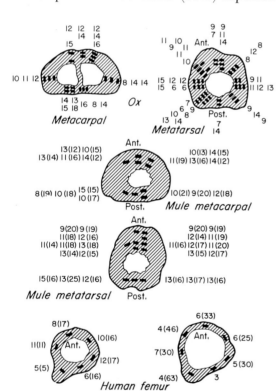

Figure 59. Directional differences in the breaking load (kg) and deflection (for 0.01 mm/5 kg load) of cortical bone. Deflections are in parentheses. (Redrawn from Olivo, Maj, and Toajari: *Boll Sci Med (Bologna)*, 1937)

directional differences in the bending strength of standardized specimens of tibial and mandibular compact bone from adult humans. The specimens were obtained from museum material, which was probably embalmed, although no data on the methods of preservation or biological history of the bones were given. Dry specimens as well as those soaked in water for half an hour were tested.

The authors found that the bending strength of the specimens was considerably greater parallel to the grain, or predominant direction of the haversian systems, than across the grain (Fig. 51; Table XX). Dry specimens were stronger than wet ones in both directions. Fracture of the specimens undoubtedly occurred from tensile stresses and strains created by bending.

TORSION PROPERTIES

Bonfield and Li (1967) also investigated the anisotropy of nonelastic flow in bone by studying microdeformations produced by torsion loading of specimens of cortical bone from tibia of cattle. The test specimens were filaments with a diameter of 0.010 inch and were prepared in the longitudinal or transverse directions with respect to the shaft of the bone (Fig. 60).

Torsional deformation in the filament was measured with an apparatus consisting

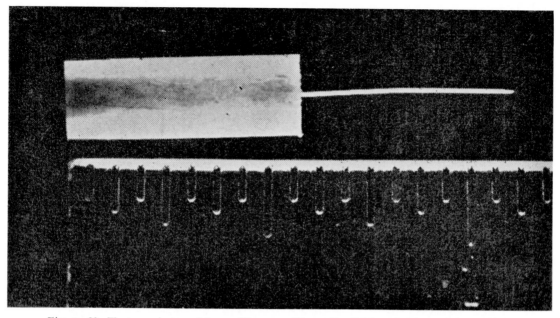

Figure 60. Test specimen of bone filament. (From Bonfield and Li: *J Appl Physics,* 1967)

of a modified Microsyn torque balance and a spectro-goniometer. Complete load-unload curves, obtained by a series of increasing torques applied to specimens of a 0.25 gauge length at a twist rate of 1°/min, were recorded on an XY plotter. The total angle of twist and residual twist after unloading were measured manually on a vernier dial. Torque and angle of twist values were converted into shear stress (σ) and strain (γ) on the surface of the specimen by use of the following formulas: (1) $\sigma = 2T/\pi r^2$ and (2) $\gamma = \theta.r/l$ in which r = radius and l = length of the test filament. Shear stress and strain had a maximum measured sensitivity of 5.6×10^{-2} lbf/in² and 4×10^{-7} in/in, respectively. The microscopic yield stress, i.e. the stress required to produce a nonelastic strain of 2×10^{-6} in/in, and the resultant nonelastic strain with stress were determined from experimental data. The values obtained for elastic modulus and microscopic yield stress were quite accurate,

except in the plastic range where the values are only approximate.

It was found that the longitudinal specimens had an initial elastic region with a shear modulus of 0.81 to 0.88×10^6 lbf/in² (562 to 619 kgf/mm²). A microscopic yield stress was typically evident at approximately 570 lbf (259 kgf) and the residual nonelastic strain after unloading increased as the amount of applied stress was raised (Fig. 61). Because the specimens were rigidly fixed in the testing apparatus, the residual nonelastic strain probably had both a permanent and an elastic component. Immediate retesting produced no significant change in the microscopic yield stress but the strain rate of hardening increased. The values for the modulus in the elastic region in the retest and the initial test were the same.

A small microscopic yield stress (about 150 lbf/in²; 132 kgf/mm²) and a lower strain rate of hardening was produced by a second immediate retest to the same stress

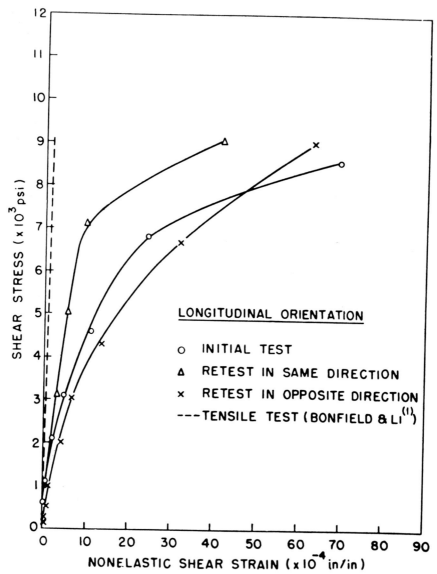

Figure 61. Variation in shear stress-nonelastic strain curves without intermediate recovery in compact bovine bone. (From Bonfield and Li: *J Appl Physics,* 1967)

level but in the opposite direction of twist. No significant change was noted in the shear modulus in the elastic range. Comparison of these results with earlier ones (Bonfield and Li, 1966) revealed that deformation occurring in tensile tests was considerably less than that in torsion tests.

These experiments showed that hardening or softening of the bone occurred with a re-

test in either the same or the opposite direction of twist and was associated with either an anelastic or a permanent strain. The difference between these effects was distinguished by repeating the experiments as before except that after each test the specimen was released from the jaws of the apparatus and allowed to remain at room temperature for twenty hours. During this time the anelastic strain would be recovered so that when the specimen was retested the effects of permanent strain alone would be assessed. It was found that retesting the specimen by twisting it in the same direction still produced a measurable hardening although the effect seemed to be reduced (Fig. 62). Retesting the specimen by twisting it in the opposite direction produced little additional effect on microscopic yield stress or hardening indicating that an intermediate recovery period considerably modified the effect of prestrain.

The experiments were extended to include investigation of the effect of continuous cycling between constant stress limits. Figure 63 is an example of typical results obtained from cycling longitudinal specimens between stress levels of $\pm 4,700$ lbf/in^2 (3.3 kgf/mm^2). It was found that the

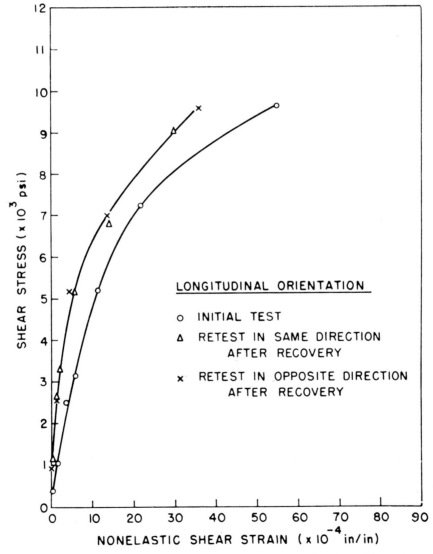

Figure 62. Variation in shear stress-nonelastic strain curves after immediate recovery in compact beef bone. (From Bonfield and Li: *J Appl Physics*, 1967)

amount of nonelastic strain at the end of each cycle decreases from a maximum value after the second cycle to approximately a constant value after five cycles (Figs. 63 and 64). After seven cycles the decrease in amplitude of each hysteresis loop appeared to be constant. Specimens cycled at stresses of $\pm 2,800$ lbf/in² (2 kgf/mm²) and $\pm 6,400$ lbf/in² (4.5 kgf/mm²) exhibited similar changes. The magnitude of the hysteresis loop depended on the stress level and specimen orientation (Table XXII).

The same experimental sequence of tests on transverse specimens, kept in the grips at all times and not allowed to recover to zero stress, gave significantly larger values for modulus of elasticity and microscopic yield stress than in the longitudinal specimens (Fig. 65). The modulus was measured at 1.83 to 2.09×10^6 lbf/in² (11,286 kgf/mm²). The yield stress of 2,600 lbf/in² (1.8 kgf/mm²), five times greater than in the longitudinal specimens, was followed by an increased strain rate of hardening.

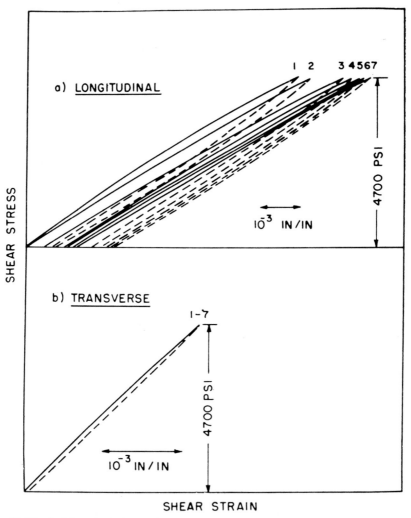

Figure 63. Typical hysteresis loops for longitudinal and transverse specimens of cortical beef bone cycled between stress limits of ± 4700 lbf/in². Only half of each loop is shown. (From Bonfield and Li: *J Appl Physics,* 1967)

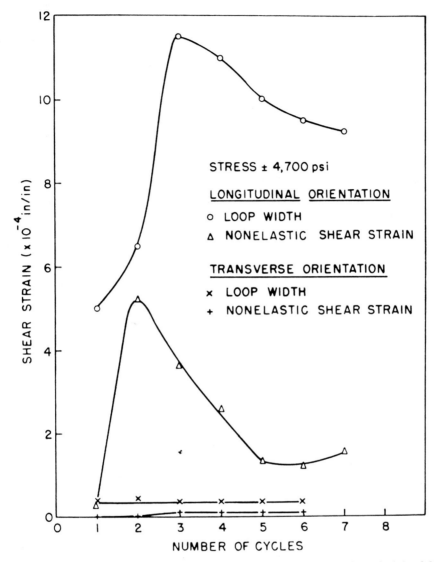

Figure 64. Dependence of loop width and nonelastic shear strain of cortical beef bone on the number of cycles. (From Bonfield and Li: *J Appl Physics*, 1967)

Bonfield and Li's studies with longitudinal specimens of cortical bone showed that a small amount of torsional stress caused a departure from elastic behavior as well as considerable amounts of nonelastic strain. Similar results had been obtained in their previous studies (1966) on microstrain in tensile tests. They also demonstrated that retesting the specimen in the same direction of twist hardened it while retesting in the opposite direction softened it. However, these effects were reduced if the specimens were allowed to recover between tests.

The authors argue that if the nonelastic strain were entirely anelastic in nature one would expect no difference between the initial test and a later retest after recovery. The presence of a measurable hardening after recovery suggests that a permanent strain had been produced.

TABLE XXII

DEPENDENCE OF HYSTERESIS LOOP WIDTH ON STRESS
AND SPECIMEN ORIENTATION IN CORTICAL BONE FROM
OX TIBIA (Bonfield and Li, 1967)

Stress Cycle (lbf/in²)	Loop Width After Seven Cycles ($\times 10^{-4}$ in/in)	
	Longitudinal	Transverse
± 2,800	4.10	0.15
± 4,700	9.21	0.35
± 6,400	12.50	0.46

The response of bone to applied stress was considered to occur in two stages. At stress levels less than the microscopic yield stress (Stage I) bone deforms in an elastic manner with the stress distributed between the hydroxyapatite crystals and the collagen fibers. When the stress exceeds the microscopic yield stress (Stage II) nonelastic deformation occurs. The residual microstrain

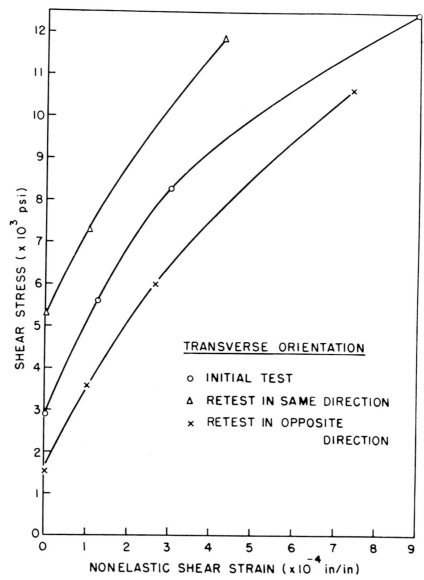

Figure 65. Variation in nonelastic strain with shear stress in transverse specimens of cortical beef bone with no intermediate recovery. (From Bonfield and Li: *J Appl Physics,* 1967)

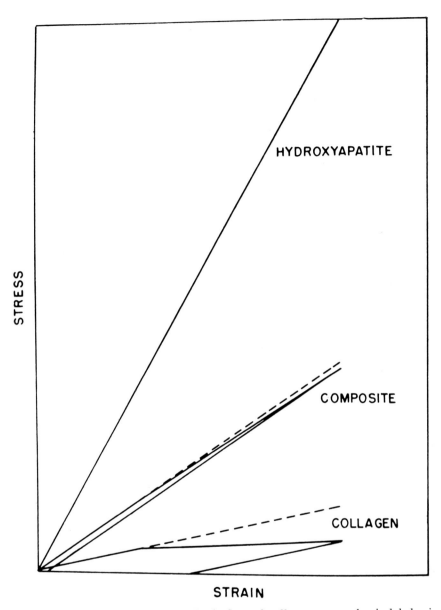

Figure 66. Diagram of effects of nonelastic flow of collagen on mechanical behavior of bone. (From Bonfield and Li: *J Appl Physics,* 1967)

found in the torsion tests results either from (1) nonelastic deformation of the collagen and/or the crystals or (2) shearing along the interfacial region between the two components. Bonfield and Li think that initial nonelastic flow in collagen is the more likely explanation. The effective "modulus" of collagen decreases so that an increasing percentage of the applied load is supported by crystals.

Bonfield and Li suggest that the strain hardening and softening found in their experiments is due to nonelastic flow in the collagen fibers during loading accompanied by continued elastic deformation of the hydroxyapatite crystals. The extended collagen fibers reach zero strain when the load is removed but the crystals are still elastically strained (Fig. 66). When immediately retested in the same direction of twist the elastic strain in the crystals must be overcome. The implication of retesting the specimen in the opposite direction of twist is that the elastic strain in the crystals assists the applied stress and leads to nonelastic flow at a lower level of applied stress. If the bone remains at zero stress the collagen fibers undergo some anelastic recovery thus allowing decrease in the elastic strain in the crystals. The internal strain in the crystals may also be relieved by local convolutions in the collagen fibers so they have a more irregular configuration.

A somewhat similar explanation was offered for the mechanical behavior of bone during cycling between constant stress levels. They believe that in the first stress cycles the collagen deforms in both an anelastic and a permanent manner. However, the collagen work hardens with continued cycling and the permanent strain produced in each cycle decreases until the bone shows an essentially elastic behavior. The approximately constant residual nonelastic strain found after five cycles corresponds to the point at which no significant permanent strain occurs during each cycle, the residual strain at this time being anelastic.

Data from tests with transverse specimens showed that the initial nonelastic yielding is anisotropic. The transverse specimens had about five times more microscopic yield strain and a much higher strain rate of hardening than the longitudinal specimens. This variation was ascribed to differences in the collagen fiber orientation which was mainly perpendicular to the long axis of the transverse specimens. Consequently, the collagen fibers in the transverse specimens could not have the extension and rotation

possible in the longitudinal ones. The small nonelastic deformation they found was attributed to some collagen fibers, or sections of fibers, inclined to the long axis of the bone at angles less than 90°. The fibers then undergo hardening or softening by a mechanism similar to that occurring in the longitudinal specimens.

IMPACT SNAPPING STRENGTH

Directional differences in the impact snapping strength of fresh wet compact bone from man and other mammals were determined by Japanese investigators (cited by Yamada, 1970) from 16-mm rods with a 3×3 mm-cross section. A 60 kg cm-capacity Izod impact machine was used to test the specimens which were fixed in the holder so that six millimeters of bone, corresponding to twice the diameter of the sides, were exposed.

It was found that the impact snapping strength in the tangential direction was only 73% as great as that in the radial direction (Table XXIII) for specimens from femurs of individuals 30 to 59 years of age. Specimens from the anterior and posterior aspects of the femur had a greater impact snapping strength than those from the medial and lateral aspects.

The impact snapping strength of fresh wet femoral specimens from horses was al-

TABLE XXIII

DIRECTIONAL DIFFERENCES IN THE IMPACT SNAPPING STRENGTH OF RECTANGULAR RODS OF FRESH WET FEMORAL CORTICAL BONE* (Data from Yamada, 1970)

Source	Direction	$kg\text{-}cm/mm^2$	lbf/in^2
Adult human .	radial	0.26 ± 0.029	12.13 ± 1.35
Adult human .	tangential	0.19 ± 0.021	8.87 ± 0.98
Horse	radial	0.22 ± 0.019	10.27 ± 0.89
Horse	tangential	0.23 ± 0.020	10.73 ± 0.93
Bovine	radial	0.21 ± 0.014	9.80 ± 0.65
Bovine	tangential	0.24 ± 0.018	11.20 ± 0.84

* The number of specimens in each case was not given.

most the same in the radial and tangential directions. Similar specimens of femoral bone from cattle had a greater impact snapping strength tangentially than radially (Table XXIII). Specimens from various aspects of the horse femurs showed no significant differences in the impact snapping strength in the radial direction. However, in the tangential direction specimens from the anterior and lateral sides of horse bone had somewhat higher values than those from the posterior and medial sides. In cattle bone the anterior side was shown to have the greatest strength in both directions.

Human bone had a 15% and 19% greater impact snapping strength in the radial direction than horse and cattle bone, respectively, but was 21% and 26% weaker in the tangential direction. There are no significant differences in the snapping strength of horse and cattle bone.

Energy Absorbing Capacity

Directional differences in the energy absorbed to failure by beef cortical bone have been reported by Bonfield and Li (1966). Although a marked temperature dependence on energy absorption was found (see Chapter 6 for discussion) both notched and unnotched longitudinal impact specimens absorbed more energy before failure than did similar transverse specimens. However, the temperature dependence of unnotched transverse specimens was considerably less

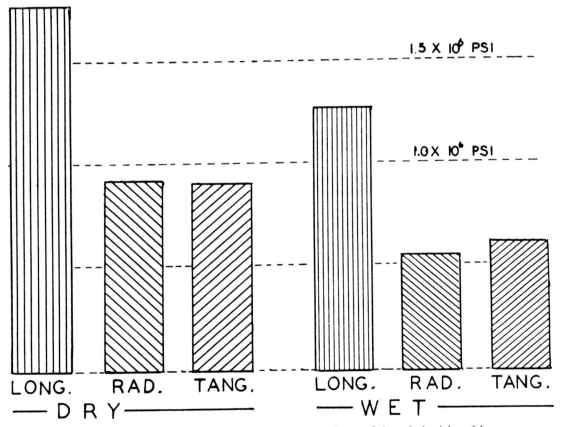

Figure 67. Directional differences in average compressive modulus of elasticity of human cortical bone. (From Dempster and Liddicoat: *Am J Anat,* 1952)

than that of comparable longitudinal specimens.

Modulus of Elasticity

The earliest investigator of the directional differences in the modulus of elasticity of compact bone was Hülsen (1896). He reported that four fresh specimens from an ox tibia had an average bending modulus of 2,634 kgf/mm² (3.7 × 10⁶ lbf/in²) in the longitudinal direction compared to an average of 1,939 kgf/mm² (2.8 × 10⁶ lbf/in²) in the transverse direction for four other specimens.

Directional differences in the compressive modulus of elasticity of bone were studied by Dempster and Liddicoat (1952). The modulus for dry and wet cubes of adult human femoral and humeral cortical bone was determined when compressed in the longitudinal, the tangential, and the radial directions with respect to the long axis of the in-

tact bone. They reported that the average modulus was approximately twice as great in the longitudinal as in the tangential or radial direction for the dry cubes and even greater for the wet cubes (Fig. 67). The average modulus for the dry cubes was slightly higher in the radial than in the tangential direction but the reverse was true for the wet specimens (Table XXIV).

Sweeney et al. (1965) determined the compressive and tensile modulus of elasticity in the longitudinal and transverse directions, with respect to the long axis of the intact bone of moist specimens, probably unembalmed, of compact bone from cattle femurs. They found that the modulus was greater in the longitudinal than in the transverse direction for both compression and tension (Table XXV). The tensile modulus in the longitudinal direction was slightly higher than the longitudinal compressive modulus but the reverse relation was found

TABLE XXIV

Modulus of Elasticity of Human Bony Cubes Compressed in Three Axes
(Data from Dempster and Liddicoat, 1952)

Longitudinal Axis			Radial Axis			Tangential Axis		
lbf/in² (× 10⁶)		*kgf/mm²* (× 10³)	*lbf/in²* (× 10⁶)		*kgf/mm²* (× 10³)	*lbf/in²* (× 10⁶)		*kgf/mm²* (× 10³)
Femur (dry)*								
1.67	(100%)	1.17	1.48	(89%)†	1.04	1.22	(73%)†	.857
1.96	(100%)	1.38	1.09	(56%)	.77	1.23	(63%)	.864
1.54	(100%)	1.08	.92	(60%)	.65	.96	(62%)	.67
1.92	(100%)	1.35	.67	(35%)	.47	.94	(49%)	.66
Humerus (dry)*								
2.05	(100%)	1.44	.83	(41%)	.58	.99	(48%)	.70
1.86	(100%)	1.31	.88	(47%)	.62	.60	(32%)	.42
1.29	(100%)	.91	.55	(43%)	.39	.95	(73%)	.67
Average (dry)								
1.756 ± 3.72	(100%)	1.23 ± .26	.916 ± .301	(52%)	.64 ± .21	.912 ± .224	(52%)	.64 ± .16
Average (wet)								
1.262 ± .231	(100%)	.89 ± .16	.546 ± .117	(43%)	.38 ± .08	.608 ± .203	(48%)	.43 ± .14
Wet bones—% of dry, longitudinal average								
	(72%)			(31%)			(35%)	
Wet bones—% of dry modulus for bone similarly compressed								
	(72%)			(60%)			(67%)	

* Each figure represents average determinations from a given bone.
† Percent of compression along longitudinal axis.

TABLE XXV

Directional Differences in the Compressive and Tensile Modulus of Elasticity of Femoral Compact Bone of Cattle (Data from Sweeney, Byers, and Kroon, 1965)

Spec. Condition	Loading Direction	lbf/in^2	kgf/mm^2
Compression			
Unembalmed (?) moist	longitudinal	2.39×10^6	1,680
Unembalmed (?) moist	transverse	1.44×10^6	1,012
Tension			
Unembalmed (?) moist	longitudinal	2.50×10^6	1,758
Unembalmed (?) moist	transverse	1.33×10^6	935

for the two types of modulus in the transverse direction. The number of specimens tested in their experiments was not stated.

Skull Bones

With few exceptions studies on the mechanical properties of bone have been made on material from the major long bones of man and other animals because suitable test specimens are more easily obtained from long bones than from flat or irregular ones. It is particularly true in tensile testing for which the specimen must be straight and long enough to be held in a testing machine or apparatus. For these reasons, relatively little research has been done on skull bone despite the importance of such data in relation to the high incidence of head injury in all kinds of vehicular accidents.

Evans and Lissner (1957) determined the tensile and compressive strength of standardized specimens of parietal bone from embalmed adult human cadavers. The test specimens (Fig. 13) were rectangular bars consisting of outer and inner tables of compact bone with intervening diploë. In order to obtain long, straight specimens for tensile testing, it was impossible to have uniform orientation of the specimens within the intact parietal bone. In the tensile tests the load was oriented tangentially with respect to the skull. Compression tests were made both lengthwise and crosswise in rela-

tion to the long axis of the specimen. All specimens were wet when tested.

The results of Evans and Lissner's study (Table XXVI) revealed that compact tabular bone, tested in the lengthwise direction or long axis of the specimen, had a compressive strength about twice that of its tensile strength. In these tests the load was primarily supported by the two layers of compact bone. In the compression tests performed crosswise to the long axis of the specimen, the diploë in addition to the two layers of compact bone were supporting the load. After failure of the diploë, the tests were continued until the layers of compact bone also failed. The data thus obtained showed that the compressive strength, in the crosswise direction, of the diploë was only about one-seventh of that of compact bone in the same direction.

The most thorough investigation of the mechanical properties of skull bones is that of McElhaney et al. (1970a), who determined the strength characteristics, the modulus of elasticity, Poisson's ratio, the energy absorption, the dry weight density, and the microhardness of standardized test specimens from human calvaria. The material consisted of embalmed specimens from the frontal, both parietals, and the occipital bones of seventeen calvaria of adults ranging from 56 to 73 years of age as well as fresh specimens from craniotomies and au-

TABLE XXVI

AVERAGE ULTIMATE STRENGTH AND RANGE OF VARIATION IN HUMAN PARIETAL BONE
(Evans and Lissner, 1957)

Bone Type	No. Spec.	Body Side	Direction of Loading	lbf/in²	kgf/mm²
Tensile Strength					
Compact	8	right	lengthwise	10,790 (7,540-15,800)	7.59 (5.30-11.11)
Compact	7	left	lengthwise	9,600 (6,030-15,150)	6.75 (4.24-10.65)
Average	15	—	lengthwise	10,230 (6,030-15,800)	7.19 (4.24-11.11)
Compressive Strength					
Compact	36	right	lengthwise	21,070 (12,400-33,900)	14.81 (8.72-23.83)
Compact	33	left	lengthwise	23,200 (13,900-47,800)	16.31 (9.77-33.60)
Average	69	—	lengthwise	22,080 (12,400-47,800)	15.52 (8.72-33.60)
Diploë	11	right	crosswise	3,660 (2,580-5,550)	2.57 (1.81-3.90)
Diploë	12	left	crosswise	3,620 (1,700-5,700)	2.54 (1.20-4.01)
Average	23	—	crosswise	3,640 (1,700-5,770)	2.56 (1.20-4.06)
Compact	28	right	crosswise	22,260 (9,800-35,500)	15.65 (6.89-24.96)
Compact	28	left	crosswise	25,870 (4,500-46,900)	18.19 (3.16-32.97)
Average	56	—	crosswise	24,280 (4,500-46,900)	17.07 (3.16-32.97)

topsies of forty individuals. A few mechanical properties were also determined on specimens from the skulls of forty rhesus monkeys.

A grid system of one-centimeter squares was drawn on the surface of the human calvaria so that the site, with respect to the coronal, sagittal, and lambdoidal sutures, from which the test specimens were obtained could be accurately recorded. Three types of test specimens were used: (1) cylinders, 10 mm in diameter, consisting of a layer of compact bone from the outer and inner skull tables separated by diploë; (2) cubes of the same component parts; and (3) flat bars, with a reduced middle region, of compact tabular bone. Type 1 specimens were used for simple shear and torsion tests,

type 2 specimens for triaxial compression tests, and type 3 for tensile tests.

During preparation the specimens were kept damp with an isotonic solution buffered with calcium and were moist when tested. Tensile specimens were loaded in a tangential direction and the compression specimens in the tangential and radial directions with respect to the skull.

McElhaney et al. found that the mean compressive strength, the modulus of elasticity, and Poisson's ratio were all greater in the tangential than in the radial direction (Table XXVII). However, the mean compressive strain and the energy absorbed to failure were greater in the radial direction. Individual (skull to skull) differences in the ultimate compressive strength and the energy absorbed to failure were statistically significant in the radial but not in the tangential direction. The compressive modulus of elasticity exhibited significant individual differences in both directions but there were no significant directional differences for the compressive strain or Poisson's ratio. Directional differences were not investigated for the tensile properties of human skull specimens nor for any mechanical properties of the monkey specimens. The Vickers hardness of the compact bone of the outer skull table was greater than that of the inner table.

In evaluating mechanical property data obtained from specimens of skull bone, it should be remembered that the specimens are essentially sandwiches consisting of strong compact bone from the outer and inner skull tables separated by weak diploë. In tests of such specimens, in a direction perpendicular to the skull surface, the diploë supports some of the load while in tests tangential to the skull surface, the load is supported by the compact tabular bone.

In compression tests perpendicular to the skull surface the diploë fails first after which, with greater loads, failure of the compact tabular bone occurs. All investigators agree that the compressive strength of the diploë is far less than that of tabular bone. Mechanical property differences between skull bone in the tangential and perpendicular (radial) directions are the result of the greater structural weakness of the diploë. Consequently, tests of skull bone are as much structural as they are mechanical property tests. The same is true of tests of cancellous bone alone because the results depend upon the orientation and distribution of the individual trabeculae as much as on their mechanical properties which, as far as I am aware, have never been determined.

The energy-absorbing capacity of diploë was confirmed by McElhaney et al. who found that the compressive energy absorbed by their skull specimens in the radial direction was almost three times greater than that absorbed in the tangential direction (Table XXVII).

TABLE XXVII

DIRECTIONAL DIFFERENCES IN THE MECHANICAL PROPERTIES OF HUMAN SKULL BONE
(Data from McElhaney et al., 1970)

Property	Direction of Loading	No. of Spec.	No. of Subj.	Mean	Standard Deviation	Mean	Standard Deviation
				$\times 10^3$ lbf/in^2		kgf/mm^2	
Ult. compressive strength	radial	237	26	10.7†	5.1	7.52	3.59
Ult. compressive strength	tangential	210	14	14.0	5.2	9.84	3.66
				$\times 10^{-3}$ in/in			
Ult. compressive strain*	radial	237	26	97.0	80.0	—	—
Ult. compressive strain	tangential	210	14	51.0	32.0	—	—
				$\times 10^5$ lbf/in^2		kgf/mm^2	
Compressive modulus	radial	237	26	3.5†	2.1	246.1	147.6
Compressive modulus	tangential	219	14	8.1†	4.4	569.4	309.3
Poisson's ratio*-compression	radial	122	14	0.19	0.08	—	—
Poisson's ratio-compression	tangential	327	18	0.22	0.11	—	—
				$in\text{-}lbf/in^3$		$kg\text{-}cm/cm^3$	
Energy absorbed-compression	radial	237	26	1,200†	700	84.39	49.22
Energy absorbed-compression	tangential	189	14	480	440	33.76	30.94

* No conversions necessary for strain or Poisson's ratio.
† Significant differences between individuals.

CANCELLOUS BONE

Long Bones

Although cancellous (spongy) bone also exhibits directional differences in its mechanical properties, they have not been studied as thoroughly as those of compact bone.

The first investigation of directional differences in the shearing strength of cancellous bone was made by Rauber (1876) who determined them from fresh specimens from an adult human tibia. Six specimens, cut parallel and loaded perpendicular to the long axis of the bone, had an average shearing strength of 1.06 kgf/mm² (1,507 lbf/in²) in contrast to an average strength of only 0.38 kgf/mm² (540 lbf/in²) for five similar specimens, cut transverse but loaded parallel to the long axis of the bone. The average shear modulus was 0.56 kgf/mm² (796 lbf/in²) perpendicular to the fiber and 0.2 kgf/mm² (284 lbf/in²) parallel to the fiber.

Directional differences in the compressive strength and modulus of elasticity of cuboidal spongy bone specimens from the femur of a 70-year-old man were reported

by Knese (1958). The highest compressive strength was found in a specimen, loaded in the anteroposterior direction, from the anterior half of the femoral head while the lowest compressive strength was recorded for a specimen, subjected to transverse loading, from the posterior half of the fibular condyle. The specimen, loaded in the anteroposterior direction, from the posterior half of the fibular condyle had the highest modulus of elasticity and the one, loaded in the transverse direction, from the same region had the lowest modulus (Table XXVIII).

The compressive strain for a tibial condyle specimen loaded in the direction of the shaft, for a specimen from the back of the fibular condyle loaded in the transverse direction, and for another specimen from the same region but loaded in the anteroposterior direction was 49.2%, 22.8%, and 60.5%, respectively. The proportional limit for the above specimens was 90%, 45.7%, and 85.8%, respectively, of the breaking load (Fig. 68).

Evans and King (1961) and Evans

TABLE XXVIII

Directional Differences in Some Mechanical Properties of Cancellous Bone* from a 70-Year-Old Man
(Data from Knese, 1958)

Region of Bone†	Direction of Loading	kgf/cm²	lbf/in²
	Ultimate Compressive Strength		
Head, anterior half	anteroposterior	116.5	1,657
Head, posterior half	direction of neck	96.3	1,369
Tibial condyle, anterior half	longitudinal	58.9	838
Fibular condyle, posterior half	transverse	28.3	402
Fibular condyle, posterior half	anteroposterior	99.1	1,409
	Modulus of Elasticity		
Head, anterior half	anteroposterior	580	8,248
Head, posterior half	direction of neck	887	12,613
Tibial condyle, anterior half	longitudinal	623	8,859
Fibular condyle, posterior half	transverse	518	7,366
Fibular condyle, posterior half	anteroposterior	1,565	22,254

* Bone assumed to be fresh, although condition not actually stated.
† One specimen from each region was tested.

(1969) made a more extensive study of the directional differences in the mechanical properties and density of cancellous bone from embalmed femurs of six adult white men, two white women, and three Negro men. Two types of test specimens were used: (1) rectangular (standard) specimens, 2.5 cm long and 0.79 cm on each side, with a slenderness ratio of about 11.4 and (2) cubes, 0.79 cm on each side. The rectangular specimens (Fig. 14) and cubes were cut and loaded in different directions with respect to the three primary axes of the intact femur. Density measurements were made on air-dried specimens to avoid the effect of moisture within the spaces of the specimens whereas various mechanical properties were determined on wet specimens which had been kept in a physiological saline solution. A total of ninety-one rectangular and sixteen cubic specimens was tested.

The specimens were slowly loaded to failure in a 5,000 lb-capacity Riehle materials testing machine calibrated to an accuracy of ±1%. In order to read the load in units of 0.5 lb on the dial of the machine, the low range scale (0-250 lb) was used. Failure was indicated by a drop in the magnitude of the recorded load. A minimum of twenty load-deformation readings was made for each specimen. From the data obtained during a test, a stress-strain curve was drawn for each specimen and used to calculate the tangent modulus of elasticity and the energy the specimen absorbed to failure. By measuring the area below the stress-strain curve with a compensating polar planimeter, the magnitude of the energy absorbed to failure was determined.

The mechanical property values obtained from rectangular specimens were considered to be more realistic than those from cubes. When a cube is tested in com-

pression, there is a tendency for the upper part of the specimen to become impacted into the lower part thus giving rise to abnormally high values for compressive stress. The increase, in turn, influences the values obtained for the compressive strain, the modulus of elasticity, and the energy absorbed by the specimen.

Evans and King found that both rec-

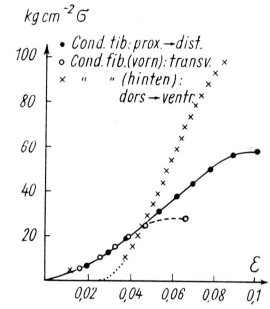

Figure 68. Directional differences in compressive stress-strain curves of human cancellous bone. (From Knese: *Zwanglose Abhandlungen aus dem Gebiet der Normalen und Pathologischen Anatomie*. Courtesy of Georg Thieme.)

tangular standard (S) and cubic (C) specimens that were cut and loaded in the lateromedial direction, regardless of the region of the femur from which they were obtained, had the highest average compressive modulus of elasticity, compressive strain, energy absorbed to failure, and density (Table XXIX). The highest average compressive strength was found for the standard specimens loaded in the long axis of the femoral neck and in the cubes loaded in the lateromedial direction.

TABLE XXIX

MEAN AND RANGE OF VARIATION IN SOME MECHANICAL PROPERTIES OF HUMAN FEMORAL SPONGY BONE ACCORDING TO THE DIRECTION OF LOADING (Data from Evans and King, 1961)

Direction	No. of Specimens	Mean (Range of Variation)	Standard Deviation	Mean (Range of Variation)	Standard Deviation
Maximum Compressive Stress		lbf/in^2		kgf/mm^2	
Sup-inf	S 30	402 (57-1,380)	296.70	2.83 (0.40-9.70)	2.09
	C 2	308 (66-550)	342.05	2.17 (0.46-3.87)	2.40
Ant-post	S 29	326 (44-798)	228.28	2.29 (0.31-5.61)	1.60
	C 11	623 (194-1,560)	390.38	4.38 (1.36-10.97)	2.74
Along neck	S 5	627 (166-989)	103.63	4.41 (1.17-6.95)	0.73
	C 0	—	—	—	—
Lat-med	S 6	599 (16-2,150)	223.00	4.21 (0.11-15.11)	1.57
	C 2	1,684 (1,063-2,305)	878.24	11.84 (7.47-16.20)	6.17
Modulus of Elasticity		lbf/in^2		kgf/mm^2	
Sup-inf	S 27	35,533 (6,220-120,000)	7,441.77	249.80 (43.73-843.60)	52.32
	C 2	18,125 (5,000-31,250)	5,652.43	127.42 (35.15-219.69)	39.74
Ant-post	S 26	30,458 (5,190-100,300)	7,083.78	214.12 (36.49-705.11)	49.80
	C 11	24,434 (8,180-50,000)	15,658.86	171.77 (57.51-351.50)	110.08
Along neck	S 5	55,960 (12,500-83,350)	29,720.36	393.40 (87.88-585.95)	208.93
	C 0	—	—	—	—
Lat-med	S 3	89,065 (5,820-141,375)	23,067.00	626.13 (40.91-993.87)	162.16
	C 2	66,425 (61,350-71,500)	7,177.05	466.97 (431.29-502.65)	50.45
Energy Absorbed		$in-lbf/in^3$		$kg-cm/cm^3$	
Sup-inf	S 28	5.34 (2.09-13.78)	2.918	0.38 (0.15-0.97)	0.21
	C 2	12.08 (1.37-22.80)	15.152	0.85 (0.01-1.60)	1.07
Ant-post	S 27	4.33 (.67-9.17)	2.448	0.30 (0.05-0.64)	0.17
	C 11	21.90 (6.20-67.70)	17.198	1.54 (0.44-4.76)	1.21
Along neck	S 5	6.98 (1.12-11.21)	2.176	0.49 (0.08-0.79)	0.15
	C 0	—	—	—	—
Lat-med	S 3	17.74 (3.01-34.00)	15.550	1.25 (0.21-2.40)	1.09
	C 2	76.40 (40.00-112.80)	51.478	5.37 (2.81-7.93)	3.62
Density		g/cm^3			
Sup-inf	S 31	.682 (.293-1.020)	.669	—	—
	C 2	.472 (.293-1.020)	.669	—	—

Direction	No. of Specimens	Mean (Range of Variation)	Standard Deviation	Mean (Range of Variation)	Standard Deviation
Ant-post	S 25	.672 (.273-1.170)	.240	—	—
	C 11	.669 (.356-.928)	.661	—	—
Along neck	S 5	.822 (.575-.980)	.163	—	—
	C 0	—	—	—	—
Lat-med	S 2	1.000 (.217-1.083)	.117	—	—
	C 2	1.000 (.917-1.083)	.117	—	—
Strain at Failure		*in/in*			
Sup-inf	S 29	.0302 (.011-.078)	.0157	—	—
	C 2	.0372 (.036-.038)	.0014	—	—
Ant-post	S 27	.0224 (.015-.039)	.0073	—	—
	C 11	.0707 (.058-.086)	.0310	—	—
Along neck	S 5	.0202 (.017-.025)	.0122	—	—
	C 0	—	—	—	—
Lat-med	S 6	.0320 (.020-.289)	.0093	—	—
	C 2	.101 (.098-.105)	.0050	—	—

S = standardized specimens, .79 cm × 2.5; C = cubic specimens, .79 cm × .79 cm.

Comparison of the directional differences for the various mechanical properties of wet cancellous specimens showed that the mean maximum compressive strength of the cubic specimens, loaded in the anteroposterior and the lateromedial directions, was higher than that of the similarly tested standard specimens (Figs. 69 and 70; Table XXIX). The strain at failure and the energy absorbed to failure for the cubic specimens were greater in all directions than those for the standard specimens, although the latter had a higher modulus of elasticity. The density of both types of specimens was identical for those cut in the lateromedial direction; the standard specimens cut in the superior-inferior direction were considerably denser than the comparable cubic specimens while they were approximately equal in the anteroposterior direction. No cubic specimens were obtained from the femoral neck.

The slope of the stress-strain curve for a standard specimen was steeper than that for a cubic specimen indicating that the former was stiffer and had a higher modulus of elasticity (Fig. 71). However, a cubic specimen absorbed considerably more energy to failure, as suggested by the larger area below the stress-strain curve. Due to the distribution of the cancellous bone within the two types of specimens, the differences may well be structural ones.

Statistical analysis of the data revealed that the differences between the mean values for the compressive stress (strength), the modulus of elasticity, and the density of standard specimens loaded in different directions were not significant. However,

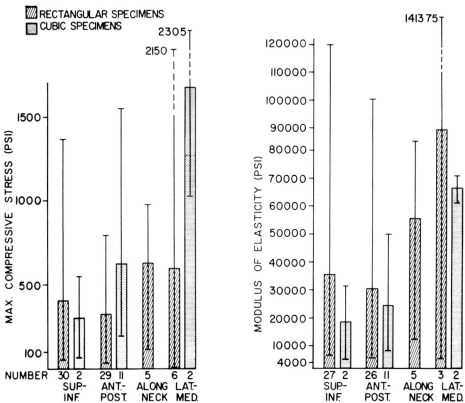

Figure 69. Directional differences in compressive strength and modulus of elasticity of human cancellous bone. (From Evans: *Artif Limbs,* 1969)

the average amount of energy absorbed by the specimens loaded in the lateromedial direction was significantly greater, at the 1% level of confidence, than that of the specimens loaded in either the anteroposterior direction or the superior-inferior direction.

Vertebrae

Directional differences in the compressive strength, the apparent density, the real density, and the percent porosity of standardized specimens of cancellous bone from the bodies of the third and fourth lumbar vertebrae were recently determined by Galante et al. (1970). The specimens,

10 mm long, were obtained at twenty-three routine autopsies performed within twenty-four hours after death of the subject. Patients with known malignant diseases were excluded. The relation between compressive strength and density was studied in seventeen specimens, the effect of specimen orientation on compressive strength in forty-six specimens, and the effect of different rates of loading on compressive strength in twenty-four specimens.

In order to minimize water loss the specimens were prepared under conditions of saturated humidity. The compression strength of the specimens was determined at a constant rate of loading with an Instron materials testing machine, ultimate strength being calculated from the highest point before failure on the load-deformation curve. A test was completed in less than a minute so that the effects of air drying would be minimal. Stress-strain relations were not investigated because, with the equipment available, it was impossible to measure strain directly in the specimen.

The real density of the specimens was calculated by dividing the wet weight by the volume of bone tissue, and the apparent density by dividing the wet weight by the total specimen volume. Prior to the mechanical property tests, the total specimen volume, including both marrow spaces and bone, was determined by mi-

crometer measurements. After these tests the bone matrix volume was determined by Arnold's method (1960) which involved washing the specimen under a high pressure stream of tap water to remove the marrow, immersion in distilled water, degassing under a vacuum, and weighing while submerged in water (submerged weight). The specimen was then blotted dry for two minutes and weighed in air (fully hydrated weight). Once the water from the surface and marrow vascular spaces was removed by centrifuging the specimen for fifteen minutes at 8,000 × g, it was again weighed to determined its wet weight. The specimen was then oven dried for twenty-four hours at 100° C and

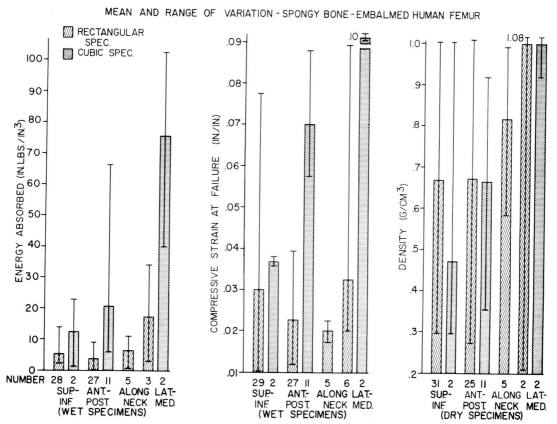

Figure 70. Directional differences in energy absorbed to failure, compressive strain at failure, and density of human cancellous bone. (From Evans: *Artif Limbs,* 1969)

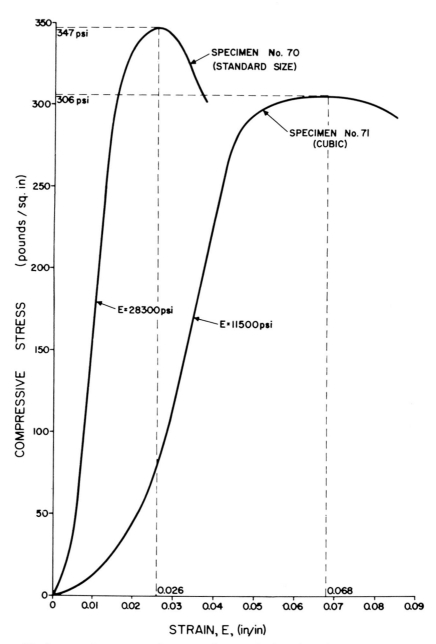

Figure 71. Compressive stress-strain curves for standard and cubic specimens of human spongy bone. Standard specimen = 2.52 cm long by 0.79 cm on each side. Cubic specimen = 0.79 cm on each side. (From Evans and King: in *Biomechanical Studies of the Musculoskeletal System.* Courtesy of Charles C Thomas, Publisher)

weighed (dry weight). The ash weight of the specimen was determined after it was ashed in a muffle furnace at 500° C for forty-eight hours. From the difference between wet and submerged weight—water density being assumed to be unity—the volume of the bone tissue, exclusive of the marrow spaces, was calculated.

The results of the tests of the forty-six specimens oriented in different directions revealed that the greatest and the lowest mean compressive strength was found in the specimens oriented in the superior-inferior direction and the lateral direction, respectively (Table XXX). The laterally oriented specimens had the highest mean real density while the greatest apparent density occurred in the laterally and the anteroposteriorly oriented specimens. Linear regressions between compressive strength and apparent density (Fig. 72) were significantly different for each direction but the slopes of the lines were not.

The mean values for the seventeen specimens used for this series of experiments was 20.99 ± 2.57 kp/cm^2 for compressive strength, 0.22 ± 0.02 g/cm^3 for apparent density, 1.79 ± 0.04 g/cm^3 for real density, and $87.21 \pm 1.37\%$ for porosity.

The real density values, calculated from the bone matrix volume after the specimens had been tested, may not be the true ones. The specimen was prepared for this determination by washing away the marrow under a high pressure stream of tap water. In this process it is very likely that any loose spicules of bone caused by crushing of the specimen during a compression test would also be washed away. Consequently, since the volume of the bone matrix in the specimen would actually be a little less than at the time of the test, the value Galante et al. obtained for the real density of their specimens is probably somewhat low.

The foam-like structure of cancellous bone and diploë is very well adapted to absorb energy. As suggested by Evans et al. (1951b), energy absorption may be the chief mechanical function of spongy bone. This function was demonstrated more than a century ago by some experiments of Dr. Physick, who, according to Wistar (1825),

. . . has pointed out another very important advantage of the cellular structure of bones, besides those of its making them nearly as strong as if they were solid, and at the same time diminishing what otherwise would have been a weight too op-

TABLE XXX

Mean Values for the Compressive Strength and Density of Fresh Cancellous Bone from Human Lumbar Vertebral Bodies (Data from Galante et al., 1970)

No. of Spec.	Spec. Orientation	kpf/cm²	lbf/in²
	(Compressive Strength)		
14	superior-inferior	20.90 ± 1.61	297 ± 23
17	anteroposterior	8.5 ± 1.27	121 ± 18
15	lateral	7.37 ± 1.05	105 ± 15
	(Apparent Density)	*g/cm³*	
14	superior-inferior	0.21 ± 0.01	
17	anteroposterior	0.23 ± 0.02	
15	lateral	0.23 ± 0.01	
	(Real Density)		
14	superior-inferior	1.83 ± 0.40	
17	anteroposterior	1.79 ± 0.40	
15	lateral	1.91 ± 0.10	

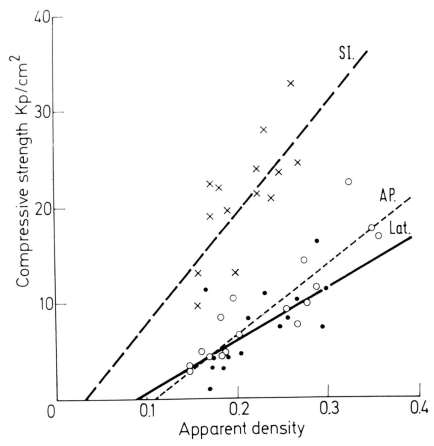

Figure 72. Compressive strength vs apparent density of cancellous bone from human vertebrae when compressed in the superior-inferior (SI), anteroposterior (AP), and bilateral (Lat) directions. (From Galante, Rostoker, and Ray: *Calcif Tissue Res*, 1970)

pressive for the muscular powers. He thinks that thereby the concussion of the brain and of the other viscera is frequently prevented; and in nearly all cases diminished, in falls and in blows. He illustrates the position by showing, first, the concussion which takes place through a series of ivory balls suspended by threads; if one be drawn to some distance from the others, and allowed to impel them by falling. The momentum in this case impels the ball at the further end of the row, almost to the distance from which the first one fell. But if a ball of the same size, composed of the cellular structure of bone, be substituted for one of the ivory balls, and the experiment be repeated, the momentum of the first ball is lost almost entirely in the cellular structure of the substitute; particularly if the latter be well soaked previously in water, so as to give it a condition in point of moisture allied to the living state.

The load applied to a cancellous bone specimen is supported by the various trabeculae composing the specimen, the proportion of the total load being borne by individual trabeculae varying with their distribution and orientation. Undoubtedly the stress in a single trabeculum is much higher than that of the entire specimen but, as far as I know, the stress (strength) and other mechanical properties of a trabeculum have never been determined. Therefore, it can be said that the values given by various investigators for the mechanical properties of cancellous bone actually represent structural as well as mechanical properties.

In the living condition cancellous bone also contains blood, fat, marrow, and hemopoietic elements which aid in the supportive functions of the bone. According to Policard and Roche (1937), the talus and calcaneum are actually composed of 80% nonosseous tissue. Living cancellous bone, therefore, represents a quasi-hydrostatic system that is well adapted to absorb energy.

SUMMARY

Bone, both compact and cancellous, is an anisotropic material whose strength and other mechanical properties have marked directional differences. The majority of studies on directional differences in mechanical properties of compact bone have been made on specimens from the principal long bones.

All investigators of the problem agree that the ultimate tensile, compressive, and bending strength as well as the accompanying modulus of elasticity of compact bone are considerably greater in a direction parallel with than perpendicular to the long axis of the bone or the predominant direction of the osteons. The impact snapping strength of human compact bone is greater radially than tangentially with respect to the long axis of the intact bone, the reverse of the relations in the compact bone of cattle. The values for horse bone are about equal in both directions. Human compact bone has a greater shearing strength perpendicular than parallel to the long axis of the bone.

The maximum compressive strength of fresh cortical beef bone is greatest in the longitudinal and least in the radial direction. However, the greatest compressive strain is in the radial direction and the least in the longitudinal direction at high stress rates of loading. At lower stress rates of loading the strain is approximately the same in both the longitudinal and circumferential directions.

The energy absorbed to failure by cortical bone from bovine femurs and tibias is greater in the longitudinal than in the transverse direction with respect to the shaft of the bone.

Compact bone from ox tibias, according to Maj and Toajari has a breaking load under bending that is three times greater in the longitudinal direction, with respect to the long axis of the bone, than that in the tangential direction and six times greater than that in the radial direction. In the tangential direction the breaking load is about twice as great as that in the radial direction. Olivo and his colleagues found that the breaking load under bending of specimens of compact bone from the same cross sections of metatarsals and metacarpals of a mule, an ox, and femurs of two women tended to increase in an anteroposterior direction while the deflection decreased. No such tendencies were evident in the lateromedial direction. Directional differences in torsional properties of compact bone appear not to have been investigated.

Cortical bone, separated by diploë, from the outer and inner tables of parietal bones from embalmed adult human cadavers has a compressive strength in the lengthwise direction (i.e. tangential to the skull surface) that is more than twice as great as the tensile strength in the same direction. However, the compressive strength in the lengthwise direction is a little less than that in the crosswise direction (i.e. radial to the skull surface). Diploë has a compressive strength in the crosswise direction that is only about one-seventh that of cortical bone in the same direction.

McElhaney et al. reported that comparable specimens, both embalmed and fresh, from adult human calvaria had a greater compressive strength, modulus of elasticity, and Poisson's ratio in the tangential than in the radial direction. The opposite relations were found for the compressive strain and energy absorbed to failure. Differences in the tensile properties of skull bone in the tangential and radial directions have not been investigated.

Directional differences in cancellous bone have not been studied as thoroughly as those in compact bone. Fresh femoral cancellous bone, according to Rauber, has a higher shearing stress and modulus in the perpendicular than in the longitudinal direction with respect to the long axis of the intact bone. Evans and King found that the same type of bone from embalmed femurs had a higher compressive strain, modulus of elasticity, and energy absorbed to failure as well as being denser in the lateromedial than in other directions with respect to the three primary axes of the bone. The compressive stress was greater in the longitudinal direction for rectangular specimens and in the lateromedial direction for cubic specimens. The energy absorbed to failure was significantly greater, at the 1% level, in the lateromedial than in the anteroposterior or the superior-inferior direction. Directional differences for the other mechanical properties and for density were not statistically significant.

Fresh cancellous bone from bodies of human lumbar vertebrae has the highest mean compressive strength in the superior-inferior direction, second highest in the anteroposterior direction, and least in the lateral direction. Longitudinal compressive strength has a positive and a negative relation with apparent density and real density, respectively, of vertebral cancellous bone.

Mechanical property tests of cancellous bone and of diploë are as much structural tests as mechanical property tests because the results obtained are primarily dependent upon the orientation and distribution of the trabeculae of the bone.

CHAPTER 8

EFFECTS OF DURATION, FREQUENCY, AND RATE OF LOADING

BRIEF INTERMITTENT LOADING

THE FIRST DEMONSTRATION that the mechanical properties of bone are influenced by the duration of the load applied to it was made by Rauber (1876) who performed a series of experiments on small elongated rods of human and beef compact bone. Intermittent bending loads of increasing magnitude but of brief duration were applied to the middle of the rods which were supported at both ends. The time between loads varied. Fresh as

TABLE XXXI

EFFECTS OF BRIEF INTERMITTENT LOADS, AT TEMPERATURES OF 15° TO 25° C, ON THE FLEXURE PROPERTIES OF FRESH MOIST HUMAN COMPACT BONE (Data from Rauber, 1876)

Source	Load (g)	Total Flex. (mm)	Residual Flex. (mm)	Elastic Flex. (mm)	Elastic Aftereffect (mm)	Elastic Flex. Increase (mm)
Tibial	200	19	—	19	—	19
specimen,	400	38.5	—	38.5	0.5	19.5
46-yr-old	600	57.5	—	57.5	0.5	19
male	800	76	0.5	75.5	0.5	18
	1000	94.5	0.5	94	1.0	18.5
	1400	132.5	1.5	131	1.5	18.5
	1600	—	—	—	—	—
	1800	—	—	—	—	—
	2000	—	—	—	—	—
	2100	360 Failure				
	Modulus of elasticity—2469 kgf/mm^2 (3.51×10^6 lbf/in^2)					
Second	200	15	—	15	—	15
specimen,	400	30.5	—	30.5	0.5	15.5
same	600	46	—	46	0.5	15.5
bone	800	61	—	61	0.5	15
	1000	76.5	0.5	76	1.0	15
	1200	93.5	0.5	93	1.0	17
	1400	110	1.0	109	1.5	16
	1600	128.5	1.5	127	1.5	18
	1800	148	2.0	146	2.0	19
	2000	—	—	—	—	—
	2200	299 Failure				
	Modulus of elasticity—2339 kgf/mm^2 (3.33 lbf/in^2)					
Humeral	200	17.5	—	17.5	—	17.5
specimen,	400	34.5	—	34.5	—	17
same	600	52	—	52	—	17.5
man	800	69	—	69	0.5	17
	1000	87.5	0.5	87	0.5	18
	1400	126.5	1.5	125	1.5	19
	1600	—	—	—	—	—
	1700	—	—	—	—	—
	1800	288 Failure				
	Modulus of elasticity—2424 kgf/mm^2 (3.45×10^6 lbf/in^2)					

well as dry specimens were tested at temperatures of 15° to 25° C. A few additional specimens were tested at 38° C.

Fresh moist specimens from the tibia of a 46-year-old man were tested with brief intermittent loads of gradually increasing magnitude. There was no residual (permanent) flexure with loads up to 600 g although the magnitude of the elastic flexure steadily increased (Table XXXI). With a load of 800 g a residual flexure appeared along with an increase in the elastic flexure and elastic aftereffect which was first observed at a load of 400 g. The values for all the mechanical properties increased with continued loading up to 1,400 g. No values were recorded for loads greater than 1,400 g until failure of the specimen occurred with a load of 2,100 g and a total flexure of 360 mm. A second specimen from the same bone, for which flexures up to a load of 1,800 g were recorded, behaved in a similar fashion.

When tested at 38° C, fresh moist specimens from the same individual exhibited a similar behavior to those tested at 15° to 25° C. However, the breaking load and the modulus of elasticity had lower values although the total flexure at failure was a little higher.

Rauber demonstrated that the flexure deformation produced in bone by brief intermittent loads showed a rapid and complete recovery after removal of the load. With smaller loads he found that the recovery occurred within a maximum of fifteen minutes, but with larger loads the recovery consisted of an instantaneous component (elastic flexure) as well as a gradual component (elastic aftereffect). With larger loads a residual of permanent deformation (flexure) was produced. The effect of stresses close to or exceeding the yield point, the point at which strain or deformation of a material continues without an increase in stress or load, was not investigated because Rauber's specimens were also used for other experiments. According to Rauber, the yield point of bone is very difficult to determine because the elastic aftereffect has a considerable range in both fresh and dry specimens.

PROLONGED LOADING

Rauber also determined the effects of prolonged loading on the flexure of dry cortical rods from the humerus and femur of a man whose age was not given. The flexure properties studied were the same as those in his intermittent loading experiments. For one of the humeral specimens he found that a 100 g load applied for 0.5 minutes produced no residual flexure or elastic aftereffect, while the same load applied for forty-eight hours caused a small residual flexure and elastic aftereffect that required forty-eight hours for its completion (Table XXXII). A second similar specimen from the same bone subjected to a 1,000-g load for 0.5 minutes al-

TABLE XXXII

EFFECTS OF PROLONGED LOADING ON THE FLEXURE PROPERTIES OF TWO DRY SPECIMENS OF HUMERAL CORTICAL BONE FROM A MAN (Data from Rauber, 1876)

Load (g)	Period of Loading	Total Flex. (mm)	Residual Flex. (mm)	Elastic Flex. (mm)	Elastic Aftereffect (mm)	Duration of Aftereffect
100	0.5 min	16	—	16	—	—
100	48 hr	19	0.5	18.5	2.0	48 hr
1,000	0.5 min	102	—	102	0.5	5 min
1,000	24 hr	127	7.0	120	19	24 hr

so had no residual flexure but an elastic flexure and an elastic aftereffect that persisted for five minutes. When a 1,000-g load was applied for twenty-four hours, a residual flexure appeared and there was an increase in the magnitude of the elastic flexure and the elastic aftereffect that endured for twenty-four hours. It is interesting to note that in prolonged loading of both specimens the time required for the completion of the elastic aftereffect was of the same length as the period of loading.

In other experiments on two dry femoral specimens from the same individual, Rauber studied the effect of gradually increasing loads, each of which was sustained for twenty-four hours before it was increased. In these experiments the total flexure as well as the immediate and complete flexure increases produced by each load were measured at the beginning and end of each 24-hour loading period. Rauber found that the total flexure produced by each load during a 24-hour period increased with the magnitude of the load applied. However, the immediate flexure increase was almost constant at all loads and the amount of complete flexure increased only slightly (Table XXXIII). Both specimens ruptured during the night. All the specimens in the prolonged loading experiments failed at a much smaller load than those under brief intermittent loads.

The effects of prolonged loading on anelasticity of wet and dry specimens of compact bone tested at various temperatures were determined by Currey (1965). Test specimens of beef metacarpals obtained from a slaughterhouse a few hours after death of the animal and beef tibias from a butcher shop were used. The tibial specimens, which had not been frozen, were presumably two or three days postmortem.

TABLE XXXIII

EFFECTS OF PROLONGED LOADING ON THE FLEXURE PROPERTIES OF TWO DRY SPECIMENS OF FEMORAL CORTICAL BONE FROM A MAN (Data from Rauber, 1876)

Load (g)	Total Flexure* (mm)		Flexure Increase* (mm)	
			Immediate	Complete
100	14	15	14	15
200	27.5	31	13.5	16
300	40.5	49	13	18
400	54.5	67.5	14	18.5
500	68	86	13.5	18.5
600	82	117	14	31
700	96	136	14	19
800	109	157	13	21
900	122	183	13	26
1,000	135	222	13	39
1,100	148	—	13	—
Ruptured at night				
100	12	13.5	12	13.5
200	24	27.5	12	14
300	36	42.5	12	15
400	48	58	12	15
500	60	73.5	12	15.5
600	72	89	12	15.5
700	84	106.5	12	17.5
800	96	124.5	12	18
900	107	142.5	11	18
1,000	119	165.5	12	20
1,100	131	182.5	12	20
1,200	143	204.5	12	22
1,300	154	—	11	—
Ruptured at night				

* Flexures were measured at the beginning and end of a 24-hour period.

Standardized specimens, kept moist and cool during their preparation, were tested by loading them like a cantilever beam. By adding weights to a swan-necked hook, the load was applied to the lower part of the specimen (Fig. 73). The deflection produced in this part of the specimen was determined by measuring, with a Baker traveling microscope, the vertical distance between reference marks on the upper (unloaded) and lower (loaded) parts of the specimen. Any deflections or rotations occurring in the supportive part of the specimen were discounted because the loaded and unloaded parts of the specimen would be equally affected.

The influence of physiological saline on

the mechanical properties of bone was one of the problems Currey investigated. It was found that no large or consistent changes were produced in the modulus of elasticity of two tibial specimens after four days of immersion in physiological saline.

The chief problem studied was anelasticity, the property of a solid in which its deformation depends upon the time rate of change in the stress or force applied to it as well as upon the magnitude of the stress. Anelasticity was demonstrated in a fresh tibial specimen to determine if extra deflection would occur. The immediate deflection was 1.66 mm compared to a deflection of 2.20 mm, a 33% increase over the original deflection, after ten days of loading.

Two minutes after removal of the load, a residual deflection of 0.55 mm was recorded. This was about the same as the extra deflection (0.54 mm) that occurred during the ten days of the experiment.

The residual deflection disappeared in an approximately exponential manner and gave a fairly straight line when plotted against logarithm time. After about sixty days, however, the curve became irregular and at one hundred days a residual deflection of 0.04 mm, approximately 8% of the extra deflection, was present (Fig. 74B). There is no reason to doubt that this small amount of deflection would eventually disappear. The experiment showed that a large part of the extra deflection produced by prolonged loading is recoverable and that the total extra deflection was not more than 30% of the original deflection.

Repeating the experiment on the same specimen for fifty-five days (Fig. 74A) produced a curve which showed an initial maximum difference from the first curve of only 5%. Later no differences between the two curves were evident. The extra deflection occurring during the second experiment was 53% of the initial deflection. Two minutes after removal of the load

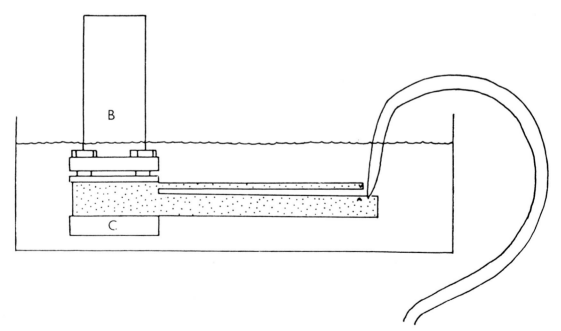

Figure 73. Apparatus for cantilever loading of bone specimens. (From Currey: *J Exp Biol*, 1965)

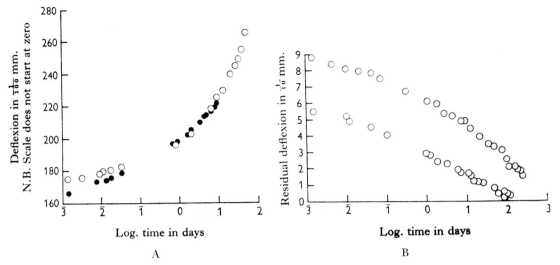

Figure 74. *A*. Deflection/time curves for same specimen illustrated in Fig. 73 loaded twice at room temperature. ● = first experiment; ○ = second experiment. (From Currey: *J Exp Biol,* 1965) *B*. Relaxation curves for same specimen loaded twice at room temperature. Lower curve = first experiment; upper curve = second experiment. (From Currey: *J Exp Biol,* 1965)

a residual deflection of 0.89 mm was found. This was similar to that of the extra deflection of 0.92 mm. After 234 days the residual deflection was 0.15 mm, 17% of that two minutes after removal of the load.

As indicated by the recovery curve after the ten days of loading, only a small amount of the residual deflection was not recoverable; a very long time would be required for full recovery. Currey's tests showed that most of the "considerable extra deflection" caused by prolonged loading is true anelasticity rather than plastic flow or the result of a change in the elastic properties of the bone. It can also be seen that the total amount of extra deflection was much greater than the 10% reported by Smith and Walmsley (1959) who only observed the deflection for half an hour. Currey admitted that there was a slight plasticity in the extra deflection.

The effect of drying on anelasticity was also investigated. A wet metatarsal speci-

men was loaded until the anelastic or extra deflection was 10% of the immediate deflection. It was then unloaded, allowed to recover nearly all of the anelastic deflection, dried at room temperature for one week, and reloaded with the same weight. The experiment was subsequently repeated. The two deflection-time curves for wet bone were similar to each other and the same was true for the two curves of dry bone. Although the curves for the wet versus dry bone were quite different (Fig. 75), Currey believes they indicate that drying does not have a very marked irreversible effect on anelasticity of bone.

Proportionality of anelasticity of bone to load was studied in a series of experiments with a single test specimen loaded three times with weights of 0.5, 1.0, 1.5, and 2.0 kg (indicated by A, B, C, and D in Table XXXIV). The specimen was loaded with a weight and the immediate deflection and the deflection after four hours were measured in millimeters. It was

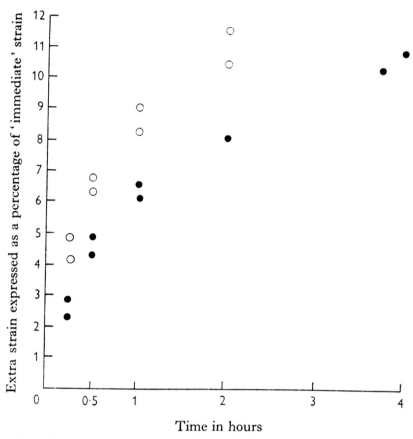

Figure 75. Deflection/time curves for same specimen loaded twice wet and twice dry with the same weight. ○ = wet loading; ● = dry loading. (From Currey: *J Exp Biol,* 1965)

then unloaded for two days after which another weight was applied. Most of the anelastic strain disappeared during the two days the specimen was unloaded. The order of application of the loads was A, B, C, D, D, C, B, A, D, C, B, A. Although there was a fair amount of spread in the results obtained, the initial deflections exhibited very good proportionality to load and the means closely approximated the expected proportionality.

In another series of experiments the effects of prolonged loading at different temperatures on the anelasticity of bone were investigated. A range of thermostatically controlled water temperatures was used. In the short-term experiments the temperature never varied more than 1° C, but in the longer experiments it occasionally varied a few degrees for a brief time.

In one experiment a specimen was loaded with the same weight ten times at temperatures of 37°, 18°, 37°, 16°, 3°, 49.5°, 2.5°, 50°, 19°, and 48° C, in that order. Each specimen was loaded for two hours and its immediate deflection and the deflection at the end of the two hours of loading were measured. After being loaded, the specimens were subjected to reversed loading for a short period to quickly decrease part of the anelastic strain and were allowed to recover for one day at room temperature.

Currey found that both elastic and anelastic deflection increased with the temperature at a rate of approximately 0.4% per degree (Fig. 76 *A* and *B*). Anelastic deflection did not increase linearly with the temperature but was greater at higher temperatures. The same was true of the immediate deflection, although Currey

TABLE XXXIV

ANELASTIC DEFLECTIONS (MM) PRODUCED IN A SINGLE PIECE OF CORTICAL BEEF BONE BY WEIGHTS OF 0.5 KG (A), 1.0 KG (B), 1.5 KG (C), AND 2.0 KG (D), EACH APPLIED THREE TIMES* (From Currey, 1965)

Weights	*A*	*B*	*C*	*D*
	0.04	0.10	0.12	0.14
	0.04	0.04	0.09	0.10
	0.03	0.08	0.10	0.16
Mean	0.037	0.073	0.103	0.133

* The specimen was unloaded for 2 days between weights.

pointed out the possibility that it may vary linearly with the temperature at first and that the nonlinear component is caused by unmeasured anelastic deflection occurring within the first two minutes.

At temperatures between 3° and 49° C the increase in immediate and anelastic deflection was about 24% and 300%, respectively. Between room temperature and blood temperature anelastic deflection increased about 100%.

Because all the tests were made on a single specimen, the possibility that after the first experiment the specimen was recovering from the previous experiments is discounted by Currey. His reasoning is that the amount of recovery between twenty-four and twenty-six hours after unloading is very small compared to the magnitude of the anelastic deflection within the first two hours of loading. None of his data from later experiments showed consistently lower values for anelastic deflection than in the earlier tests.

Although Currey's data show that anelasticity in bone is primarily a function of temperature, there is no indication whether raising the temperature increases the rate at which final equilibrium is approached or the rate of the strain at equilibrium. Furthermore, the data do not prove if equilibrium exists. As Currey

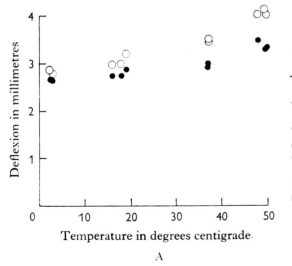

A

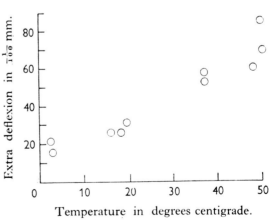

B

Figure 76. *A*. Deflection/temperature curves. ● = immediate deflection; ○ = deflection at end of 2 hours. (From Currey, *J Exp Biol,* 1965) *B*. Extra deflection/temperature curve after 2 hours of loading at different temperatures. (From Currey: *J Exp Biol,* 1965)

points out, it may be very difficult to determine the actual equilibrium value at which anelastic movement stops.

In an attempt to solve the latter problem, Currey investigated the behavior of a test specimen loaded for fifty-four days at a temperature of 37° C. The initial deflection was 2.53 mm compared to 5.99 mm at the end of the fifty-four days, an increase of 136%. A deflection versus logarithm time curve (Fig. 77) showed no indication of having reached the expected point of bending, if equilibrium were being approached. Currey speculated that the final deflection at equilibrium would probably be about twice the observed deflection if it were all recoverable. However, if the strain were partially plastic, the bone specimen would continue bend-

ing until failure. The recovery as seen in the illustration indicated recovery of a considerable part of the large deflection produced during the experiment.

A similar experiment on another specimen loaded for just twenty-four hours at 37° C showed that the extra deflection appeared more rapidly than in the previous experiment. At the end of the experiment it was 40.6% of the original deflection (Fig. 78). When the experiment was discontinued after seventy-nine days, 92% of the extra deflection had been recovered and it was assumed that eventually all of it would have been recovered.

The significance of anelasticity in bone with respect to resistance to impacts was discussed by Currey who pointed out that the resistance of a material to impact is in-

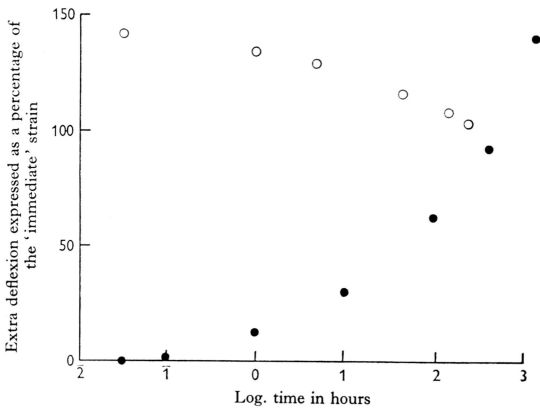

Figure 77. Prolonged loading at 37° C. ● = loading curve; ○ = relaxation curve. (From Currey: *J Exp Biol,* 1965)

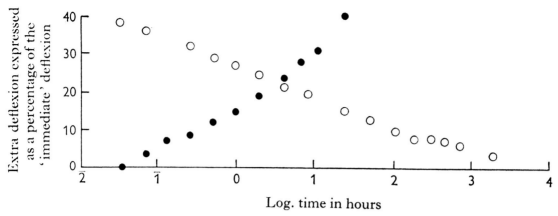

Figure 78. Loading for 24 hours at 37° C. ● = loading curve; ○ = relaxation curve. (From Currey: *J Exp Biol,* 1965)

versely proportional to its modulus of elasticity. Consequently, if bone exhibits anelastic effects for a few minutes, any values of modulus calculated from strain, seen a second or so after loading, may be far too low. It is possible that bone is very stiff, i.e. has a high modulus of elasticity, for a very short time but quickly shows a reversible, further strain or deformation. The effects of anelasticity in static loading of bones, e.g. bones of a bird roosting on one leg, or in cyclical loading, e.g. foot bones of a running animal or wing bones of a flying bird, are also discussed.

REPETITIVE LOADING

During daily activities the bones of the skeleton, individually and collectively, are subjected repeatedly to a variety of force systems most of which tend to bend the bones. The capacity of a bone to resist repeated loadings without breaking is an important factor to be considered in fracture mechanisms. This is especially true with respect to the so-called fatigue, stress, or march fractures, which most frequently occur in the metatarsal bones, although they have been reported elsewhere. They were called "march" fractures since it was believed that they arose from repetitive loading of the bones during marching. This type of fracture appears in x-ray films as a hair-line fracture and there is usually no history of trauma to account for it. Despite the importance and frequency of repetitive loading during normal daily activity, a search of the available literature revealed only a few publications dealing with the fatigue life of bone or its behavior under repetitive loading.

The first investigation of the strength of cortical bone under repetitive loading was made by Evans and Lebow (1957) who determined the fatigue life (the number of repetitions or cycles to failure) of standardized specimens of unembalmed femoral, tibial, and fibular bone from above-knee amputations of five adult men. One of the men was a paraplegic but the others had been active up to a short time before the leg was amputated for vascular difficulties of the foot.

Specimens designed as cantilever beams (Fig. 8D ②) were tested wet in a Model SF-2 Sonntag flexure fatigue machine at a stress of 5,000 lbf/in² (3.52 kgf/mm²) and a rate of 1,800 repetitions per minute.

Fatigue failure, probably the result of tensile stresses and strains created within the specimen by bending, occurs at a lower stress than in pure static tension; therefore, a stress of 5,000 lbf/in² was chosen because it was approximately one-half the tensile strength of human compact bone under pure tension. The rate or number of repetitions per unit time at which a fatigue test is made has no effect on the results of the test, fatigue life being dependent upon the total number of repetitions rather than on how fast they occurred. During a flexure test the amplitude of the bending of a specimen is not usually monitored because it has no influence on the fatigue life of the specimen. Further details on the method are given in Chapter 2.

The average fatigue life (repetitions or cycles to failure) was 1,982,650 for forty-seven tibial specimens; 1,188,453 for fifteen femoral specimens; and 2,841,400 for five fibular specimens.

In a second study Lease and Evans (1959) determined the fatigue life of intact metatarsals II through V from eight embalmed adult men and three women. Nine of the individuals were white and two were Negroes. No gross pathology was evident in the bones, ten of which were tested wet and forty-one dry. The age of the white men varied from 60 to 100 and the white women from 56 to 90 years of age. The Negro man was 54 and the woman 65 years of age. The specimens were tested with 10, 12, and 15-lb loads in the same Sonntag fatigue machine used previously.

Among the wet metatarsals tested with a 15-lb load, the third had the longest (10,384,000 cycles to failure) and the fifth the shortest (358,000 cycles to failure) average fatigue life. The second metatarsal, the one most frequently in-

volved in "march" fractures, had the second longest average fatigue life (6,152,666 cycles to failure) among the wet tested bones. When tested dry with the same load the fifth metatarsal had the longest (1,788,125 cycles to failure) and the second metatarsal the shortest (324,858 cycles to failure) average fatigue life. No consistent relations were found between the fatigue life and bone size or age of the individual from whom the specimens were taken.

In a third study King and Evans (1967) determined the fatigue life of 248 uniform specimens of cortical bone (Fig. 8D①) from the various thirds and quadrants of the shaft of the femurs of seventeen embalmed adult human cadavers. The specimens, designed as cantilever beams clamped at one end and loaded at the other, were tested with three precalibrated Sonntag flexure fatigue machines at alternating loads with a zero mean stress. Cool air was blown on the specimens during machining to prevent their being heated. Drying of the specimens during preparation was prevented by wetting them with normal saline solution. The specimens were stored in test tubes of saline solution until tested and were moistened with the solution during a test.

On the basis of previous experience, the specimens were tested at twelve stress levels varying from 4,375 to 11,250 lbf/in² at 625 lbf/in² intervals (3.08 to 7.91 kgf/mm² at 0.44 kgf/mm² intervals). In order to eliminate the influence of human judgment in the selection of specimens, about twenty were preassigned to each stress level before testing. The specimens were tested at a rate of 1,800 repetitions (cycles) per minute. If failure had not occurred after 10,000,000 repetitions, the test was stopped on the assumption that

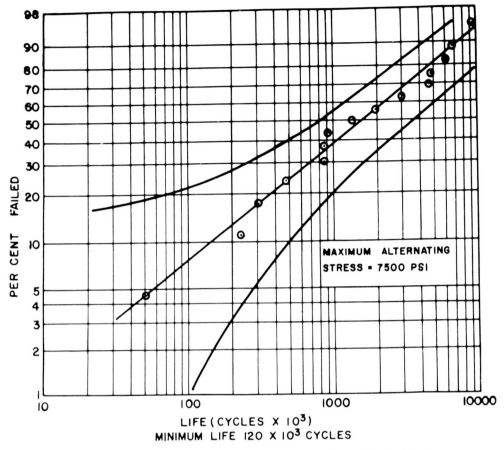

Figure 79. Weibull lines with 90% confidence limits for fatigue life of adult human cortical bone. (From King and Evans: in *Digest of the Seventh International Conference on Medical and Biological Engineering.* Stockholm, 1967)

the specimen would have gone to infinity under the conditions of the test.

The results of the tests were analyzed by assuming the Weibull probability distribution. Specimens from each of the twelve stress levels were arranged according to the length of their fatigue life and a percentage of failure (median rank) assigned to each one. By plotting the fatigue life against the percentage of failure on Weibull paper, a straight line (Fig. 79) was obtained. The slopes of the Weibull lines were approximately equal to zero. An S-N (Stress-Number of cycles) diagram was obtained from the twelve Weibull

lines (Fig. 80). From this diagram the fatigue life at 10%, 50%, and 90% failures were read off along with the 90% confidence band values at 50% failed.

The authors found the Weibull method suitable for analyzing fatigue data from compact bone although it was primarily designed for certain engineering materials. The endurance limit of human femoral cortical bone is about 4,000 lbf/in² (2.81 kgf/mm²) and the ultimate strength is more than 12,000 lbf/in² (8.44 kgf/mm²) at 50% failed. King and Evans are the only investigators who have given an S-N diagram for bone.

A search of the available literature revealed that the only investigation of the behavior of living bone under repetitive loading was made by Seireg and Kempke (1969) who determined the fatigue life of the tibia of living male rats about eighty days old. A load fluctuating between 0 and 0.2 lb (0 and 90.72 g) was applied to the right bone at a rate of 1,725 cycles per minute. The necessity of sustaining a load indefinitely determined the magnitude of the maximum load. The cyclic load was applied for three to four hours per day for several weeks. The remainder of the time the rats were free of the restraining jig. A typical long duration load wave-form is seen in Figure 81. Short duration tests with relatively high loads were also made.

At the end of the experiments the rats were sacrificed and the cleaned tibias cooked in a serological bath at 80° C for thirty-eight hours to remove tissue from the bones. The fat was extracted from the bones by putting them in jars with an ether-alcohol solution and vibrating the jars for twenty minutes in a *Son Blaster.* After the bones had been air dried, the effects of cyclic loading with respect to bone weight, mineral content, and density were determined. A Sartorius Electronic Balance was used to determine the weight while the mineral content and width of the bones were obtained with the scanning technique developed by Sorenson and Cameron (1967). Scans were taken at a distance of $\frac{1}{4}$, $\frac{3}{8}$, $\frac{1}{2}$, $\frac{5}{8}$, $\frac{3}{4}$, and $1\frac{1}{4}$ inches from the distal end of the bone. In some cases scans were taken at intervals of 0.050 inch over the entire length of the bone. Several scans were taken at each site and from this data averages and standard deviations were computed. Standard deviations for mineral content were within 2%

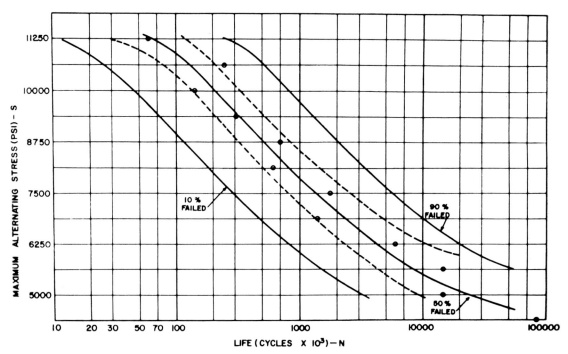

Figure 80. S-N diagram for fatigue life of adult human cortical bone. (From King and Evans: in *Digest of the Seventh International Conference on Medical and Biological Engineering,* Stockholm, 1967)

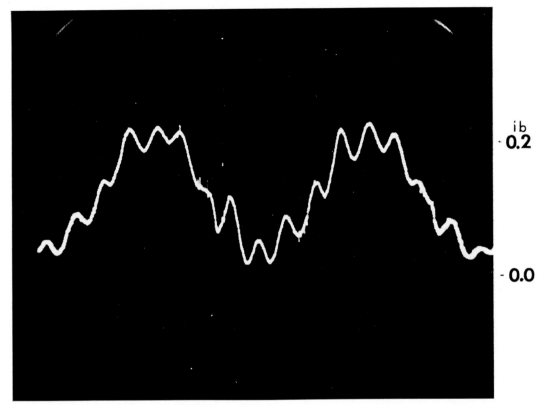

Figure 81. Typical long duration wave form for cyclic loading of living rat tibia. (From Seireg and Kempke: *J Biomech,* 1969)

of the average value. The total mineral content of each bone was determined by ashing it at 1,500° F and weighing the remnants.

The data from the long duration tests at relatively small loads (Table XXXV) showed no conclusive evidence of a change in the mineral content or between the bone weight and ashed weight ratios. Except for the animals used in tests 2 and 4, all the rats lost weight during the experiments. The most significant weight loss occurred during tests 7 and 8 when the rats were kept in the restraining jig throughout the entire test period. In tests 2 and 4 the rats exhibited an increase in the mineral content of the loaded tibia. The food intake of the animals was not regulated and may have affected the results

of the experiments. The authors admit that certain psychological or physiological factors, not controlled or measured in their experiments, were probably involved.

In other studies the maximum bending loads that the rat tibias could support were determined from static tests. Then successively smaller, fluctuating loads of short duration were applied until fracture occurred. Figure 82 is a typical example of the type of short duration load wave-form obtained. The load applied in each test varied between 0.6 lb (272.16 g) and a predetermined maximum. The smaller loads were applied at a rate of 1,725 cycles per minute and the larger ones at a rate of 190 cycles per minute. Results obtained from applying loads at both rates showed no sensitivity to the cycling rate. The ani-

TABLE XXXV

FATIGUE LIFE OF RAT TIBIAS *In Vivo* (Data from Seireg and Kempke, 1969)

Test No.	Test Days*	Week Period	Total No. of Cycles	Peak Load (lbs)	Initial Subject Weight (g)	Final Subject Weight (g)	Bone Weight Ratio	Ashed Weight Ratio	Width Ratio	Mineral Content Ratio As Measured	Normalized
1	Control		0	0	315	383	1.019	1.017	1.012	1.026	1.013
2	13	3	5,100,000	0.2	315	335	0.978	0.993	1.017	1.033	1.017
3	13	3	5,100,000	0.2	318	303	0.953	0.933	1.007	0.979	0.990
4	14	3	6,500,000	0.2	270	315	N.A.	N.A.	1.170	1.067	0.912
5	9	2	3,600,000	0.2	295	290	0.950	0.946	1.034	1.030	0.990
6	9	2	3,600,000	0.2	303	285	0.941	0.956	0.987	0.959	0.972
7	8	8	2,000,000	0.2	300	235	N.A.	N.A.	0.970	0.969	1.000
8	9	9	3,500,000	0.2	305	230	0.962	0.968	0.940	0.946	1.012

N.A. = Not available.
* Tests were run several hours per day for a test period of 2 to 9 weeks.

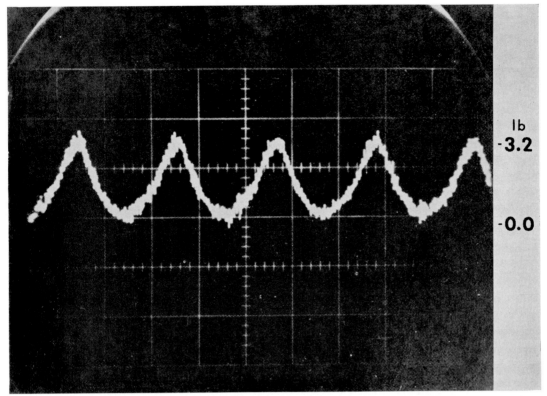

Figure 82. Typical short duration wave form for cyclic loading of living rat tibia. (From Seireg and Kempke: *J Biomech*, 1969)

mals were anesthetized with sodium nembutal during the tests to eliminate muscular activity and thus obtain a more accurate measurement of load.

A crackling sound accompanied each fracture whose exact site was later verified by gross dissection. The load-cycle curve (Fig. 83) had a sharp bend at about 4,000 cycles which established the endurance limit of the specimen. Below this limit, which was approximately 42% of the static fracture load, the load could be applied indefinitely without producing a fracture.

The authors believe that their experiments showed that other variables with different magnitudes than those used in their tests may play a significant role in any bone growth attributable to cyclic mechanical stress. The loads used in the long duration tests were of the same order of magnitude as those imposed by the weight of the animals and were about one-fifteenth of the safe endurance loads. It was felt that the relatively small number of cycles necessary to reach the endurance limit suggests that muscle fatigue may be an important factor in fractures produced by cyclic loading. The cyclic loading studies by Evans and Lebow and by King and Evans would seem to indicate that human compact bone has a relatively high resistance (fatigue life) to repetitive bending loads.

Recently, Evans and Riolo (1970) determined the fatigue life of forty-seven standardized specimens of unembalmed cortical bone from tibias of above-knee amputations of seven adult men. The specimens were tested at a stress of 344.7×10^6 dynes/cm^2 (5,000 lbf/in^2)

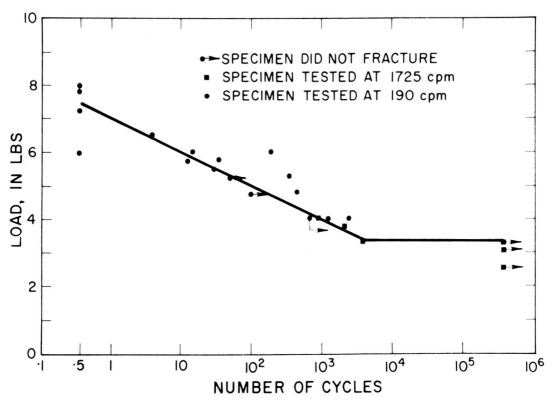

Figure 83. Load-cycle curves for short duration tests of fatigue life of living rat tibia. (From Seireg and Kempke: *J Biomech,* 1969)

in the same Sonntag fatigue machine (Figs. 18 and 19) used by Evans and Lebow (1957) and by Lease and Evans (1959). Specimen shape and dimensions were the same as those tested by Evans and Lebow. All specimens were tested wet at a rate of 1,800 repetitions per minute.

The average fatigue life of thirty randomly selected specimens whose structure was analyzed histologically was 2,350,000 ± 2,029,000 cycles to failure. The large standard deviation was explained on the basis of variations in the histological structure, as revealed by cross sections of the specimens at the fracture site, between specimens with a short (less than 500,000 cycles to failure) and a long (more than 4,000,000 cycles to failure) fatigue life.

The fatigue properties of cortical bone from fresh femurs of twenty-two sub-

jects, 35 to 98 years of age, were recently investigated by Swanson et al. (1971). The femurs were obtained at routine autopsies and stored at −20° C until they were used. Test specimens were machined to a standardized size and shape from the various quadrants of the middle region of the shaft of the bone. Usually eight specimens, but sometimes as many as sixteen, were obtained from a single bone. A total of sixty-eight specimens from fourteen men and thirty-nine from seven women were tested. The long axis of the specimen and the bone coincided.

The test specimens were spindles, 20 mm long and 3 mm in diameter at the ends, with a reduced central region 1.77 mm in diameter. The fatigue life of the specimens was determined with a Wöhler rotating fatigue machine by loading them to failure at a rate of 70 cycles/second. During a test the specimen was loaded like a cantilever beam. The lathe motor rotated the specimen during a test so that all elements in the specimen were subjected to alternating tensile and compressive stresses about a mean zero stress. At all times during preparation and testing the specimens were kept moist and cool with Ringer's solution.

In addition to fatigue life the amplitude of the bending stress at the top and the bottom surface of the reduced area of the specimen was calculated. A correction was made for the fact that the maximum stress was not is the reduced region but a short distance nearer the chuck. Effect of surface finishing was investigated in specimens from a 69-year-old man by preparing specimens with a standard, a coarse, or a fine finish.

Swanson et al. found a mean fatigue life of 15,000 cycles to failure at an amplitude of 12,180 lbf/in² (84 MN/m²), a mean of 350,000 cycles at an amplitude of 8,700 lbf/in² (60 MN/m²), and a mean of 4,500,000 cycles to failure at an amplitude of 6,670 lbf/in² (46 MN/m²).

Seven specimens with a standard surface finish (0.5 mm radius tool, 5 μm feed) had an average of 279,986 (68,900 to 778,000) cycles to failure, four specimens with a coarse surface finish (0.5 mm radius tool, 50 μm feed) had an average of 26,923 (7,900 to 136,000) cycles to failure, and three specimens with a fine surface finish (polished with 320 grit Carborundum paper) had an average of 78,867 (12,200 to 156,000) cycles to failure.

As the authors point out, the standard finish tool used for all specimens except those of the 69-year-old man in which variation in surface finish was specifically studied, made a mark with a crest-to-trough depth of approximately 6×10^{-9} m which is comparable to the size of an osteocyte lacuna. Consequently, the effect of surface finish in these specimens was controlled by natural features of the microscopic anatomy of the specimen and not by tool marks. Thus, it is not surprising that the fatigue life of specimens with a coarse or a fine surface finish is in the same range as those with the standard surface finish.

VARIOUS RATES OF LOADING

Long Bones

The first to investigate the effects of high strain rates of loading on the mechanical properties of bone were McElhaney and Byars (1965) and McElhaney (1966). For their experiments a special testing machine capable of constant-velocity compression tests at strain rates up to 4,000/sec was developed. The machine had adjustable stops so that predetermined strain rates could be applied. High frequency response instrumentation utilizing a piezoelectric load cell and a capacitance transducer were also used. The data were

recorded on a Tektronix Model 555 dual-beam oscilloscope.

Specimens of cattle and human cortical bone were tested. Cattle specimens, $0.175 \times 0.175 \times 0.250$ inch long, were taken from the right femur of a 3-year-old steer and all tests, except for the highest strain rate ones, were completed less than five days after death of the animal. During this time the specimens were submerged in water and refrigerated. The human specimens were obtained from the right femur of a 24-year-old man who died of acute cardiac failure. The body from which the femur was taken had been em-

TABLE XXXVI

Effects of Various Strain Rates of Loading on the Mechanical Properties of Cortical Bone
(Data from McElhaney, 1966)

Material	Strain Rate (in/in/sec)	Ultimate Compressive Strength (lbf/in²)	Ultimate Compressive Strength (kgf/mm²)	Energy Absorption Capacity (in-lb/in³)	Energy Absorption Capacity (kg cm/cm³)	Elastic Modulus (×10⁵ lbf/in²)	Elastic Modulus (kgf/mm²)	Maximum Strain to Failure (%)	Poisson's Ratio*	Number of Tests
Fresh bovine femur	0.001	25,500 (19,300-28,500)	17.93 (13.57-20.04)	350	24.67	2.7 (1.8-3.2)	1,898 (1,265-2,250)	1.88 (1.37-2.89)	.30	10
	0.01	30,000 (24,500-36,300)	21.09 (17.22-25.52)	416	29.32	2.9 (2.2-3.8)	2,039 (1,547-2,671)	1.82 (1.40-2.05)	—	10
	0.1	33,500 (24,600-37,000)	23.55 (17.29-26.01)	420	29.60	3.5 (2.7-4.7)	2,461 (1,898-3,304)	1.75 (1.41-2.15)	.28	10
	1.0	36,500 (32,000-38,000)	25.66 (22.50-26.71)	260	18.32	4.0 (3.3-5.0)	2,812 (2,320-3,515)	1.25 (.90-1.50)	—	5
	300	41,000 (38,000-46,000)	28.82 (26.71-32.34)	230	16.21	4.8 (4.6-5.1)	3,374 (3,234-3,585)	1.00 (.80-1.50)	.26	5
	1500	53,000 (47,000-58,000)	37.26 (33.04-40.77)	220	15.50	6.1 (5.0-7.0)	4,288 (3,515-4,921)	0.90 (.65-1.30)	—	5
Embalmed human femur	0.001	21,800 (18,000-23,000)	15.33 (12.65-16.17)	270	19.03	2.2 (1.6-2.7)	1,547 (1,125-1,898)	1.65 (1.10-2.65)	—	5
	0.01	26,000 (21,000-28,000)	18.28 (14.76-19.68)	310	21.85	2.5 (1.9-3.2)	1,758 (1,336-2,250)	1.75 (1.30-2.91)	—	3
Embalmed human femur	0.1	29,000 (24,000-32,000)	20.39 (16.87-22.50)	340	23.96	2.6 (2.0-3.5)	1,828 (1,406-2,461)	1.80 (1.42-3.20)	—	5
	1.0	32,000 (27,000-36,000)	22.50 (18.98-25.31)	350	24.67	3.2 (2.7-3.9)	2,250 (1,898-2,742)	1.78 (1.60-3.2)	—	3
	300	40,500 (36,000-42,000)	28.47 (25.31-29.53)	300	21.14	4.3 (3.3-4.8)	3,023 (2,320-3,374)	1.10 (.96-1.30)	—	3
	1500	46,000 (39,000-58,000)	32.34 (27.42-40.77)	260	18.32	5.9 (4.8-7.0)	4,148 (3,374-4,921)	0.95 (.91-1.16)	—	5

* Measured within the elastic limit of dry specimens.

balmed with a mixture of formalin, phenol, alcohol, and glycerin.

It was found that the ultimate compressive stress and the modulus of elasticity of the specimens progressively increased with high strain rates (1.0 in/in/sec or greater) while the maximum strain at failure and energy-absorbing capacity decreased (Table XXXVI). Poisson's ratio, determined at three different strain rates, decreased progressively with increasingly high strain rates of loading. These investigators were the first to demonstrate that certain mechanical properties of compact bone are rate-sensitive.

The decreased energy-absorbing capacity of bone at high strain rates of loading is of special interest with respect to fracture.

Most fractures arise from impacts, in which the fracturing force is applied at a high strain rate, and involve energy absorption by the bone itself as well as all the surrounding tissues. Thus, the increased energy-absorbing capacity of bone at high strain rates of loading is a safety factor in reducing the possibility of fracture.

As mentioned in Chapter 7, Bird et al. (1968) reported that the compressive stress and modulus of elasticity of cortical bone from beef femurs, cut and loaded in the longitudinal, circumferential, and tangential directions with respect to the intact bone, are rate sensitive. The increase in average failure stress as a function of loading rate was quite marked for longitudi-

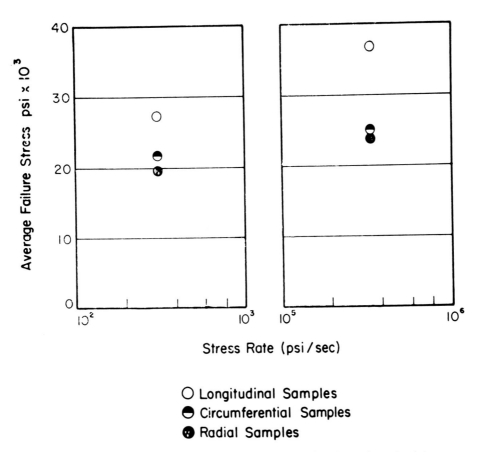

O Longitudinal Samples
● Circumferential Samples
◉ Radial Samples

Figure 84. Average compressive failure stress in fresh cortical bone from beef femurs as a function of loading rate. (From Bird, Becker, Healer, and Messer: *Aerosp Med,* 1968)

nal and circumferential specimens but less so for radial ones (Fig. 84). Similar rate sensitive effects were found for the modulus of elasticity of the different types of specimens (Fig. 85).

The approximately identical values for mechanical properties of the circumferential specimens was explained on the basis of specimen size, since the length of the specimen represented a significant angular sector of the cross section of the bone. Variations in the values for mechanical properties of specimens was attributed to differences in histological structure of the bone.

Skull Bones

Melvin et al. (1969a) determined the effect of different strain rates of loading on some of the mechanical properties of diploë from plugs, three-fourths inch in diameter, of bone removed from human skulls at autopsy. At the time of removal the orientation of the plugs within the calvarium as well as their distance from the sagittal, coronal, and lambdoidal sutures were recorded. Within thirty minutes after removal, the fresh plugs were placed in a freezer at −10° C. If desired, a clinical history of the subject from whom the plugs were taken could be learned from

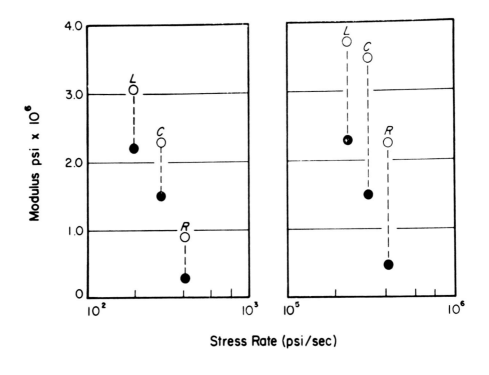

L = Longitudinal Sample
C = Circumferential Sample
R = Radial Sample

○ Elastic Modulus
● Tangent Modulus

Figure 85. Average compressive modulus of elasticity of fresh cortical bone from beef femurs as a function of loading rate. (From Bird, Becker, Healer, and Messer, *Aerosp Med,* 1968)

the autopsy number. The compressive strength, the modulus of elasticity, and the specific weight were determined for all the specimens which were moist when tested. Data were obtained from fifty-two specimens from five individuals.

Compressive tests of the specimens were made with an Instron TT-C testing machine at strain rates of 0.22 sec^{-1} and 2.2 sec^{-1}. Specimen load was measured with a piezoelectric Kistler 937A force link load cell with a maximum compressive capacity of 45,000 lbs (30,412 kg) in compression, a resolution of 0.1 lb, and a resonant frequency of 22.5 KHz. Specific weight was calculated from the specimen weight as determined with a Voland 640-D balance. A Tektronix Type 564 Storage Oscilloscope was used to record the tests and a permanent record obtained by photographing the trace with a Polaroid camera.

Data from the tests revealed the human diploë had a compressive strength varying from 1,820 to 11,350 lbf/in^2 (1.28 to 7.98 kgf/mm^2) and a modulus of elasticity from 0.57×10^5 lbf/in^2 to 3.99×10^5 lbf/in^2 (40.07 to 280.50 kgf/mm^2). Because of the web-like structure of the diploë, in contrast to that for cortical bone, failure occurred as a localized tearing of the trabeculae. A direct positive linear relationship was found between the modulus of elasticity of diploë and its specific weight. No strain rate effects were found.

In another study Roberts and Melvin (1969) investigated some of the dynamic properties of fresh human skull bone obtained from plugs of bone removed at autopsy as in the experiments just discussed. Preliminary impact penetration tests on whole calvaria indicated the feasibility of performing tension, compression, and shear tests on the specimens. The same methods employed by Melvin et al.

(1969a) for recording the site of the plugs before removal from the skull and for storing the specimens until tested were used.

Tensile properties, in a direction tangent to the skull surface, were determined for flat tensile specimens from the outer and the inner tables of cortical skull bone. Care was exercised to prevent heating or drying of the specimens during their preparation.

Tests at low strain rates (up to 20 in/min; 50.8 cm/min) were made with the Instron testing machine and at high (dynamic) strain rates with a Model 591-U Plastechon high speed testing machine. The Plastechon machine has a movable crosshead and a ramp speed from 20 in/min to 10,000 in/min (25,400 cm/min) in the closed model and up to a speed of 30,000 in/min (76,200 cm/min) with the open loop model using a 2,500-lb (1,134 kg) capacity ram. Except for the tensile tests load transducing was accomplished with a Kistler 937A piezoelectric load cell in union with a Kistler 503 electrostatic charge amplifier. The load cell had a maximum compression load capacity of 45,000 lbf (20,412 kg), a resolution of 0.1 lb, a frequency response flat to 5,000 Hz, and a resonant frequency of 22.5 KHz.

Most of the compression tests were made on cubes of diploë approximately 0.15 inch on a side. The specimens were compressed between two plattens in a direction perpendicular (radial) to the skull. The lower platten was attached to the ram and the upper one was a low mass attachment to the load cell. Because of the low stiffness of the diploë ram motion was an adequate indication of deformation and compressive strain. At speeds up to 5,000 in/min (12,700 cm/min) ram travel and compressive strain were limited by a mechanical stop.

Shear tests were also made on fresh and embalmed cylindrical specimens of diploë about 0.375 inch in diameter. Direct transverse shearing strength was determined by using the specimen as a shear pin between two sliding blocks with the diploë centered on the sliding plane. One block was attached to the load cell and the other one to the ram which was allowed to reach a constant velocity by a ball and socket mechanism. Tests were performed at speeds up to 2,000 in/min (508 cm/min). The only recorded data obtained in the tests was peak load.

The load on the specimen was measured with a Kistler 937A load cell with a tensile capacity of 1,000 lb (453.6 kg) and a resonant frequency of 70 KHz. Tensile strain was measured with two foil gauges with a 0.0625-inch grid length bonded to the specimen with Eastman 910 adhesive. Test velocities up to 5,000 in/min (12,700 cm/min) were routinely used. In tests up to a speed of 200 in/min (508 cm/min) data were recorded as a load-strain curve with a z-axis modulation as the time base (Fig. 86). At higher strain rates all data were recorded with open shutter oscillophotography and stress-strain curves obtained by cross plotting load-time and

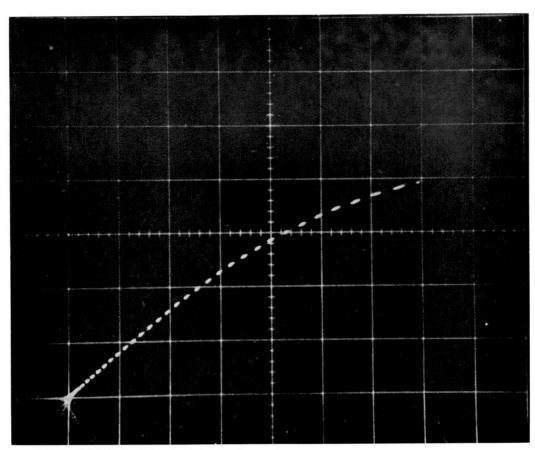

Figure 86. Tensile load-strain curve for standardized fresh specimens of bone from adult human calvaria. Crosshead speed = 20 in/min; vertical scale = 10 lb/div; horizontal scale = 1500 in/in/div; intensity modulation frequency = 1200 Hz. (From Roberts and Melvin: *Appl Polymer Symposia,* 1969)

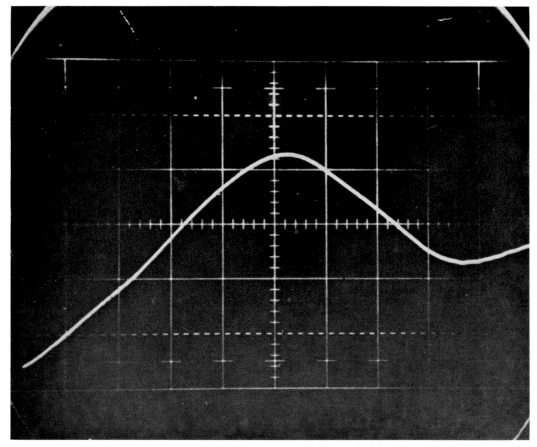

Figure 87. Load-time curve in compression for fresh diploë from adult human calvariae. Ram speed = 5000 in/min; vertical scale = 2516/div; horizontal scale = 20 sec/div. (From Roberts and Melvin; *Appl Polymer Symposia,* 1969)

strain-time traces. Figure 87 is a typical high speed load-time curve.

A summary of the tensile tests of cortical bone in a direction tangent to the calvaria surface is illustrated by stress-strain curves for low and high strain rates of loading (Fig. 88). The curves show significant strain rate effects over the four orders of magnitude range illustrated and that the bone behaves as a brittle nonlinear material.

A frequency distribution curve of penetration force data separated by test speed, based on preliminary skull penetration tests, showed a marked difference between zero mph (20 in/min) and 20 mph (32.18 kmh) tests but not between 10 mph (16.09 kmh) and 20 mph tests (Fig. 89). A mean penetration force of 810, 1,320, and 1,350 lb (367, 598, 612 kg) was found for speeds of 20 in/min, 10 mph, and 20 mph, respectively. Tests made at 20 mph had a tendency to produce plugs with steeper sides and smaller diameter bases for the inner skull table of bone than tests at slower speeds. In one of the 20-in/min tests the strain near the penetration points was recorded with a radially oriented strain gauge. A peak penetration strain of 4,600 μin/in with a time to failure of 230 msec was found. Application of this information to high speed tests in-

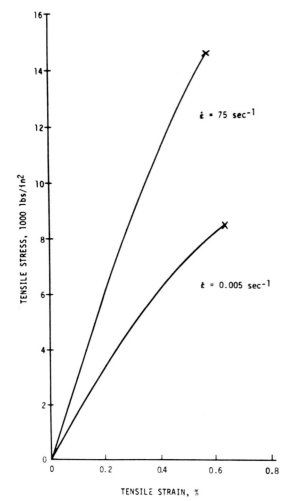

Figure 88. Typical low and high speed tensile stress-strain curves for fresh cortical bone from adult human calvariae. (From Roberts and Melvin: *Appl Polymer Symposia, 1969*)

dicates a strain rate of 20 sec⁻¹ in the outer skull table at a 20-mph impact velocity.

Data from radial compression tests indicated that at low strain rates of loading, diploë behaved like a dense open cell foam whose mechanical properties were closely related to its porosity. The compressive strength of the diploë ranged from below 2,000 lbf/in² (1.41 kgf/mm²) to yield strength values of more than 30,000 lbf/in² (21.09 kgf/mm²). A typical load-time curve for diploë with a

specific weight ranging from 0.030 to 0.055 lb/in³ (0.830 to 1.522 g/cm³) is seen in Figure 87. In this specific weight range there is a linear relation between strength and modulus of elasticity.

Test results at compressive strain rates up to 555 sec⁻¹ showed that the linear relation between strength and modulus was valid for dynamic rates, but a shift, to a limited extent, was evident in the relations between the mechanical properties and the specific weight. Because of the porosity effects, the compressive modulus of the diploë can vary from 6.0 × 10⁴ lbf/in² (42.18 kgf/mm²) up to the modulus value for cortical bone which is 2.0 or 3.0 × 10⁶ lbf/in² (1,406-2,109 kgf/mm²). At specific weights above 0.055 lb/in³ compressive failure occurred as a form of yielding instead of an abrupt collapse, essentially the same behavior as for cortical bone whose specific weight is 0.069 lb/in³ (1.910 g/cm³). Strain rates in this specific weight range would probably be similar to those reported by McElhaney (1966) for cortical bone in compression.

The shear strength of diploë also had a wide range in values due to structural variations in the diploë itself. Fresh diploë had an average shear strength of 3,272 lbf/in² (2.30 kgf/mm²) at a strain rate of 6.66 sec⁻¹ and of 4,386 lbf/in² (3.08 kgf/mm²) at a strain rate of 66.6 sec⁻¹.

Investigation of rate sensitive differences in tensile properties of cortical bone from adult human calvariae was continued by Wood (1971) who tested more than one hundred specimens from individuals ranging from 25 to 95 years of age. The specimens were obtained at autopsies which were usually performed within twelve hours after death of the subject. No specimens were taken from subjects with contagious diseases nor diseases known to affect the mechanical properties of bone.

Test specimens were taken from circular plugs, 0.75 inch or 1.5 inches in diameter, from the frontal, temporal, and parietal bones. Before the plugs were removed, their sites were marked on the skull with a cross whose long axis was parallel to the sagittal suture and whose short axis, crossing the anterior end of the long axis, was parallel to the coronal suture. In order to record the site of the plug, the distance from the edge of the hole of the above sutures was measured. Usually, only one plug was obtained from an individual although two small plugs were removed in a few cases. Depending upon the size of each plug, seven to nine tensile speci-

mens were machined to a standard size and shape. To prevent drying, the specimens were put into small test tubes with cork stoppers and stored in a freezer at a temperature of −10° to −20° C. All the specimens were tested at room temperature and normal humidity.

Tests at a slow strain rate of loading (0.02 to 20 in/min) were made with the Instron testing machine and at dynamic or high strain rates of loading with the Plastechon high speed testing machine previously described. The ram rate of the Plastechon machine was not affected by loads up to 2,000 lb, a rate much lower than that applied to the bone specimens which failed at loads of 50 lb or less.

Strain occurring in the specimens was

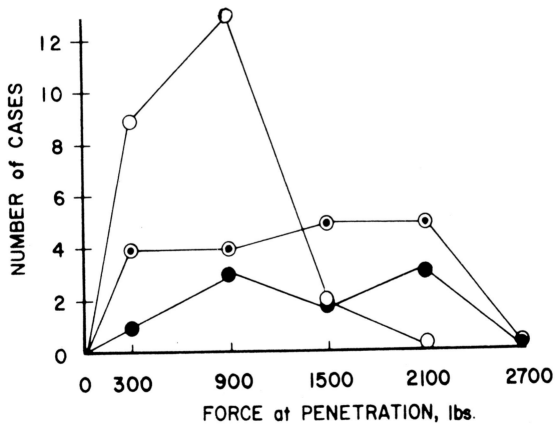

Figure 89. Frequency distribution for forces required to penetrate adult human calvaria separated by impact velocity. (From Roberts and Melvin: *Appl Polymer Symposia*, 1969)

measured with two metal foil strain gauges applied directly to the bone, one on each side of the specimen. Every specimen was tested within ten minutes after installation of the strain gauge. Static tests were made at a strain rate of 0.0003 in/in/sec (sec⁻¹) and dynamic tests at a rate of 150 sec⁻¹. The latter rate was chosen on the basis of data from skull penetration studies of Melvin et al. (1969b), suggesting that strain rates of more than 100 sec⁻¹ would rarely occur in automobile accidents. Higher strain rates would probably be found with bullet impacts.

Tensile data of compact cranial bone were obtained from 123 specimens, the breaking strength of the coronal suture from six specimens, and the approximate tensile strength of the diploë from eight specimens consisting entirely of diploë (Table XXXVII).

Poisson's ratio for lateral contraction in the radial direction with respect to the head was determined for two specimens used in tensile tests. All mechanical property data were calculated from oscilloscopic load versus strain or load and strain versus time curves (traces) obtained at different strain rates. Because the ram required about one inch of travel to attain the selected constant rate, there was some slack in the system and the slope of the stress-time curve was less constant at higher speeds of loading. However, no tests had more than about a two to one ratio of final strain rate to initial strain rate. For

technical details of the testing and recording apparatus, the reader should consult the original references.

The initial part of the load and strain versus time curve was lost at high strain rates of loading because of the preselected level of the oscilloscope. Therefore, to achieve greater consistency, the secant modulus of elasticity, based on 0.02% strain, was used instead of the tangent modulus more commonly employed in bone studies. The stress-strain curve is usually straight for the first 0.3% strain but shows a steadily increasing curvature up to failure. For strains less than 0.3% the secant modulus approximates the initial tangent modulus.

Wood's first test series was designed to reveal the scatter to be expected in data obtained from five parallel specimens from a single bone plug that were all tested at the same (nominal) strain rate of loading (Fig. 90). In this case, and twenty-four others in which the two or more parallel specimens were tested at the same strain rate, the modulus of elasticity of specimens from a single bone plug were always within ±6% of the average modulus value for that plug. However, considerable variation was found in breaking strength within each subject.

The scatter to be expected in data obtained from perpendicular specimens from a single bone plug and tested at one strain rate was also determined. Data from fifteen specimens showed that modulus of

TABLE XXXVII
TENSILE PROPERTIES OF HUMAN DIPLOË AND THE CORONAL SUTURE (Data from Wood, 1969)

	No. of Spec.	U.T.S. (lbf/in²)	U.T.S. (kgf/mm²)	Secant Modulus (×10⁵ lbf/in²)*	Secant Modulus (kgf/mm²)*	Tensile Strain (%)*
Diploë	8	4940	3.47	8.9	625.67	0.73
Coronal suture	6	2140	1.50	—	—	—

U.T.S. = ultimate tensile strain; secant modulus = secant modulus of elasticity.
* Approximate values.

elasticity values were still within ±6% (usually much less) of the mean value for all the specimens from the plug. Although some variation was found when the stress-strain curves for perpendicular specimens (dashed lines, Fig. 91) were compared with those from specimens in the opposite direction (solid lines, Fig. 91) the modulus data for all specimens from a single bone plug seemed consistent enough for the modulus value to be used as an indicator for strain rate.

Failure of the specimens occurred in a plane approximately transverse to their long axis. The fracture surface was very

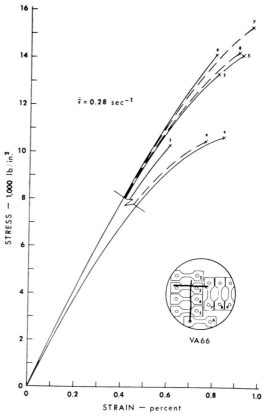

Figure 91. Tensile strain curves for perpendicular specimens, tested at the same strain rate, from a single plug of fresh cortical bone from adult human calvaria. (From Wood: *J Biomech,* 1971)

jagged, probably because of a tendency of the initial crack to follow regions of microscopic weakness such as cement lines and lamellae. At all strain rates used in the study, the fracture surface was similar and showed no correlation with more gross anatomical structures such as blood vessels. No significant differences were found among mechanical properties of specimens from different bones nor among specimens tested in different directions tangent to the skull.

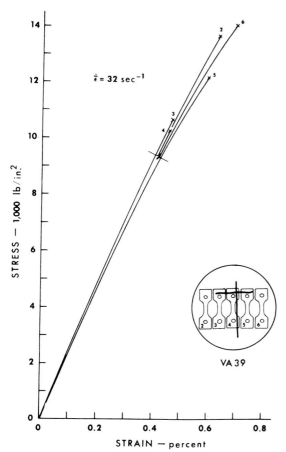

Figure 90. Tensile stress-strain curves for parallel specimens, tested at the same strain rate, from a single plug of fresh cortical bone from adult human calvaria. (From Wood: *J Biomech,* 1971)

Wood compared his tensile data with mechanical property data reported by others for cortical bone from long bones. Mc-Elhaney (1966) found that the compressive modulus of bovine and human femoral bone both increased in an approximately linear manner with the logarithm of strain rate for speeds between 0.001 sec⁻¹ and 100 sec⁻¹. The actual value for the compressive modulus of human femoral bone varied from 2.1×10^6 lbf/in² (1,476 kgf/mm²) at a low strain rate to 4.1×10^6 lbf/in² (2,882 kgf/mm²) at a high strain rate. Wood also found that the modulus of elasticity of his specimens increased linearly with respect to the logarithm of strain rate from about 1.5×10^6 lbf/in² (1,055 kgf/mm²) in the "static" test range to approximately 3.0×10^6 lbf/in² (2,109 kgf/mm²) at the highest strain rates. The average breaking stress

of his specimens varied from 9,000 lbf/in² (6.33 kgf/mm²) at low strain rates to about 14,000 lbf/in² (9.84 kgf/mm²) at high strain rates. Comparable values for average breaking strain (percentage elongation) were 76% and 54% at low and high strain rates, respectively.

From a simple linear regression analysis of his data Wood demonstrated that the modulus of elasticity and breaking stress of cortical bone from adult human calvaria increased but the breaking strain decreased with increasing strain rates of loading. Energy absorbed to failure was not rate sensitive.

The major difference found between mechanical properties of cortical bone from adult human calvariae and that from long bones is that the former is isotropic in all directions tangent to the skull, while, as demonstrated by many investigators, cortical bone from long bones is highly anisotropic. Wood points out that this variation may be the result of functional and structural differences in the two kinds of bone. Long bones, which are usually weight bearing, typically consist of well developed haversian bone whose osteons (haversian systems) exhibit rather definite orientation parallel to the long axis of the bone. In the calvaria, which is not weight bearing, the osteons are randomly oriented. As a consequence of this variation in osteon orientation, well defined split-line patterns parallel to the long axis of the bone can be obtained in long bones but only a very random split-line pattern can be demonstrated in the calvarium.

From his data (Fig. 92) Wood concluded that the modulus of elasticity of compact cranial bone is biaxially orthotropic. Because of the scarcity of material he was unable to determine all mechanical properties of specimens from each plug at all

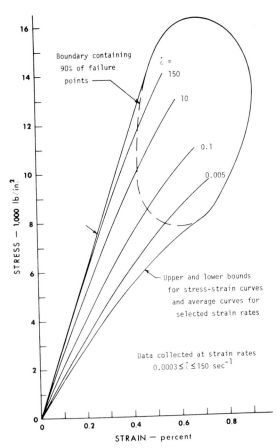

Figure 92. Summary of tensile properties of fresh cortical bone from adult human calvariae. (From Wood: *J Biomech,* 1971)

strain rates, but data were obtained from specimens tested at two or three different strain rates.

The low value Wood found for the tensile strength of the coronal suture, in comparison with that of the surrounding compact bone of adult calvariae, would lead one to conclude that the suture is a site of weakness where fractures or separations readily occur. However, such is not the case; fractures through the coronal suture rarely occur in intact skulls.

IMPACT LOADING

Long Bones

The energy absorbing capacity of notched and unnotched standardized impact specimens of beef cortical bone from femurs and tibias, cut in different directions and tested at various temperatures, was investigated by Bonfield and Li (1966). Energy of 5.1 in-lb was applied to the midpoint of the specimen by a modified Charpy impact tester. The surface of the specimen was estimated to have a strain rate of 60 sec^{-1} at the moment of impact.

The results of their study (Figs. 93 and 94) showed that the maximum energy was absorbed at zero degrees centigrade and decreased as the temperature was raised or lowered. At all temperatures the longitudinal specimens absorbed significantly more energy than the transverse specimens. For further details of this study see Chapter 6.

In order to investigate the relation between mode of failure and impacter particle velocity Bird et al. (1968) made impact tests on specimens of cortical bone from fresh beef femurs. A special impact test jig (Fig. 95), in which the specimen was placed in direct contact with a steel impacter the opposite end of which was struck with a cylindrical lead projectile, was developed for the tests. The amplitude of the impact transferred to the test specimen was controlled by changing the length of the steel impacter.

After impact the specimen passed between photoelectric gates whose generated impulses were imposed upon the oscilloscope. Once the bone specimen velocity was decided, the secant modulus of elasticity, as a function of loading rate, was determined from the gate spacing and the oscilloscopic trace. Bone specimen velocity was taken to be two times the effective stress wave particle velocity of the impacter, 2v. After the impact the specimen was caught in soft cotton waste so it could be used for photomicrographic examination.

The impact strain in each specimen was calculated from the formula,

$$\xi_s = V \ (e/E_t) \frac{1}{2}$$

where ξ_s is the specimen strain, V is the particle velocity of the impacter, e is the mass density, and E_t is the failure tangent modulus of elasticity obtained from the quasi-static stress-strain curve. The validity of the relation is dependent upon the small e/E_t of bone in comparison to that of the impacter.

Impact test results (Fig. 96) were classified as (a) survival, (b) microcracking, and (c) gross failure. Survival meant no observable evidence of cracks when the specimen was examined at 100× magnification. Microcracking was defined as the presence of continuous cracks varying from 1×10^{-3} to 1×10^{-2} inches in width when the specimen was examined at magnification of 50× and 100×. Gross failure was fracture of the specimen into two or more pieces. Many of the microcracks tended to follow the contours of osteons (haversian systems) which suggest the

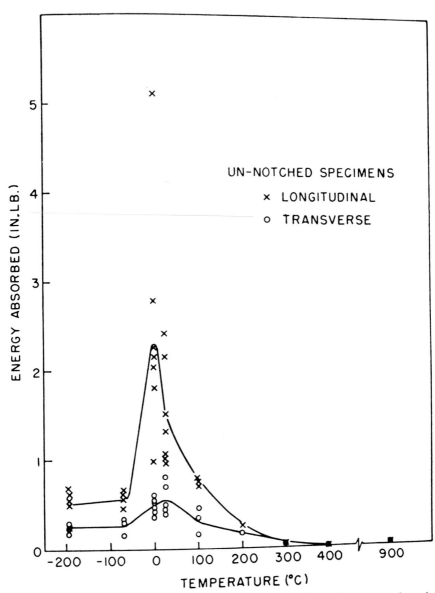

Figure 93. Energy absorbed during impact by longitudinally and transversely oriented unnotched specimens of beef cortical bone tested at different temperatures. (From Bonfield and Li: *J Appl Physics*, 1966)

presence of stress concentration factors greater than unity.

Data from the impact tests established an approximate relationship between the threshold for failure strain with impact loading and quasi-static failure strains at high strain rates of loading. Impact failure strain data show more scatter but do not fall below this threshold. The threshold for impact damage to bone was indicated by microcrack failure.

Tsuda, cited by Yamada (1970), determined the impact bending strength of unembalmed cortical bone from the femur of a 37-year-old Japanese man. Standardized specimens with a 2.5 mm-square cross section, a span-side ratio of 16:1, and expanded ends 3 mm long were tested with

a Charpy impact tester. The long axis of the specimen was parallel with that of the intact bone. An average impact bending strength of 0.14 ± 0.018 kg.cm/mm² was found for wet specimens and 0.12 ± 0.23 kg.cm/ mm² for air-dried ones.

The impact snapping strength of wet standardized specimens of femoral cortical bone from three adult Japanese subjects was determined by Takezono, Yasuda, and Maeda (cited by Yamada, 1970). Specimens 16 mm long with a square cross section 3 mm on each side were tested with an Izod impact tester. During a test the specimen was held with a drill chuck on an adjustable stand. Specimens were tested in the radial and in the tangenital direction with respect to the shaft of the bone.

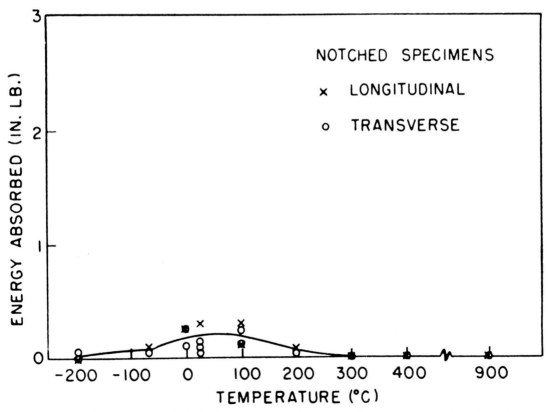

Figure 94. Energy absorbed during impact by longitudinally and transversely oriented notched specimens of beef cortical bone tested at different temperatures. (From Bonfield and Li: *J Appl Physics*, 1966)

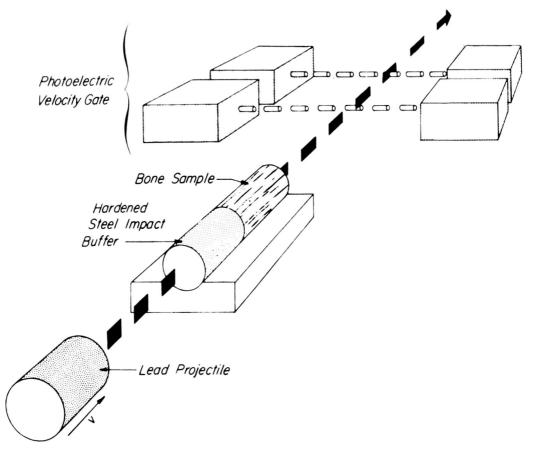

Figure 95. Schematic diagram of impact test jig for cortical bone. (From Bird, Becker, Healer, and Messer: *Aerosp Med,* 1968)

An average snapping strength of 0.26 ± 0.029 kg.cm/mm² in the radial direction and of 0.19 ± 0.021 kg.cm/mm² in the tangential direction was found. Specimens from the anterior and posterior aspects of the shaft had a much higher impact snapping strength than specimens from the lateral and medial aspects.

Skull Bones

Impact penetration tests on embalmed adult human calvariae and on 1.5 inch diameter bone plugs taken from embalmed and fresh (autopsy) skulls were made by Melvin et al. (1969b). The autopsy plugs were frozen within twelve hours and test-

ed within two weeks after death of the subject. Tests at speeds of zero mph (20-50 ipm) were made with the Instron and at speeds of 10 and 20 mph (16.09 and 32.18 kph, respectively) with the Plastechon testing machine already described. Load was measured with a Kistler 937A piezoelectric load cell and a 503 charge amplifier fed into an oscilloscope. Load-time curves were photographed with a Polaroid camera.

Impacts were applied to the calvaria via a penetrator which was screwed into a load cell mounted on the cross heads of the testing machine. The skull cap (calvaria) was put into a holder consisting of a circular mold over which the calvaria was placed, its cut edge being fixed with Castone. After the calvaria was in the holder on the ram of the testing machine it was fired upward into the penetrator at the speeds mentioned above. In order to have complete penetration at a constant velocity the cross head placement was adjusted according to ram travel. Test data were recorded as a load-time trace.

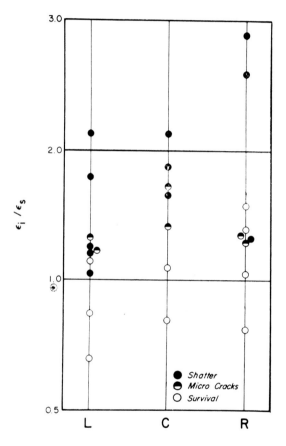

ϵ_s = Average Quasistatic Failure Strain
ϵ_i = Impact Failure Strain
ϵ_i = $V(\rho/E_t)^{\frac{1}{2}}$

Figure 96. Summary of experimental results of impact tests on fresh cortical bone from beef femurs. L= longitudinal specimens; C = circumferential specimens; R = radial specimens. (From Bird, Becker, Healer, and Messer: *Aerosp Med*, 1968)

The impacts were applied to the frontal and parietal regions of the calvaria. Great care was taken to ensure that the penetrator was perpendicular to the surface of the calvaria.

Three penetrators, essentially flat-ended cylinders, were used. Penetrator No. 1 was hollow with a ring-shaped end and a cross-sectional area of 0.147 in². Penetrators No. 2 and No. 3 were solid with flat ends and cross-sectional areas of 0.147 in² and 0.294 in², respectively.

The effects of fixation of the calvaria in the skull holder were evaluated by comparison of data obtained from a strain gauge mounted on the unrestrained calvaria near the point of application of a 600-lb force and data from a similar test on the same calvaria when fixed in the skull holder. Strain in the fixed calvaria was about 10% less than that in the unrestrained condition, but this was not considered to be a significant difference because the calvaria of the intact skull is fixed.

A special jig was developed to hold the bone plugs during a test because preliminary experiments revealed that unsupported plugs shattered at impact, whereas in whole calvariae penetration occurred without shattering or linear fractures. The jig provided edge conditions for the plug similar to those in whole calvariae so that data from fresh plugs could be compared with similar data from embalmed plugs or from embalmed whole calvariae. Penetration forces for embalmed plugs were found to be equivalent to those for whole embalmed calvariae.

The influence of the scalp on energy absorption or the force required for calvaria penetration was evaluated by covering the impact area with fresh pork shoulder 0.25 inch thick. A 10% difference was found between the force necessary for penetration with and without the presence of the pork. Therefore, the authors do not believe that the scalp significantly affects the magnitude of the force necessary for skull penetration.

Data obtained from tests on twenty calvariae (Figs. 97 and 98) indicated that the magnitude of the force required for penetration at different velocities is more or less independent of penetrator size. Furthermore, the penetration is quite localized. It was also pointed out that the thickness, curvature, and elasticity of the skull significantly affect the magnitude of the force necessary for penetration of the outer skull table (Fig. 99).

Linear fractures generally do not accompany calvaria penetration which usually occurs in the following five steps:

1. An initial load build-up as the entire skull structure is loaded by the penetrator.

2. A sudden penetration of the outer skull table with an abrupt drop in load with a primary tensile fracture approximating the circumference of the penetrator.

3. Compression of the diploë.

4. A cone-shaped region of shear failure of the diploë progressing to the inner skull table.

5. Fracture of the inner skull table occur-

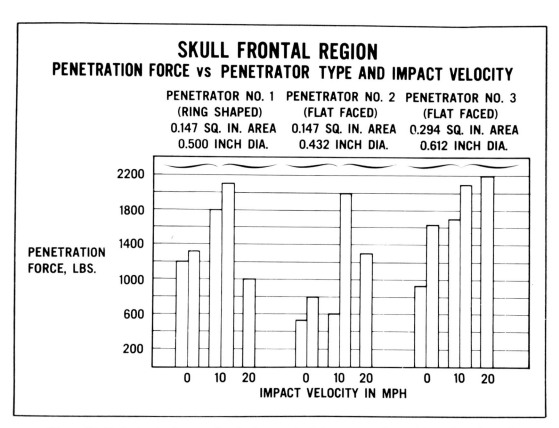

Figure 97. Variation in force and velocity required for penetration of frontal region of adult human calvariae. (From Melvin, Fuller, Daniel, and Pavliscak: Courtesy of Society of Automotive Engineers publication, 1969)

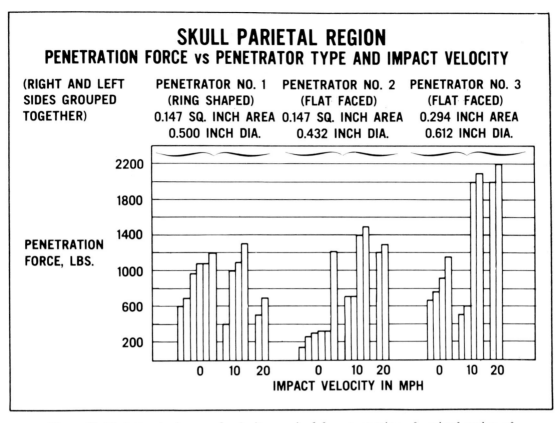

Figure 98. Variation in force and velocity required for penetration of parietal region of adult human calvaria. (From Melvin, Fuller, Daniel, and Pavliscak: Courtesy of Society of Automotive Engineers publication, 1969)

ring as a plug with a diameter larger than that of the penetrator. The internal surface geometry of the skull influences, to some extent, the shape of the plug.

In the authors' opinion their data do not accurately indicate tolerance levels for living bone. However, they believe their data provide a basis for preliminary determination of the approximate response values needed for development of the necessary instrumentation for research on skull penetration in relation to trauma.

SUMMARY

Stress-strain characteristics of cortical bone from adult human long bones are influenced by the duration as well as the magnitude of the load. Definite elastic aftereffects occur with prolonged loading.

Fresh cortical bone from beef tibias and metacarpals exhibits considerable, largely anelastic, strains that continue for at least fifty-four days with an extra deflection that may amount to 13% of the original deflection. The rate of anelastic deflection appears to be proportional to applied stress. A 300% increase in the rate of appearance of anelastic deflections oc-

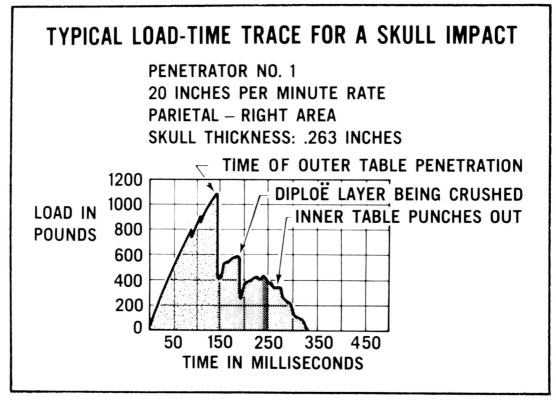

TYPICAL LOAD-TIME TRACE FOR A SKULL IMPACT

PENETRATOR NO. 1
20 INCHES PER MINUTE RATE
PARIETAL – RIGHT AREA
SKULL THICKNESS: .263 INCHES

TIME OF OUTER TABLE PENETRATION
DIPLOË LAYER BEING CRUSHED
INNER TABLE PUNCHES OUT

LOAD IN POUNDS

1200 1000 800 600 400 200 0

50 150 250 350 450

TIME IN MILLISECONDS

Figure 99. Load-time trace of impact penetration of adult human calvaria. (From Melvin, Fuller, Daniel, and Pavliscak: Courtesy of Society of Automotive Engineers publication, 1969)

curs at temperatures between 2° C and 50° C. Drying does not irreversibly affect the anelastic properties of bone.

Standardized specimens of wet unembalmed cortical bone from the femur (distal fourth only), tibia, and fibula from above-knee amputations of five adult men, tested at a stress of 5,000 lbf/in² (3.52 kgf/mm² or 344.7 × 10⁶ dynes/cm²) had an average flexure fatigue life of 1,982,650 repetitions or cycles to failure for the forty-seven tibial specimens, 1,188,453 cycles for the fifteen femoral specimens and 2,841,400 for the five fibular specimens. There is a difference in the histological structure of specimens with a long fatigue life (more than 4,000,000 cycles to failure) and those with a short fatigue life (less than 500,000 cycles to failure).

Data from similar flexure fatigue tests on 248 standardized specimens of cortical bone from femurs of seventeen embalmed adult human cadavers can be analyzed by the Weibull method and an S-N diagram obtained. The specimens had an endurance limit of about 4,000 lbf/in² (2.81 kgf/mm²) and an ultimate strength of more than 12,000 lbf/in² (8.44 kgf/mm²) at 50% failed.

Long duration cyclic loading of the tibia of living male rats about eighty days old provided no conclusive evidence of a change in mineral content or between bone weight and ashed weight ratios. Fractures were produced by loads varying between 0.6 lb (272.16 g) and a predetermined maximum. Smaller loads applied at a rate of 1,725 cycles/min and larger loads at a rate of 190 cycles/min revealed no sensitivity to cycling rate. The endurance limit occurred at about 4,000 cycles, approximately 42% of the static fracture load. Below this limit the rat tibias supported the load indefinitely.

Some mechanical properties of bone are rate-sensitive. The ultimate compressive stress and the modulus of elasticity of compact bone increase with increasing strain rates of loading, but the maximum strain at failure, the energy-absorbing capacity, and Poisson's ratio decrease.

The tensile properties of compact bone from fresh adult human skulls are also rate-sensitive although they exhibit no significant directional differences tangent to the skull. The average values at low (0.005 sec^{-1}) and high (150 sec^{-1}) strain rates vary from 9,000 lbf/in^2 (6.33 kgf/mm^2) to about 14,000 lbf/in^2 (9.84 kgf/mm^2), respectively, for the breaking stress; from 76 to 54% for the tensile strain; and from about 1.5 × 10^6 lbf/in^2 (1,055 kgf/mm^2) to about 3.0 × 10^6 lbf/in^2 (2,109 kgf/mm^2) for the modulus of elasticity. The breaking stress and the modulus increase, whereas the breaking strain decreases with increasing strain rates. However, the energy absorbed by fresh compact bone from adult human skulls is not rate-sensitive.

The average tensile strength of the coronal suture is 2,140 lbf/in^2 (1.50 kgf/mm^2). Two fresh compact bone specimens had an average Poisson's ratio of 0.43. The latter values were obtained for radial contraction with respect to the intact head.

Fresh cortical bone from beef femurs, tested at a low strain rate (1 × 10^2 lbf/in^2/sec) has marked directional differences in its mechanical properties. The greatest compressive stress and modulus but lowest compressive strain are found in the longitudinal direction, while the lowest compressive stress but highest strain occur in the radial direction. Mechanical property values in the circumferential direction are intermediate in value but more uniform than those in the longitudinal or radial direction. Comparable specimens tested at high strain rates of loading (5 × 10^5 lbf/in^2/sec) have similar mechanical property characteristics, but the magnitudes of failure stress and strain and of elastic and secant moduli are significantly higher.

Human diploë has an average compressive stress, perpendicular to the skull surface, of 1,820 lbf/in^2 (1.28 kgf/mm^2) and an average compressive modulus of 0.57 × 10^5 lbf/in^2 (40.07 kgf/mm^2), both of which are much less than similar properties of compact bone.

Fresh diploë of adult human skulls has an average tensile strength of 4,940 lbf/in^2 (3.47 kgf/mm^2), a breaking strain of 73%, and a modulus of elasticity of 8.9 × 10^5 lbf/in^2 (625.67 kgf/mm^2).

The shear strength of fresh human diploë is also rate-sensitive with values of 3,272 lbf/in^2 (2.30 kgf/mm^2) at a shear rate of 6.66 sec^{-1} and of 4,386 lbf/in^2 (3.08 kgf/mm^2) at a strain rate of 66.6 sec^{-1}.

The energy absorbing capacity of beef cortical bone, tested by impact loading, is greatest at 0° C and decreases as the temperature is raised or lowered. Longitudinal specimens at all temperatures absorbed significantly more energy than transverse specimens. Bone is sensitive to notch effects. Data for failure strain in impact tests show reasonably good agreement with those from quasi-static tests at high strain rates of loading although the impact strain data are more scattered.

The impact bending strength of unembalmed femoral bone of human adults is 0.14 ± 0.018 kg.cm/mm² for wet bone and 0.12 ± 0.023 kg.cm/mm² for dry bone. The impact snapping strength for wet femoral cortical bone is 0.26 ± 0.029 kg.cm/mm² in the radial direction and 0.19 ± 0.021 kg.cm/mm² in the tangential direction with respect to the long axis of the bone.

Load required for penetration of the adult human calvaria at different velocities is independent of penetrator size and the penetration is quite localized.

CHAPTER 9

TOPOGRAPHIC DIFFERENCES

CORTICAL (COMPACT) BONE

THE MECHANICAL PROPERTIES of bone are affected not only by nonbiological variables such as those previously discussed but also by the anatomical site or location from which the test specimens were obtained. Thus, values for mechanical properties of bone vary from one bone to another as well as within different regions of the same bone. Unless otherwise stated these values were obtained under static loading in the direction of the long axis of the bone at normal room temperature and humidity.

Topographic Variation Among Bones

The classic and most thorough study ever made on the strength and elasticity of human bone is that of Messerer (1880) who determined these mechanical properties for five hundred bones or bone combinations from ninety cadavers. All bones were tested in the completely fresh condition shortly after removal from the body. During the interval between removal and testing, the bones—which still had their periosteum—were wrapped in wet cloths or pieces of meat to keep them moist. All tests were made at room temperature (20° to 25° C).

Only intact bones were tested and usually just the breaking load (kg) was recorded. Consequently, most of the results of Messerer's excellent study are beyond the scope of this book which is concerned with bone as a material rather than as a structural member. However, the few cases in which the strength (kg/cm²) of the bones is given will be included in the present discussion.

Tensile Properties

UNEMBALMED HUMAN LONG BONE

Strength (Table XXXVIII). All investigators who have studied the tensile strength of standardized specimens of bone have reported that its average value varied with the bone from which the specimens were obtained. Wertheim (1847) found that the average tensile strength of fresh fibular bone of adult men was greater than that of femoral bone; however, only two specimens from each bone were tested. Rauber (1876), who determined the tensile strength of fresh humeral, femoral, and tibial specimens, reported that the tibial specimens were the strongest and the femoral ones the weakest. Hülsen (1896) also noted that fresh femoral specimens were stronger than humeral ones, although the difference was not great.

The most extensive study of tensile strength of standardized fresh specimens of cortical bone from the major long bones was made by Ko, cited by Yamada (1970), who determined it for specimens from the femur of thirty-six people—the leg bones of five people, the humerus of fourteen people, and the forearm bones of five people. He demonstrated that in people 20 to 30 years of age, radial bone had the highest average tensile strength followed, in descending order of strength, by ulnar, fibular, tibial, humeral, and femoral bone.

TABLE XXXVIII

Variation Among Bones in Average Tensile and Compressive Strength, in the Longitudinal Direction, of Wet Unembalmed Standardized Specimens of Adult Human Cortical Bone

	Author	No. of Spec.	Humerus	No. of Spec.	Radius	No. of Spec.	Ulna	No. of Spec.	Femur	No. of Spec.	Tibia	No. of Spec.	Fibula	Unit of Measurement
Tensile Strength	Wertheim (1847)								7.77 / 11,049			4	8.23 / 11,703	kgf/mm^2 / lbf/in^2
	Rauber (1876)	11	10.24					8	9.74 / 13,850	19	12.4 / 17,633			kgf/mm^2 / lbf/in^2
	Hülsen (1896)	4	10.55 / 15,002								10.58 / 15,045			kgf/mm^2 / lbf/in^2
	Yamada (1970)	15-20	12.5 ± 0.08 / 17,775 ± 114	15-20	15.2 ± 0.14 / 21,614 ± 199	15-20	15.1 ± 0.15 / 21,472 ± 213	15-20	12.4 ± 0.11 / 17,633 ± 156	15-20	14.3 ± 0.12 / 20,335 ± 171	15-20	14.9 ± 0.15 / 21,188 ± 213	kgf/mm^2 / lbf/in^2
	Evans*	73	9.71 / 13,813					209	6.51 / 9,262	23	9.02 / 12,824	23	10.21 / 14,522	kgf/mm^2 / lbf/in^2
Compressive Strength	Rauber (1876)	13	13.93 / 19,808					7	14.36 / 20,420		16.79 / 23,875			kgf/mm^2 / lbf/in^2
	Hülsen (1896)	2	20.42 / 29,037								20.92 / 29,748			kgf/mm^2 / lbf/in^2
	Calabrisi & Smith (1951)							2	21.2 / 30,146		15.54 / 22,098			kgf/mm^2 / lbf/in^2
	Yamada (1970)	15-20	13.5 / 19,197			15-20	12.0 / 17,064	15-20	17.0 / 24,174	15-20	16.2 / 23,036	15-20	12.5 / 17,775	kgf/mm^2 / lbf/in^2
	Evans*							77	8.63 / 12,269		11.22 / 15,956	9	13.01 / 18,500	kgf/mm^2 / lbf/in^2

* Previously unpublished material.

Studies made in this laboratory on differences in the tensile strength of wet unembalmed standardized specimens from the major long bones of the lower limb showed that the fibular ones were the strongest and the femoral ones the weakest. An analysis of variance revealed that the mean tensile strength of the fibular and tibial specimens were both significantly greater, at better than the 0.01 level, than that of the femoral ones. The strength of the fibular specimens was also significantly greater, at the 0.05 to 0.01 level, than that of the tibial specimens.

Because our material was obtained from above-knee amputations, only the distal fourth or so of the femur was available for specimens. This may account for their low tensile strength in comparison with values reported by others, because, as will be shown later, the distal third of the femur is weaker than the middle third, the region of the bone from which other investigators took their specimens.

Strain (Table XXXIX). Japanese investigators, cited by Yamada (1970), have also demonstrated that tensile strain varied in fresh specimens from different bones of people 20 to 39 years of age. Fibular bone had the highest tensile strain followed, in descending order, by radial and tibial bone (same value), ulnar, humeral, and femoral bone.

Tensile strain data obtained in this laboratory from wet unembalmed cortical specimens from the major long bones of the lower limb showed that it was highest in fibular and lowest in femoral specimens. However, an analysis of variance revealed that the mean strain for specimens from the three bones was not significantly different.

Modulus of Elasticity (Table XL). The modulus of elasticity of fresh cortical human bone was first determined by Wertheim (1847) who reported that fibular bone had a higher modulus of elasticity than femoral bone (Table XL). Rauber (1876) and Hülsen (1896) also found that fresh tibial bone was stiffer than femoral bone. However, only a few specimens from each bone were tested by these investigators. Yamada (1970) cited some work by Ko which showed that the tensile modulus of elasticity was greatest in radial and fibular bone (same value), followed in descending order by ulnar, tibial, femoral, and humeral bone.

TABLE XXXIX

AVERAGE STRAIN, IN THE LONGITUDINAL DIRECTION, OF
STANDARDIZED SPECIMENS OF WET, UNEMBALMED
ADULT HUMAN CORTICAL BONE

Bone	Tensile Strain (% Elongation) Yamada (1970)	Evans*	Compressive Strain (% Contraction) Yamada (1970)	Evans*
Humerus	1.45		1.90	
Radius	1.50		2.00	
Ulna	1.49		2.00	
Femur	1.41	1.47	1.80	0.61
Tibia	1.50	1.70	1.90	1.53
Fibula	1.59	1.79	2.10	1.25

* Previously unpublished material.

Topographic differences have also been found in this laboratory for the modulus of elasticity of standard specimens from wet unembalmed cortical bone from the major long bones of the lower extremity. Tibial specimens were the stiffest while femoral ones were most flexible. An analysis of variance showed that the modulus of both the tibial and the fibular specimens was significantly greater, at the 0.01 or better significance level, than that of the femoral specimens. The difference between the modulus of the tibial and fibular specimens was not significant.

HUMAN SKULL BONE

The first study on the strength of cortical bone from adult human skulls appears

TABLE XL

MODULUS OF ELASTICITY OF WET UNEMBALMED STANDARD SPECIMENS OF ADULT HUMAN CORTICAL BONE IN
LONGITUDINAL TENSION

Bone	Wertheim (1847)		Hülsen (1896)		Yamada (1970)		Evans*	
	kgf/mm^2	lbf/in^2	kgf/mm^2	lbf/in^2	kgf/mm^2	lbf/in^2	kgf/mm^2	lbf/in^2
Humerus					1,750	2.49×10^6		
Radius					1,890	2.69×10^6		
Ulna					1,880	2.67×10^6		
Femur	2,264	3.2×10^6	1,735	2.47×10^6	1,760	2.50×10^6	1,195	1.70×10^6
Tibia			1,762	2.51×10^6	1,840	2.62×10^6	1,701	2.42×10^6
Fibula	2,384	3.4×10^6			1,890	2.69×10^6	1,540	2.19×10^6

* Previously unpublished material.

to be that of Evans and Lissner (1957) who reported that fifteen specimens of parietal bone (Fig. 13) from embalmed cadavers had an average tensile strength, in the direction of the long axis of the specimen, of 10,230 lbf/in² (7.19 kgf/mm²) with a range of variation from 6,030 to 15,800 lbf/in² (4.24 to 11.11 kgf/mm²). These values are within the range of variation for tensile strength of cortical specimens from human long bones (Tables XXXVIII and XLI).

Recently the tensile properties of 120 fresh standardized specimens from the frontal, parietal, and temporal bones of thirty adult human subjects were determined by Wood (1971). The specimens were loaded in a direction tangential to the skull surface at strain rates varying from 0.005 to 150 sec⁻¹. Breaking stress and modulus of elasticity increased but breaking strain decreased with increasing

strain rates of loading. Energy absorbed to failure was not rate sensitive.

Wood found no important variation in the tensile properties of his specimens when analyzed with respect to bone, body side, or subject age. In contrast to long bones, his specimens were transversely isotropic. At a strain rate of 0.01 sec⁻¹ Wood reported an average tensile strength of 10,000 lbf/in² (7.03 kgf/mm²) almost the same value found by Evans and Lissner (1957). The average tensile strength of Wood's specimens varied approximately from 10,000 to 14,000 lbf/in² (7.03 to 9.84 kgf/mm²), the modulus of elasticity from 1.8 to 2.9 × 10⁶ lbf/in² (1,265 to 2,039 kgf/mm²), and failure strain from 0.7% to 0.55%. The average energy absorbed to failure was 42.6 in-lb/in³ (2.99 kg-cm/cm³), most of the data varying from 20 to 80 in-lb/in³ (1.41 to 5.62 kg-cm/cm³).

TABLE XLI

MEAN VALUES FOR TENSILE PROPERTIES, IN THE LONGITUDINAL DIRECTION, OF WET CORTICAL BONE FROM EMBALMED
ADULT HUMAN FEMURS, TIBIAS, AND FIBULAS

Mechanical Property	No.	Femur	No.	Tibia	No.	Fibula	Unit of Measurement
Tensile strength	405	$11,358 \pm 2,856$	193	$13,438 \pm 2,931$	32	$13,425 \pm 2,751$	lbf/in²
		7.98 ± 2.01		9.45 ± 2.06		9.44 ± 1.93	kgf/mm²
Tensile strain	366	1.46 ± 0.66	175	1.77 ± 0.78	30	1.71 ± 1.28	% elongation
Modulus of elasticity	383	$2,100 \pm 0.499$	188	2.303 ± 0.491	30	2.529 ± 0.441	$\times 10^6$ lbf/in²
		$1,476 \pm 351$		$1,619 \pm 345$		$1,778 \pm 310$	kgf/mm²

Wood demonstrated that fresh cortical bone from adult human calvaria was transversely isotropic. There were no significant differences in breaking stress, strain, or energy absorbed to failure according to subject age, body side, or bone type. Modulus of elasticity decreased with age but exhibited no significant relations with body side or bone type. Some of the variation in mechanical properties could not be explained on the basis of strain rate differences. Diploe had a low tensile strength but the mechanical properties of the cortical bone were intermediate between those of specimens from long bones when tested in the longitudinal and the transverse directions.

Wet Embalmed Human Long Bone (Table XLI)

Differences in the tensile properties of standardized specimens of wet cortical bone from adult embalmed human femurs, tibias, and fibulas have been studied in this laboratory. Embalmed material was used because intact unembalmed femurs, tibias, and fibulas were not available.

It was found that tibial specimens had the highest and femoral specimens the lowest mean tensile strength and strain (Table XLI). Fibular bone exhibited the highest and femoral bone the lowest modulus of elasticity.

An analysis of variance revealed that the greater tensile strength, strain, and modulus of elasticity of the tibial specimens as compared to the femoral ones were significant at better than the 0.01 level. The tensile strength and modulus of elasticity of the fibular specimens were likewise greater, at better than the 0.01 signicance level, than the same properties of the femoral specimens. Fibular specimens also had a modulus of elasticity that was greater, at the 0.05 to 0.01 significance level, than that of tibial specimens.

The average ultimate tensile strength in the longitudinal direction of seventy-three humeral specimens was 13,813 lbf/in² (9.71 kgf/mm²) which is higher than that of similarly tested femoral, tibial and fibular specimens (*cf.* Table XLI). This agrees with the reports of Japanese investigators that upper extremity bone specimens have a higher tensile strength than similar specimens from lower extremity bones.

Forty-three humeral specimens had an average longitudinal tensile strain of 61% and forty-nine specimens an average tensile modulus of 2.79×10^6 lbf/in² (1,961 kgf/mm²). The tensile strain was less than that of specimens from any of the three major bones of the lower limb but the modulus was greater (*cf.* Table XLI).

Density (Table XLII). Although density is not a mechanical property, in the strict sense, it is an important variable to be considered. The behavior of any body subjected to a load or force is a function of the amount of material in the body as well as its mechanical properties, size, and distribution. Thus, a more dense body will behave differently under a given load than will a less dense body even though the external dimensions of the two bodies may be the same.

For the above reason, we determined the density of our specimens from embalmed femurs, tibias, and fibulas. All the specimens were dried before their density was determined in order to avoid any effects of moisture trapped within the spaces in the specimens. A special apparatus and technique was developed for the density determinations (see Chapter 2 for details).

Density was greatest in the tibial speci-

TABLE XLII

DENSITY (G/CM³) OF DRY ADULT HUMAN CORTICAL BONE

| | | Differences Among Bones | | McElhaney, Alem |
Bone	No.	Evans	No.	& Roberts (1970)
Femur	127	1.88 ± 0.08	160	1.85 ± 0.75
Tibia	115	1.91 ± 0.10		
Fibula	18	1.82 ± 0.14		
Cranial full section			240	1.41 ± 0.53
Cranial alone			27	1.88 ± 0.19
Vertebral body			288	0.47 ± 0.19

| | | Differences Within Bones | | | |
Region	No.	Femur	No.	Tibia	No.	Fibula
Proximal third	39	1.86 ± 0.07	37	1.86 ± 0.12	5	1.82 ± 0.10
Middle third	48	1.89 ± 0.09	39	1.94 ± 0.09	7	1.81 ± 0.15
Distal third	40	1.88 ± 0.07	39	1.92 ± 0.08	6	1.83 ± 0.19
Anterior quadrant	32	1.85 ± 0.08	30	1.85 ± 0.12		
Lateral quadrant	34	1.87 ± 0.07	29	1.93 ± 0.08		
Medial quadrant	31	1.88 ± 0.09	27	1.92 ± 0.07		
Posterior quadrant	30	1.90 ± 0.09	29	1.92 ± 0.12		

mens, next in the femoral ones, and lowest in the fibular specimens (Table XLII). A statistical analysis of the data showed that the density of the tibial specimens was greater, at the 0.01 or better significance level, than that of the femoral or fibular specimens. The density of the fibular specimens was significantly greater, at between the 0.05 and the 0.01 level, than the density of the femoral specimens. The significantly greater density of the tibial specimens may partially explain their significantly higher tensile strength, strain, and modulus of elasticity when compared with the femoral ones. A similar explanation may account for the significantly greater tensile strength and modulus of elasticity of the fibular specimens as compared with the femoral specimens.

Coefficients of correlation between density and each of the mechanical properties were also calculated. Among the femoral specimens a positive correlation, at the 0.01 or better significance level, was found between density and Rockwell superficial hardness. No other significant correlations were found but density data were only available for seventeen specimens.

Among more than seventy tibial specimens, positive correlations—at the 0.001 significance level—were found between density and tensile modulus of elasticity, between density and ultimate tensile strength, and between density and Rockwell hardness. A positive correlation, at the 0.05 significance level, was found between density and single (punching) shear strength.

Positive correlations at the 0.001 significance level were found, in more than twenty fibular specimens, between density and single shear strength and density and Rockwell hardness. Tensile strain (% elongation) and density had a negative correlation at the 0.001 significance level.

McElhaney et al. (1970a) determined the density of 160 femoral specimens, twenty-seven specimens of cortical cranial bone alone, 240 full sections of cranial bone, and 288 vertebral bodies. The full section cranial specimens were composed of the outer and inner tables of cortical bone separated by diploë. Their femoral specimens were slightly less dense than ours but cranial bone alone was a little more dense than femoral bone (Table XLII).

TABLE XLIII

AVERAGE VALUES FOR STRENGTH, IN THE LONGITUDINAL DIRECTION, OF FRESH NONHUMAN CORTICAL BONE (Data from Yamada, 1970)

	Humerus		*Radius*		*Femur*		*Tibia*	
	kgf/mm^2	lbf/in^2	kgf/mm^2	lbf/in^2	kgf/mm^2	lbf/in^2	kgf/mm^2	lbf/in^2
Tensile Strength								
Horse	10.2 ± 0.13	14,504 ± 185	12.0	17,064	12.1 ± 0.18	17,206 ± 256	11.3	16,069
Cattle	10.1 ± 0.07	14,362 ± 100	13.5 ± 0.16	19,197 ± 228	11.3 ± 0.21	16,069 ± 299	13.2 ± 0.28	18,770 ± 398
Wild boar	10.2 ± 0.56	14,504 ± 796	12.1 ± 0.71	17,206 ± 1,010	10.0 ± 0.21	14,220 ± 229	11.8 ± 0.53	16,780 ± 754
Pig	8.8 ± 0.73	12,514 ± 1,038	10.0 ± 0.34	14,220 ± 483	8.8 ± 0.15	12,514 ± 213	10.8 ± 0.39	15,358 ± 555
Deer	10.5 ± 0.42	14,931 ± 597	12.5 ± 0.36	17,775 ± 512	10.3 ± 0.30	14,647 ± 427	12.0 ± 0.30	17,064 ± 427
Ostrich					7.1 ± 0.26	10,096 ± 370		
Compressive Strength								
Horse	15.4	21,899	15.6	22,183	14.5 ± 0.16	20,619 ± 228	14.5	20,619
Cattle	14.4 ± 0.13	20,477 ± 185	15.2 ± 0.15	21,614 ± 213	14.7 ± 0.11	20,903 ± 156	15.9 ± 0.14	22,610 ± 199
Wild boar	11.0 ± 0.15	15,642 ± 213	12.3 ± 0.16	17,491 ± 228	11.8 ± 0.11	16,780 ± 156	13.3 ± 0.22	18,913 ± 313
Pig	10.2 ± 0.16	14,504 ± 228	10.7 ± 0.12	15,215 ± 164	10.0 ± 0.07	14,220 ± 100	10.6 ± 0.20	15,073 ± 284
Deer	13.6 ± 0.13	19,339 ± 185	13.5 ± 0.22	19,197 ± 313	13.3 ± 0.15	18,913 ± 213	14.1 ± 0.20	20,050 ± 284
Ostrich					12.0 ± 0.28	17,064 ± 398		

TABLE XLIV

STRAIN, IN THE LONGITUDINAL DIRECTION, IN FRESH NONHUMAN CORTICAL BONE (Data from Yamada, 1970)

	Humerus	Radius	Femur	Tibia
	Tensile Strain (% Elongation)			
Horses	0.65 ± 0.005	0.71	0.75 ± 0.008	0.70
Cattle	0.76 ± 0.006	0.79 ± 0.009	0.88 ± 0.020	0.78 ± 0.008
Wild boar	0.77 ± 0.029	0.78 ± 0.053	0.79 ± 0.017	0.86 ± 0.033
Pig	0.70 ± 0.033	0.73 ± 0.032	0.68 ± 0.010	0.76 ± 0.028
Deer	0.72 ± 0.026	0.81 ± 0.022	0.76 ± 0.016	0.78 ± 0.016
Ostrich			0.65 ± 0.017	
	Compressive Strain (% Contraction)			
Horses	2.0 ± 0.03	2.3	2.4	2.2
Cattle	1.8 ± 0.02	1.8 ± 0.02	1.7 ± 0.02	1.8 ± 0.02
Wild boar	1.8 ± 0.02	1.8 ± 0.02	1.8 ± 0.02	1.8 ± 0.02
Pig	1.9 ± 0.02	1.9 ± 0.02	1.9 ± 0.02	1.9 ± 0.02
Deer	1.7 ± 0.02	1.7 ± 0.02	1.8 ± 0.03	1.6 ± 0.03
Ostrich			2.1 ± 0.02	

Full section cranial bone was considerably less dense than femoral, tibial, or fibular cortical bone. The density of the vertebral bodies will be discussed with cancellous bone.

FRESH NONHUMAN LONG BONE

Tensile Strength (Table XLIII). Hülsen (1896) was one of the first to report that nonhuman cortical bone also exhibits topographic differences in its tensile strength in the longitudinal direction. He found that four wet specimens from an ox tibia

had an average tensile strength of 11.80 kgf/mm^2 (16,780 lbf/in^2) compared to an average strength of 10.64 kgf/mm^2 (15,130 lbf/in^2) for four similar specimens of femoral bone.

A similar but more extensive study of tensile properties of standard specimens of cortical bone from the major long bones of different animals was made by Japanese investigators (cited by Yamada, 1970). They demonstrated (Table XLIII) that in each species except the horse, in which femoral bone was stronger than tib-

TABLE XLV

MODULUS OF ELASTICITY OF FRESH NONHUMAN CORTICAL BONE (Data from Yamada, 1970)

	Humerus		Radius		Femur		Tibia	
	kgf/mm^2	× 10^6 lbf/in^2	kgf/mm^2	× 10^6 lbf/in^2	kgf/mm^2	× 10^6 lbf/in^2	kgf/mm^2	× 10^6 lbf/in^2
	In Tension							
Horses	1,780	2.53	2,280	3.24	2,550	3.63	2,380	3.38
Cattle	1,830	2.60	2,590	3.68	2,500	3.56	2,450	3.48
Wild boar	1,570	2.23	1,550	2.20	1,500	2.13	1,480	2.10
Pig	1,460	2.08	1,580	2.25	1,490	2.12	1,720	2.45
Deer	1,850	2.63	1,900	2.70	1,750	2.49	1,800	2.56
Ostrich					1,390	1.98		
	In Compression							
Horses	900	1.28	840	1.19	940 ± 47	1.34 ± 0.07	850	1.21
Cattle					870	1.24		
Wild boar	900	1.28	630	0.90	600	0.85	670	0.95
Pig	500	0.71	530	0.75	490	0.70	510	0.73
Deer	750	1.07	780	1.11	720	1.02	800	1.14
Ostrich					540	0.77		

ial bone, the tensile strength of specimens from the distal bones (radius and tibia) was greater than that of specimens from the proximal bones (humerus and femur). However, no consistent trends were evident when specimens from each species were arranged in order from strongest to weakest.

Tensile Strain (Table XLIV). According to data given by Yamada (1970) tensile strain of fresh nonhuman cortical bone varied with the bone from which the specimen was taken. In the foreleg of all species studied, radial bone had a greater strain than humeral bone (Table XLIV) but such uniformity between proximal and distal bones was not evident in the hind legs of the same species. In horses and cattle, femoral bone had a higher strain than tibial bone, but the reverse condition occurred in wild boars, pigs and deer.

Modulus of Elasticity (Table XLV). Topographic differences also occur in the tensile modulus of elasticity of fresh nonhuman cortical bone (Yamada, 1970). In the forelimbs radial bone had a higher modulus of elasticity than humeral bone in horses, cattle, pigs, and deer but the reverse situation was found in wild boars (Table XLV). In the hind limbs femoral bone was stiffer than tibial bone in horses, cattle, and wild boars but the opposite condition prevailed in pigs and deer.

Compressive Properties

Unembalmed Human Long Bone

Strength (Table XXXVIII). Topographic differences are likewise found for the compressive properties of adult human unembalmed cortical bone. Rauber (1876) who compared the compressive strength of human femoral, tibial and humeral bone, reported that it was greatest in tibial and least in humeral bone. Hülsen (1896), too, found that tibial bone had a higher com-

pressive strength than humeral bone although the differences were slight. However, only two humeral and four tibial specimens were tested. In contrast to these results, Calabrisi and Smith (1951) reported that two femoral specimens had a greater average compressive strength than two tibial specimens.

A more extensive investigation of the compressive strength of material from all the major long bones was made by Yokoo (1952b), who determined it for specimens from the humerus and femur of twenty-six people and the forearm and leg bones of seven people. He found that femoral bone had the greatest average strength, followed in descending order by tibial, humeral, fibular, ulnar, and radial bone.

The relative compressive strength—arranged in decreasing order of magnitude—of our wet, unembalmed specimens was fibula, tibia, and femur. The low value for compressive strength of our femoral specimens is probably due to the fact that all of them were obtained from above-knee amputations so that only the distal fourth or less of the bone was available. As will be shown later this is the weakest area of the bone and also the part where the cortex is quite thin, so that it was difficult to obtain many suitable test specimens. Most of the other investigators obtained their specimens from the middle of the shaft, the strongest region.

It is interesting to note that Yamada reported that femoral and tibial bone, representing the major weight supporting bones of the lower limb, both have a greater compressive strength than fibular bone or that from any of the major long bones of the upper limb. This relationship is in contrast to the tensile strength of these bones, which is less in specimens from lower limb bones than in those from upper limb bones. These differences may be related to the fact that the upper limb bones are primarily tension members while those of the lower limb are compression members.

Comparison of the data according to the relative size of the bone from which the specimens were obtained, revealed some interesting relations. Specimens from larger bones had a greater compressive strength than ones from smaller bones. The reverse was found for compressive strain, specimens from smaller bones having a higher strain than those from larger bones.

Strain (Table XXXIX). According to data given by Yamada (1970), the compressive strain of fresh cortical bone from people 20 to 39 years of age is greatest in fibular bone, followed, in decreasing order of magnitude, by radial and ulnar bone (the same value), humeral and tibial bone (the same value), and femoral bone.

We found for wet unembalmed specimens that compressive strain was greatest in tibial bone (seventy-five specimens), next in fibular bone (nine specimens), and least in femoral bone (seven specimens).

The low value for compressive strain of our specimens may be a function of their shape ($3 \times 0.190 \times 0.70$ inches) and the special compression jig (Fig. 11) which reduced buckling or decrease in height of the specimen during a test. The data reported by Yamada was obtained from round bars, 2, 3 or 4 mm in diameter with a length-diameter ratio of 2:1. Thus, in his specimens there was probably a greater tendency for the upper part of the specimen to become impacted into the lower part, resulting in higher strain values than in our specimens.

The compressive stress (strength) and strain data were all determined in the direction of the long axis of the specimen which coincided with that of the intact bone. It is interesting to note that strain (both tensile and compressive) is greater in specimens from smaller bones than in those from larger bones. The reverse situation is true for tensile and compressive strength.

No definite conclusions can be drawn on compressive strain in our femoral and fibular specimens because only a few of them were tested.

Modulus of Elasticity. Although the modulus of elasticity for a given specimen of bone is the same in tension and compression, variations occur in the value for the compressive modulus of elasticity of specimens from different bones. Thus, we found that the modulus of elasticity of wet unembalmed specimens of cortical bone tested in compression, was 2.69×10^6 lbf/in² (1,891 kgf/mm²) for seventy-seven tibial and nine fibular specimens, compared to a modulus of 2.15×10^6 lbf/in² (1,511 kgf/mm²) for seven femoral specimens from the distal fourth of the bone. Specimens from smaller bones had a higher modulus than those from larger bones. The data from femoral and fibular specimens were too scanty for valid conclusions to be drawn from them.

EMBALMED HUMAN BONE (Table XLVI)

Strength and Modulus of Elasticity. Topographic differences occur in the mechanical properties of embalmed adult human cortical bone. Carothers et al. (1949) reported that tibial bone had a greater compressive strength and modulus of elasticity than femoral bone. However, only a few specimens were tested.

A much more extensive study of the compressive properties of moist specimens of cortical bone was made by McElhaney et al. (1970a) who determined the compressive strength, modulus of elasticity, and Poisson's ratio of 160 femoral specimens (tested in the long axis) from thirty-two individuals, of twenty-seven cranial cortical bone specimens from seven individuals, of 237 full section cranial bone specimens (tested in the radial direction) from twenty-six individuals, and of 210 similar specimens (tested in the tangential direction) from fourteen individuals. The full section cranial specimens consisted of the outer and inner tables of cortical bone separated by the cancellous diploë. The full section cranial specimens tested in the radial direction were loaded perpendicular to the skull surface while the others were tested in a direction tangential to the skull surface. The femoral specimens were obtained from embalmed cadavers while the skull material was obtained from embalmed bodies, craniotomies, and autopsies.

McElhaney et al. found that cranial cor-

tical bone alone had the highest mean compressive strength, full section cranial bone tested in the tangential direction was second, full section cranial bone tested in the radial direction was third, but femoral bone was first (Table XLVI). Full section cranial bone tested in the tangential direction had the highest modulus of elasticity, followed, in descending order, by full section cranial specimens tested in the radial direction, femoral, and cranial bone alone. This variation in stiffness is evident from stress-strain curves for the four types of specimens (Fig. 100). The mean compressive strength of their femoral specimens was greater but their modulus of elasticity less than the values reported by Carothers et al. (1949) for their femoral specimens.

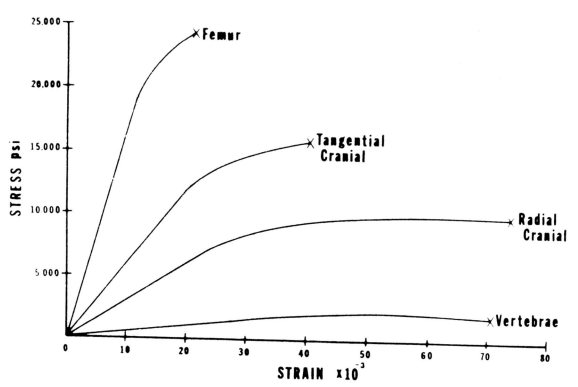

Figure 100. Stress-strain curves for human bone in compression. Tangential and radial refer to the direction, with respect to the intact skull, in which the specimens were loaded. (From McElhaney, Alem, and Roberts: Courtesy of Amer Soc Mech Eng publication, 1970)

TABLE XLVI

COMPRESSIVE PROPERTIES OF MOIST EMBALMED ADULT HUMAN CORTICAL BONE

| Author | Bone | Strength | | | | Modulus of Elasticity | | | Poisson's Ratio |
		No.	lbf/in²	kgf/mm²	No.	lbf/in²	kgf/mm²	No.	
Carothers, Smith & Calabrisi, 1949	Femur	8	25,350	17.82	7	2.55×10^6	1,793		
	Tibia	5	26,300	18.49	7	2.82×10^6	1,982		
McElhaney, Alem & Roberts, 1970	Femur (long axis)	160	26,000 ± 6,100	18.28 ± 4.29	160	$1.84 \pm 0.4 \times 10^6$	1,294 ± 28.12	7	0.3 ± 0.06
	Cranial cortical	27	20,900 ± 6,800	14.69 ± 4.78	27	$1.81 \pm 0.6 \times 10^6$	1,272 ± 42.18	7	0.28 ± 0.04
	Cranial full section								
	a. radial	237	10,700 ± 5,100	7.52 ± 3.59	237	$3.5 \pm 2.1 \times 10^5$	246 ± 147.6	14	0.19 ± 0.08
	b. tangential	210	14,000 ± 5,200	9.84 ± 3.66	219	$8.1 \pm 4.4 \times 10^5$	569 ± 309.3	18	0.22 ± 0.11
Evans*	Femur	23	17,025	11.97	23	2.24×10^6	1,575		
	Tibia	15	14,755	10.37	15	2.29×10^6	1,610		
	Fibula	5	12,774	8.98	4	2.095×10^6	1,473		

* Previously unpublished.

Results obtained in this laboratory from tests of twenty-three femoral, fifteen tibial, and five fibular specimens from the embalmed body of a 66-year-old man showed that the compressive strength of all three types of specimens was considerably lower than that found by Carothers et al. and by McElhaney et al. However, the modulus of elasticity was greater than McElhaney et al. found for their femoral and cranial cortical bone specimens; a little less than Carothers et al. reported for their femoral and tibial specimens; and a great deal lower than McElhaney et al. give for their full section cranial specimens.

Poisson's Ratio (Table XLVI). McElhaney et al. (1970a) are the only investigators, as far as I am aware, who have determined Poisson's ratio for bone. They found that it was highest in femoral bone, second in cranial bone alone, third in full section cranial bone tested in the tangential direction, and fourth in full section cranial bone tested in the radial direction.

FRESH NONHUMAN LONG BONE

Strength (Table XLIII). Topographic differences in compressive properties of fresh, nonhuman cortical bone have been investigated most extensively in Japan (see Yamada, 1970 for review). In each species, compressive strength varies among the different bones and there is no overall consistency from one species to another. In cattle, wild boars, and pigs the strength of specimens from distal extremity bones exceeds that of specimens from proximal extremity bones. Radial specimens in horses were stronger than humeral ones but femoral and tibial specimens had the same strength. Humeral specimens in deer were stronger than radial ones and tibial specimens stronger than femoral ones.

Strain (Table XLIV). Compressive strain exhibited less topographic variation than stress, being the same for all four

bones of wild boars and pigs and for three of the four bones of cattle. In deer the compressive strain was greater in specimens from the proximal bones than in those from the distal bones, but a similar relation was not found for horses.

Modulus of Elasticity (Table XLV). Specimens from the distal bones of wild boars, pigs, and deer had a higher modulus of elasticity than similar specimens from the proximal bones, but the reverse was true for horses. The modulus was only determined for femoral bone of cattle.

All the compressive data was obtained from quasi-static loading conditions and at normal room temperature and humidity.

Shearing Properties

HUMAN BONE

Strength (Table XLVII). Data on the shearing strength of bone are more scarce than those on tensile and compressive strength, probably because of the great difficulty of insuring that the shearing force is uniformly distributed over the cross-sectional area of the test specimen. In some of the shearing studies the test specimen is put through a hole in two plates and the shearing force applied by moving the plates in opposite directions. In these tests the specimen is treated like a rivet. In other tests a piece of bone is simply punched out of the specimen. This is called a punching shear test. In our studies, a special tool fabricated for that purpose was used. Shearing properties have been determined generally in a direction perpendicular to the long axis of the bone.

Ibuki (cited by Yamada, 1970) determined the shearing strength of standardized specimens of fresh cortical bone from all the major long bones of five people. According to him, femoral bone had the greatest shearing strength, followed, in descending order of magnitude, by ulnar,

TABLE XLVII

SHEARING PROPERTIES, PERPENDICULAR TO THE LONG AXIS, OF ADULT HUMAN CORTICAL BONE

		Shearing Strength					
		Fresh Bone (Yamada, 1970)				Embalmed Bone (Evans)*	
Bone	*No.*	*kgf/mm²*	*lbf/in²*	*Bone*	*No.*	*kgf/mm²*	*lb/in²*
Humerus	15-20	7.5 ± 0.27	10,665 ± 384	Femur	229	7.20 ± 1.07	10,239 ± 1,518
Radius	15-20	7.2 ± 0.08	10,238 ± 114	Tibia	116	8.06 ± 0.90	11,471 ± 1,282
Ulna	15-20	8.3 ± 0.18	11,803 ± 256	Fibula	26	7.70 ± 1.55	10,952 ± 2,205
Femur	15-20	8.4 ± 0.18	11,945 ± 256				
Tibia	15-20	8.2 ± 0.19	11,660 ± 270				
Fibula	15-20	8.2 ± 0.59	11,660 ± 839				

Ultimate Displacement (mm) (Data from Yamada, 1970)

Humerus	*Radius*	*Ulna*	*Femur*	*Tibia*	*Fibula*
0.64 ± 0.012	0.68 ± 0.040	0.71 ± 0.030	0.60 ± 0.015	0.66 ± 0.014	0.69 ± 0.018

* Previously unpublished.

then tibial and fibular bone (the same value), humeral, and radial bone. Except for the fibula, the shearing strength of specimens from the lower limb bones exceeded that of specimens from upper limb bones.

Wet specimens of embalmed adult human cortical bone tested in our laboratory showed that the average shearing strength was greatest in tibial bone, next in fibular bone, and least in femoral bone. An analysis of variance revealed that the mean shearing strength of the tibial and fibular specimens was significantly greater, at the 0.01 and between the 0.05 and 0.01 levels, respectively, than the strength of the femoral specimens. The difference between the shearing strength of the tibial and fibular specimens was not significant.

Ultimate Displacement (Table XLVII). According to Yamada, Ibuki reported that ultimate displacement during shearing was greatest in ulnar bone, followed in descending order by fibular, radial, tibial, humeral, and femoral bone.

FRESH NONHUMAN BONE

Shearing Strength (Table XLVIII). Topographic differences in the shearing strength of standardized specimens of cortical bone of nonhuman animals have been reported by Ibuki, cited by Yamada

(1970). In his tests the specimens were loaded in a direction perpendicular to their long axis.

Examination of the data in Table XLVIII shows considerable variation but no consistency in the relative shearing strength of the various bones either within or among the different species from which the test specimens were obtained.

Ultimate Displacement (Table XLIX). Nonhuman cortical bone, according to data given by Yamada (1970), shows considerable topographic variation with respect to different bones in the same species as well as in different species without any consistent relationships being evident.

Bending Properties

UNEMBALMED HUMAN LONG BONE

Strength (Table L). Rauber (1876) appears to have been the first one to determine the bending strength, perpendicular to their long axis, of standardized test specimens of human cortical bone from different subjects and bones. However, his data cannot be used for demonstration of topographic differences because his specimens were tested at different temperatures with some of them dry and others fresh.

Messerer (1880) measured the bending strength of femoral, tibial, and humeral

TABLE XLVIII

SHEARING STRENGTH, IN THE PERPENDICULAR DIRECTION, OF FRESH NONHUMAN CORTICAL BONE (Data from Yamada, 1970)

Bone	Horses		Cattle		Wild Boars		Pigs	
	kgf/mm^2	lbf/in^2	kgf/mm^2	lbf/in^2	kgf/mm^2	lbf/in^2	kgf/mm^2	lbf/in^2
Humerus	9.0 ± 0.17	12,798 ± 242	8.6 ± 0.11	12,229 ± 156	7.8 ± 0.83	11,092 ± 1,180	5.9 ± 0.20	8,390 ± 285
Radius	9.4 ± 0.33	13,367 ± 469	9.3 ± 0.18	13,225 ± 256	8.1 ± 0.33	11,518 ± 469	6.4 ± 0.32	9,101 ± 455
Ulna			8.2 ± 0.45	11,660 ± 640	7.4 ± 0.52	10,523 ± 739	4.8 ± 0.38	6,826 ± 540
Femur	9.9 ± 0.15	14,078 ± 213	9.1 ± 0.16	12,940 ± 228	8.7 ± 0.23	12,371 ± 327	6.5 ± 0.19	9,243 ± 270
Tibia	8.9 ± 0.27	12,656 ± 384	9.5 ± 0.20	13,509 ± 284	9.0 ± 0.34	12,798 ± 483	7.1 ± 0.28	10,096 ± 398
Fibula			7.6 ± 0.12	10,807 ± 171	8.7 ± 0.63	12,371 ± 896	6.2 ± 0.57	8,816 ± 811

TABLE XLIX

TABLE XLIX

Ultimate Displacement (mm) in Shearing Perpendicular to the Long Axis of Wet Cortical Nonhuman Bone (Data from Yamada, 1970)

	Humerus	Radius	Ulna	Femur	Tibia	Fibula
Horse	0.54 ± 0.017	0.58 ± 0.017		0.54 ± 0.020	0.58 ± 0.018	—
Cattle	0.51 ± 0.027	0.64 ± 0.017	0.66 ± 0.043	0.51 ± 0.009	0.47 ± 0.015	0.59 ± 0.004
Wild Boar	0.53 ± 0.003	0.59 ± 0.015	0.58 ± 0.020	0.53 ± 0.050	0.59 ± 0.014	0.51 ± 0.010
Pig	0.42 ± 0.021	0.48 ± 0.026	0.43 ± 0.026	0.43 ± 0.078	0.55 ± 0.018	0.40 ± 0.027

specimens of seven men from 18 to 78 years of age and of six women from 20 to 82 years of age. Examination of his data reveals that the average bending strength was highest in femoral, next in tibial, and lowest in humeral bone from men. In women the tibial specimens had the highest, the femoral ones were next, and the humeral specimens had the lowest average bending strength.

Tsuda (cited by Yamada, 1970) measured the bending strength of fresh cortical bone from twenty-eight subjects. He found that radial, ulnar, and fibular bone (all with the same value) had the highest average bending strength, tibial bone was second, humeral bone was third, and femoral bone was last.

The discrepancy between the data for bending strength, not only with respect to various bones but also the magnitude of the value for strength, given by Messerer and by Yamada, is probably a reflection of the test methods employed by each. Mes-serer used intact bones and calculated their bending strength from the breaking load and a cross-sectional area of the bones at the fracture site. The area of the cross sections was determined by measuring, with an Amsler moment planimeter, an outline of the cross section stamped on paper. Prints were made by covering the surface of the cross section with printer's ink and then pressing them on a paper. Thus, Mes-serer was actually measuring the bending strength of intact bones.

Tsuda, on the other hand, used test specimens with a 2.5 mm square cross section, expanded ends 3 mm long, and a span-side ratio of 16:1. The long axis of his specimens coincided with that of the intact bone. Thus, Tsuda determined the bending strength of cortical bone tissue. The higher bending strength reported by Tsuda may be the result of a racial factor because all of his material was obtained from Japanese subjects while Messerer's

TABLE L

Average Bending Strength of Fresh Adult Human Cortical Bone

Bone	No. of Spec.	Messerer (1880)		No. of Spec.	Yamada (1970)	
		kgf/mm²	lbf/in²		kgf/mm²	lbf/in²
Humerus	7 M	14.36	20,420	15-20	19.5	27,729
	6 F	13.82	19,652			
Radius				15-20	22.1	31,426
Ulna				15-20	22.1	31,426
Femur	7 M	17.80	25,312	15-20	17.7 ± 1.1	25,169 ± 1,564
	6 F	15.73	22,368			
Tibia	7 M	16.57	23,563	15-20	20.9	29,720
	6 F	16.28	23,150			
Fibula				15-20	22.1	31,426

was probably from Europeans although this is not definitely stated.

Ultimate Specific Deflection. Tsuda, according to Yamada, reported that the ultimate specific deflection was greatest in radial and ulnar bone, second in fibular bone, third in humeral and tibial bone, and least in femoral bone. No quantitative data were cited by Yamada.

Bending Modulus of Elasticity (Table LI). Messerer (1880) reported that the bending modulus of elasticity of the right humerus of a 32-year-old man was greater than that of the right femur but the reverse was true for the humerus and femur from the left side of the same subject. His information was obtained from intact bones.

The bending modulus of elasticity of fresh specimens of cortical bone 80 mm long, 2.6 to 3.6 mm wide, and 1.5 to 1.8 mm thick from the femur and tibia of a 46-year-old man was determined by Rauber (1876), who reported that the average modulus for nine tests on femoral specimens was greater than that for five tests on tibial specimens from the same man. Rauber's values for bending modulus of elasticity are higher than Messerer's.

TABLE LI

BENDING MODULUS OF ELASTICITY OF FRESH
HUMAN BONE

Bone	Intact Bones 32-Year-Old Man (Messerer, 1880)	
	kgf/mm²	lbf/in²
Right Humerus	1,800	2.56 × 10⁶
Left Humerus	1,523	2.17 × 10⁶
Right Femur	1,500	2.13 × 10⁶
Left Femur	1,536	2.18 × 10⁶

Bone	Standardized Specimens 46-Year-Old Man (Rauber, 1876)	
	kgf/mm²	lbf/in²
Femur	2,324	3.30 × 10⁶
Tibia	2,245	3.19 × 10⁶

EMBALMED HUMAN SKULL BONE

Recently, the resistance to bending and shear deflection was determined by Hubbard (1971) for eight parietal bone specimens, taken at a distance of 1 to 2.5 inches on either side of the sagittal suture, from four adult human embalmed cadavers. The long axis of the specimens was parallel with the suture. To prevent drying the specimens were stored in glass bottles with damp gauze sponges. In preparation of the specimens care was taken to insure that all cutting was perpendicular to the bone tables which were not modified more than necessary. The specimens were not of uniform width.

The specimens were subjected to three-point bending tests, at quasi-static loading rates and at spans varying from 0.750 to 1.875 inches in 0.125 inch steps. Deflection was monitored with a linear variable differential transformer. The load was measured with an Instron 1,000-lb capacity tension-compression load cell and the results displayed on a trace storing oscilloscope against the mid-span deflection.

Tests were made with the specimens in the "normal" and "inverted" position. In the normal position the specimen was supported on the inner skull table and loaded at the mid-span point on the outer skull table. In the inverted position the specimen was reversed. Beam widths, layer thickness, and total thickness were measured at seven points spaced 0.25 inch apart along the specimen. In order to apply the layered beam theory to analysis of the results the specimens were considered to be three-layered beams.

Strains on the tables of specimens loaded to failure by four-point bending were measured with strain gauges bonded to the inner and outer mid-regions of the specimens. The data thus collected allowed study of the behavior of layered cranial bone when loaded to failure and verification of the moment-strain relationship during the process. In these tests the load was applied to the specimen through a block, which was free to rotate, thus insuring that the mid-region of the specimen was subjected to pure bending action. Specimens were loaded then unloaded while the compression strain and load were monitored against fixture displacement. The specimens were then loaded to failure with the tensile gauge and load monitored against fixture displacement.

Hubbard reported that the bending stiffness of his specimens varied from 514 to 2,770 lbf/in² (0.36 to 1.95 kgf/mm²), the equivalent elastic modulus from 1.13 to 2.22 × 10⁶ lbf/in² (794 to 1,561 kgf/mm²), the shear stiffness from 3.71 to 12.1 × 10⁶ lbf/in² (2,608 to 8,506 kgf/mm²), the equivalent shear modulus from 3.1 to 108 × 10³ lbf/in² (2.2 to 75.9 kgf/mm²), and the core shear modulus from 20 to 100 × 10³ lbf/in² (14.1 to 70.3 kgf/mm²).

Except for one specimen, the elastic modulus Hubbard found for parietal bone is less than the values given by Messerer and by Rauber for long bone. There are no comparable long bone data to which the other mechanical properties determined by Hubbard can be compared.

WET FRESH NONHUMAN LONG BONE

According to Yamada (1970) the ultimate bending strength of femoral, tibial, and metatarsal bone of cattle are equal but the specific deflection for tibial and metatarsal bone is 1.4 times and 1.6 times, respectively, that for femoral bone.

Torsion Properties

FRESH HUMAN BONE

Apparently the first to determine the torsion strength of bone was Rauber (1876). Rods with a cylindrical middle region 80 mm long and ends with a quadratic cross section for gripping were used. The specimens were tested with a special jig designed for that purpose. Rauber reported a torsion strength of 7.097, 9.307, 7.097, and 7.8 kgf/mm² (10,092, 13,235, 10,092, and 11,092 lbf/in²), with a mean of 7.9 kgf/mm² (11,234 lbf/in²) for the four specimens tested. However, no conclusions regarding possible topographic differences in torsion strength can be drawn from his data because all of his specimens were obtained from the humerus of a 30-year-old man.

Hazama, cited by Yamada (1970), found a mean torsion strength of 5.82 ± 0.11 kgf/mm² (8,276 ± 156 lbf/in²) and an elastic modulus of 350 kgf/mm² (497,700 lbf/in²) for specimens of fresh femur taken from people 20 to 39 years of age, the age at which both mechanical properties have their maximum value. Specimens from a total of twenty-two people, varying from 20 to 80 years of age, were tested.

WET EMBALMED HUMAN BONE

The torsion properties of 415 specimens of cortical bone from embalmed femurs of adult men have been determined in this laboratory. Specimens of standardized size and shape were tested in a jig (Fig. 16) especially designed for that purpose. The details of the method were described in Chapter 2.

Analysis of the data obtained in our tests showed a mean torsional shear strength of 6,476 lbf/in² (4.52 kgf/mm²), a mean shear modulus of 0.869 × 10⁶ lbf/in² (610 kgf/mm²), and a mean break energy of 18.71 in-lb/in² (3.33 kg-cm/cm²). Comparisons of our data with that of Hazama for fresh femoral bone shows that the torsion strength and shear

TABLE LII

TORSION PROPERTIES OF FRESH CORTICAL BONE OF HORSES (Data from Yamada, 1970)

Bone	Torsion Strength		Angle of Twist	Modulus of Elasticity	
	kgf/mm²	*lbf/in²*		*kgf/mm²*	*lbf/in²*
Humerus	5.11 ± 0.07	7,266 ± 100	0.016 ± 0.0015	450	639,900
Radius	5.71 ± 0.15	8,120 ± 213	0.019 ± 0.008	450	639,900
Metacarpal	6.65 ± 0.10	9,456 ± 142	0.024 ± 0.005	430	611,460
Femur	5.11 ± 0.08	7,266 ± 114	0.018 ± 0.0007	370	526,140
Tibia	5.91 ± 0.14	8,404 ± 199	0.023 ± 0.0019	380	540,360
Metatarsal	6.93 ± 0.07	9,854 ± 100	0.028 ± 0.0019	410	583,020

modulus of human femoral bone are reduced by embalming. There is also the possibility that the differences are racial because all of Hazama's material was obtained from Japanese subjects whereas ours was not.

FRESH NONHUMAN BONE (Table LII).

Data on the torsional properties of horse bone, cited by Yamada (1970), showed that torsion strength was greatest in metatarsal bone followed in order from strongest to weakest, by metacarpal, tibial, radial, humeral, and femoral bone. The angle of twist, from highest to lowest, was metatarsal, metacarpal, tibial, radial, femoral, and humeral bone. Humeral and radial bone (with the same value) had the highest modulus of elasticity, followed in order of decreasing value by metacarpal, metatarsal, tibial, and femoral bone.

Examination of the data (Table LII) shows that the value for each of the torsional properties increased progressively from the proximal to the distal bones of each limb. Except for humeral and femoral bone, which had the same value, the torsional strength of specimens from the hind leg and foot bones exceeded that of specimens from the homologous bones of the foreleg and foot. The angle of twist of specimens from the hind leg bones was greater than that of specimens from the homologous foreleg bones. However, the reverse situation was found for the modulus of elasticity.

Cleavage Properties

Japanese investigators determined the cleavage properties of rectangular bars of cortical bone 6 mm thick (length of side perpendicular to the wedge) and 6 mm long (see Yamada, 1970). The specimens were cut parallel with the shaft of the bone.

Tests were made in an Amsler 100-kg-capacity compression machine by applying a load to a wedge with a top angle of 30°. The edge of the wedge was placed perpendicular to the midline of the thickest side of the specimen. A basic load of 1 kg was applied to the wedge and its penetration measured by a dial gauge with graduations of 0.01 mm and a range of zero to 20 mm.

WET HUMAN BONE

Strength. Yamada (1970) cites an average value of 8.3 kgf/mm² (11,803 lbf/in²) for adult tibial bone which he states is generally less than that for femoral bone. However, no specific value is given for femoral bone.

WET FRESH NONHUMAN BONE (Table LIII)

According to data given by Yamada (1970) the cleavage strength for horses and cattle is greatest in humeral bone, second in femoral, third in tibial (horses)

TABLE LIII

CLEAVAGE PROPERTIES, IN THE RADIAL DIRECTION, OF WET, FRESH CORTICAL BONE
(Data from Yamada, 1970)

Bone	Cleavage Strength				Ultimate Penetration (mm)	
	Horses		Cattle		Horses	Cattle
	kgf/mm^2	lbf/in^2	kgf/mm^2	lbf/in^2		
Humerus	9.0 ± 0.27	$12,798 \pm 384$	11.6 ± 0.46	$16,495 \pm 654$	0.56 ± 0.018	0.65 ± 0.024
Radius	7.6 ± 0.23	$10,807 \pm 327$	8.4 ± 0.31	$11,945 \pm 441$	0.57 ± 0.011	0.64 ± 0.024
Femur	8.8 ± 0.37	$12,514 \pm 526$	8.7 ± 0.18	$12,371 \pm 256$	0.54 ± 0.022	0.50 ± 0.009
Tibia	7.9 ± 0.23	$11,234 \pm 327$	8.2 ± 0.28	$11,660 \pm 398$	0.50 ± 0.016	0.56 ± 0.024

and radial (cattle), and fourth in radial (horses) and tibial (cattle) bone. In horses, ultimate penetration was greatest in radial bone followed by humeral, femoral and tibial bone. In cattle, ultimate penetration from greatest to least, was in humeral, radial, tibial, and femoral bone.

Fatigue Life

The fatigue life, or strength as it is sometimes called, of unembalmed specimens of cortical bone from above-knee amputations of adult men has been investigated in this laboratory. Fifteen femoral specimens had an average of 1,188,467 cycles to failure compared to an average of 2,398,207 cycles for fifty-eight tibial specimens and 2,841,400 cycles for five fibular specimens. All specimens were tested at a constant load (stress) of 5,000 lbf/in² (344.7 × 10⁶ dynes/cm²) in a Model SF-2 Sonntag flexure fatigue machine. For further details see Chapter 2. An analysis of variance showed that the differences between the means were not statistically significant.

Hardness

WET HUMAN LONG BONE

Japanese investigators, according to Yamada (1970), found an average Rockwell hardness number of 40 (using the H scale) for wet adult human femoral bone. Conversion of the Rockwell number into the Brinell system gave an average Brinell hardness number of 24. The hardness tests were made on cross sections, the medial side excluded, of the femur. Femoral and tibial bone were the hardest, followed, in descending order, by radial and fibular (the same value), humeral, and ulnar bone. Large bones were generally harder than small ones.

Wet, unembalmed adult human bone tested in this laboratory had an average Rockwell superficial hardness value of −1.5 for twenty femoral, −3.2 for 133 tibial, and −9.5 for nineteen fibular specimens. An analysis of variance between the means revealed that the average hardness of the fibular specimens was significantly greater, at the 0.05 to 0.01 level, than that of either the femoral or tibial specimens. All the material was obtained from above-knee amputations so only the distal fourth or so of the femur was available, consequently only a small number of femoral specimens were obtained. The small size of the fibula also reduced the number of specimens obtainable for testing.

Comparison of our hardness values with those obtained by the Japanese investigators shows that our specimens were considerably softer than theirs. However, the differences may be due, in part, to the fact that they used a Rockwell hardness tester while we used a Rockwell superficial hardness tester. We both used the H scale of the machines but, according to Davis, Troxell and Wiskocil (1964), the superficial tester is especially designed to determine the hardness of a specimen close to its surface. The "superficial" tester operates upon the same principle as the regular Rockwell tester, but used lighter minor and major loads (45 kg, the load used in our tests) and has a more sensitive depth measuring system. Another factor that may be responsible for the values we obtained is that our specimens were stored in tap water before testing and thus may have been wetter than those tested by the Japanese. Furthermore, the water was not buffered so some of the calcium in our specimens may have been removed. There is also the possibility that the differences might be partially racial in origin since our material was Caucasian and theirs was Japanese.

WET SKULL BONE

The squamous part of the human temporal bone, according to some Japanese studies cited by Yamada (1970), has an average Vickers hardness of 14.4 ± 0.90 in transverse sections compared to an average hardness of 16.4 ± 0.58 in tangential sections.

WET EMBALMED HUMAN BONE

Rockwell superficial hardness tests made in this laboratory on wet specimens from embalmed adult human cadavers revealed an average Rockwell hardness number of 13.2 for 292 femoral, 11.5 for 115 tibial, and 7.6 for twenty-five fibular specimens. An analysis of variance between the means show that the differences were not statistically significant.

Comparison of these hardness values with those obtained for our unembalmed specimens suggests that embalming may increase the hardness of bone. However, our values for embalmed specimens are less than those reported by the Japanese for wet, unembalmed specimens.

The smaller hardness values of our specimens in comparison with the Japanese ones may be related to differences in the direction of loading during a test. In our hardness tests the load was applied to the widest side of a specimen in a direction perpendicular to its long axis while in the Japanese studies the force was applied to a cross section of a specimen in a direction parallel to its long axis.

Right Side Vs Left Side

UNEMBALMED WET TIBIA

Data obtained in this laboratory reveal significant differences between some of the mechanical properties of right and of left bones. Thus, the mean tensile strain (% elongation) of 161 wet unembalmed specimens from left adult tibias was greater, at better than the 1% significance level, than that of thirty-three similar specimens of right tibias. Single shearing strength of five right tibial specimens was higher, at the 1% or better significance level, than that of 121 left tibial specimens. Ultimate tensile strength and modulus of elasticity of right tibial specimens were both higher, at the 5% to 1% significance level, than in similar specimens from left tibias. All specimens were obtained from above-knee amputations. Most of them happened to be left legs which accounts for the predominant number of specimens from that side. However, any conclusions drawn from this data must be tentative because of the great disparity in sample size in the comparisons.

EMBALMED WET FEMUR

Rockwell superficial hardness of 136 left femoral specimens was greater, at better than the 1% significance level, than the hardness of 132 specimens from right femurs.

Embalmed Wet Tibia

The modulus of elasticity of 120 specimens from left tibias of adult white men was higher, at the 5% to 1% significance level, than that of 101 specimens from right tibias.

Embalmed Wet Skull Bone

Evans and Lissner (1957) found that the tensile strength, in the lengthwise direc-tion, of parietal cortical bone was greater in specimens from the right than in those from the left side of the skull, while the opposite was true for compressive strength (Table XXVI). When tested in the cross-wise direction the compressive strength was greater on the left than on the right side. Diploë had a greater crosswise compressive strength in specimens from the right side.

Topographic Variation Within Bones

Specimens from different parts of the same bone also exhibit differences in their

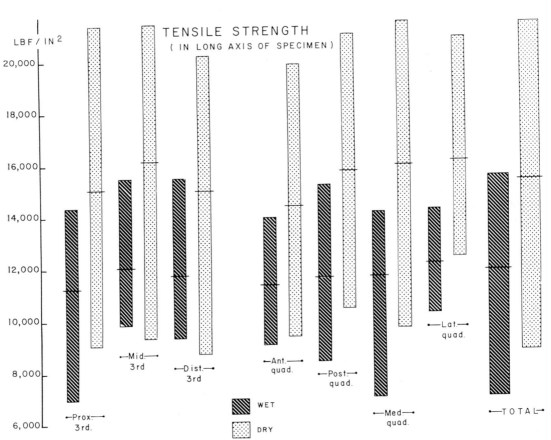

Figure 101. Average and range of variation in the tensile strength of 121 wet- and 121 dry-tested specimens of cortical bone from different regions of embalmed femurs of 6 adult men. Abbreviations for Figs. 101-104: Prox. 3rd = proximal third of shaft; Mid. 3rd = middle third of shaft; Dist. 3rd = distal third of shaft; Post. quad. = posterior quadrant of shaft; Med. quad. = medial quadrant of shaft; Lat. quad. = lateral quadrant of shaft; Ant. quad. = anterior quadrant of shaft. (Based on data from Evans and Lebow: *J Appl Physiol,* 1951)

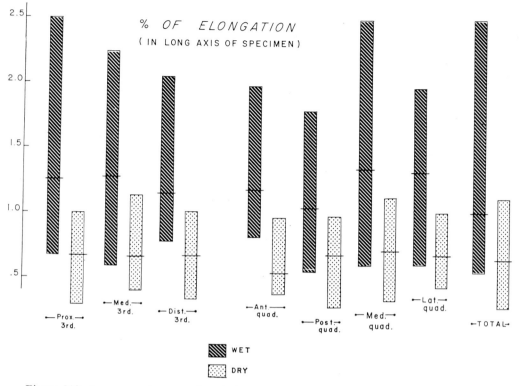

Figure 102. Average and range of variation in the percent of elongation (tensile strain) of 121 wet- and 121 dry-tested specimens of cortical bone from different regions of embalmed femurs of 6 adult men. (Based on data from Evans and Lebow: *J Appl Physiol,* 1951)

mechanical properties. However, these differences have not been investigated as thoroughly as those among bones.

Tensile Properties

WET EMBALMED FEMORAL BONE

The first extensive investigation on differences in the mechanical properties of various regions of a single bone was made by Evans and Lebow (1951) who determined certain mechanical properties of standardized specimens (Fig. 8) of cortical bone from various thirds and quadrants of the shaft of the femurs of six adult men. Embalmed material was used because intact unembalmed femurs were not available. A total of 242 specimens, half of them wet and half dry, were tested.

Their data showed that the average ultimate tensile strength in both the wet and the dry condition was highest in specimens from the middle third and lateral quadrant and lowest in those from the proximal third and anterior quadrant of the shaft (Fig. 101). All dry specimens, regardless of the region of the shaft from which they were taken, had a higher total average ultimate tensile strength than similarly tested wet specimens.

Wet specimens from the middle third and medial quadrant of the shaft had the greatest percent elongation (tensile strain) while those from the distal third and posterior quadrant had the least (Fig. 102). Dry specimens from the medial quadrant had the highest and those from the anteri-

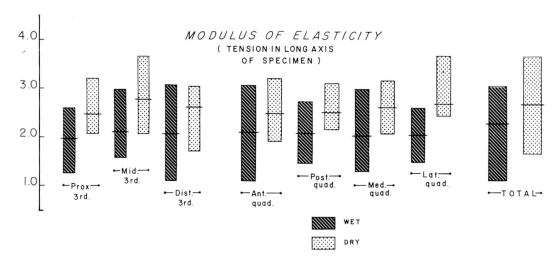

Figure 103. Average and range of variation in the modulus of elasticity (stiffness) of 121 wet- and 121 dry-tested specimens of cortical bone from different regions of embalmed femurs of 6 adult men. (Based on data from Evans and Lebow: *J Appl Physiol*, 1951)

or quadrant the lowest tensile strain. Little regional difference was noted for dry specimens from various thirds of the shaft. The total average tensile strain for all wet specimens, regardless of region, was higher than that for dry specimens.

Both wet and dry specimens from the middle third of the shaft were the stiffest, i.e. had the highest modulus of elasticity, while those from the proximal third were the most flexible (Fig. 103). Comparison of the modulus according to the quadrant of the shaft from which the specimens were taken revealed that dry specimens from the lateral quadrant were slightly

stiffer than those from other quadrants. Wet specimens exhibited little difference in the average modulus of elasticity according to quadrant. Dry specimens combined had a higher total modulus of elasticity than wet ones.

Wet specimens from embalmed adult human femurs studied in this laboratory also exhibited regional differences in their tensile properties (Table LIV). Mean tensile strength was greatest in specimens from the middle third and lateral quadrant of the shaft and lowest in those from the proximal third and the anterior quadrant. Specimens from the middle third and

TABLE LIV

TOPOGRAPHIC DIFFERENCES IN MEAN TENSILE PROPERTIES OF WET EMBALMED
CORTICAL BONE FROM FEMURS OF ADULT MEN

Region	No.	Tensile Strength lbf/in^2	kgf/mm^2	No.	Modulus of Elasticity $\times 10^6 lbf/in^2$	kgf/mm^2	No.	% Elongation
Proximal third	131	$11,013 \pm 2,658$	$7,742 \pm 1.87$	129	1.99 ± 0.45	$1,399 \pm 316$	118	1.55 ± 0.68
Middle third	135	$11,961 \pm 2,753$	8.41 ± 1.94	130	2.19 ± 0.43	$1,540 \pm 302$	122	1.45 ± 0.63
Distal third	128	$11,014 \pm 2,658$	7.743 ± 1.87	120	2.09	1,469	116	1.37 ± 0.64
Anterior quadrant ..	100	$11,076 \pm 3,174$	7.79 ± 2.23	96	2.00 ± 0.51	$1,406 \pm 359$	94	1.48 ± 0.70
Lateral quadrant ..	106	$11,610 \pm 2,875$	8.16 ± 2.02	99	2.10 ± 0.46	$1,476 \pm 323$	94	1.56 ± 0.65
Medial quadrant ...	102	$11,577 \pm 2,912$	8.14 ± 2.05	97	2.15 ± 0.57	$1,511 \pm 401$	91	1.53 ± 0.71
Posterior quadrant ..	95	$11,081 \pm 2,462$	7.79 ± 1.73	89	2.14 ± 0.45	$1,504 \pm 316$	84	1.26 ± 0.56

medial quadrant had the highest and those from the proximal third and anterior quadrant the lowest modulus of elasticity. Proximal third and lateral quadrant specimens showed the highest and those from the distal third and posterior quadrant the lowest tensile strain (percent elongation).

The mean tensile strength and modulus of elasticity of the specimens from the middle third of the bone were significantly greater, at better than the 0.01 level, than the same properties for proximal third specimens. Specimens from the distal third had a mean tensile strength greater, at between the 0.05 and the 0.01 significance level, than that of specimens from the proximal third. Differences between the tensile properties of the middle and distal thirds of the bone were not significant.

A similar analysis of tensile properties with respect to quadrants of the shaft showed that the mean percent elongation of specimens from the lateral and medial quadrants was greater, at the 0.01 or better significance level, than that of specimens from the posterior quadrant. Specimens from the anterior quadrant also had a tensile strain significantly greater, at between the 0.05 and 0.01 level, than posterior quadrant specimens. The reverse relations were found for the modulus of elasticity. No other significant differences appeared in tensile properties of specimens from different quadrants.

Wet Embalmed Tibial Bone (Table LV)

We have also found that wet specimens from the middle third and anterior quadrant of the tibia have the greatest while those from the proximal third and medial quadrant have the least tensile strength. Modulus of elasticity is greatest in specimens from the distal third and lateral quadrant but lowest in those from the proximal third and anterior quadrant. Specimens from the middle third and anterior quadrant have the highest percent elongation while the lowest is found in specimens from the proximal third and posterior quadrant.

The tensile strain of specimens from the middle third of the shaft was significantly greater, at between the 0.05 and the 0.01 level, than that of proximal third specimens but there were no other significant differences according to thirds. Anterior quadrant specimens had a tensile strain significantly greater, at the 0.05 to 0.01 level, than that of lateral and medial quadrant specimens. The greater strain of the anterior quadrant specimens in comparison with that of the posterior quadrant was significant at better than the 0.01 level. Anterior quadrant specimens also had a ten-

TABLE LV

TOPOGRAPHIC DIFFERENCES IN MEAN TENSILE PROPERTIES OF WET CORTICAL
BONE FROM EMBALMED TIBIAS OF ADULT MEN

Region	No.	Tensile Strength		No.	Modulus of Elasticity		No.	% Elongation
		lbf/in^2	kgf/mm^2		$\times 10^6 lbf/in^2$	kgf/mm^2		
Proximal third	59	13,134 ± 2,519	9.23 ± 1.77	57	2.25 ± 0.46	1,582 ± 323	49	1.57 ± 0.62
Middle third	68	13,628 ± 3,000	9.58 ± 2.11	67	2.30 ± 0.47	1,617 ± 330	66	1.88 ± 0.76
Distal third	65	13,623 ± 3,108	9.58 ± 2.18	64	2.35 ± 0.54	1,652 ± 380	59	1.78 ± 0.88
Anterior quadrant	47	13,900 ± 2,650	9.77 ± 1.86	47	2.17 ± 0.35	1,526 ± 246	44	2.09 ± 0.75
Lateral quadrant	47	13,648 ± 3,290	9.59 ± 2.31	47	2.37 ± 0.56	1,666 ± 394	45	1.68 ± 0.94
Medial quadrant	47	12,665 ± 3,108	8.90 ± 2.18	46	2.31 ± 0.48	1,624 ± 337	45	1.75 ± 0.72
Posterior quadrant	49	13,521 ± 2,547	9.51 ± 1.79	48	2.36 ± 0.54	1,659 ± 380	45	1.55 ± 0.61

TABLE LVI

TOPOGRAPHIC DIFFERENCES IN MEAN TENSILE PROPERTIES OF WET EMBALMED
CORTICAL BONE FROM FIBULAS OF ADULT MEN

| Region | No. | Tensile Strength | | No. | Modulus of Elasticity | | No. | % Elongation |
		lbf/in^2	kgf/mm^2		$\times 10^6\ lbf/in^2$	kgf/mm^2		
Proximal third	10	$14{,}328 \pm 2{,}632$	10.07 ± 1.85	9	2.44 ± 0.49	$1{,}715 \pm 344$	9	1.91 ± 1.32
Middle third	14	$13{,}340 \pm 2{,}946$	9.38 ± 2.07	14	2.57 ± 0.27	$1{,}807 \pm 190$	14	1.78 ± 1.42
Distal third	8	$12{,}445 \pm 2{,}493$	8.75 ± 1.75	7	2.56 ± 0.66	$1{,}800 \pm 464$	7	1.33 ± 0.94

sile strength significantly greater, at the 0.05 to 0.01 level, than that of medial quadrant specimens. Modulus of elasticity of lateral quadrant specimens was significantly greater, at the 0.05 to 0.01 level, than the modulus of the anterior quadrant specimens.

WET EMBALMED FIBULAR BONE
(Table LVI)

Because of its small size, mechanical properties of the fibula were only analyzed according to various thirds of the bone. The maximum and minimum values for tensile strength were found in specimens from the proximal and distal thirds, respectively. However, the greatest modulus of elasticity and tensile strain occurred in middle and proximal third specimens, respectively. Specimens from the proximal third had the lowest modulus and those from the distal third the least strain. None of the differences were statistically significant.

WET EMBALMED HUMERAL BONE
(Table LVII)

Comparison of the tensile properties of specimens from various thirds of the humerus made in our laboratory showed that tensile strength and strain (percent elongation) were greatest in specimens from the distal and middle thirds, respectively, and least in those from the proximal third of the shaft. Modulus of elasticity was maximum in distal third specimens and minimal in middle third ones.

When the data were analyzed according to quadrants it was seen that the posterior quadrant specimens had the highest and the medial quadrant specimens the lowest average tensile strength. Specimens from the lateral quadrant had the highest and those from the anterior quadrant the lowest average modulus of elasticity. Tensile strain (percent elongation) was maximum in specimens from the lateral quadrant and minimum in those from the medial

TABLE LVII

TOPOGRAPHIC DIFFERENCES IN MEAN TENSILE PROPERTIES OF WET EMBALMED
CORTICAL BONE FROM THE HUMERUS OF ADULT HUMANS

| Region | No. | Tensile Strength | | No. | Modulus of Elasticity | | No. | % Elongation |
		lbf/in^2	kgf/mm^2		$\times 10^6\ lbf/in^2$	kgf/mm^2		
Proximal third	21	11,785	8.28	13	2.45	1,722	12	0.53
Middle third	20	12,781	8.99	19	2.36	1,659	19	0.65
Distal third	17	13,164	9.25	13	2.54	1,786	10	0.63
Anterior quadrant	16	12,524	8.80	13	2.34	1,645	11	0.63
Lateral quadrant	9	13,112	9.22	9	2.58	1,814	7	0.65
Medial quadrant	17	11,946	8.40	11	2.39	1,680	8	0.49
Posterior quadrant	17	14,965	10.52	16	2.39	1,680	15	0.64

TABLE LVIII

TOPOGRAPHIC DIFFERENCES IN MEAN TENSILE PROPERTIES OF WET UNEMBALMED
CORTICAL BONE FROM THE TIBIA OF ADULT WHITE MEN

Region	No.	Tensile Strength		No.	Modulus of Elasticity		No.	% Elongation
		lbf/in^2	kgf/mm^2		$\times 10^6\ lbf/in^2$	kgf/mm^2		
Proximal third	53	$12,532 \pm 3,065$	8.81 ± 2.15	52	2.4 ± 0.72	$1,687 \pm 506$	46	1.50 ± 0.83
Middle third	78	$13,425 \pm 2,913$	9.44 ± 2.05	81	2.50 ± 0.63	$1,758 \pm 443$	75	1.73 ± 0.86
Distal third	78	$12,420 \pm 2,939$	8.73 ± 2.07	79	2.3 ± 0.68	$1,617 \pm 478$	73	1.71 ± 0.79
Anterior quadrant ...	55	$12,386 \pm 3,628$	8.71 ± 2.55	54	2.40 ± 0.87	$1,687 \pm 612$	48	1.76 ± 0.79
Lateral quadrant	50	$13,574 \pm 2,584$	9.54 ± 1.82	49	2.41 ± 0.56	$1,694 \pm 394$	47	1.73 ± 0.85
Medial quadrant	46	$12,672 \pm 2,767$	8.91 ± 1.95	49	2.59 ± 0.59	$1,821 \pm 415$	41	1.73 ± 0.94
Posterior quadrant ..	58	$12,711 \pm 2,743$	8.94 ± 1.93	60	2.41 ± 0.61	$1,694 \pm 429$	58	1.50 ± 0.79

quadrant. Because of the small total number of specimens tested, the data were not subjected to statistical analysis.

WET UNEMBALMED FEMORAL BONE

According to studies by Ko, cited by Yamada (1970), the ultimate tensile strength and percentage elongation (tensile strain) of fresh wet femoral bone of adults are slightly greater in the middle part and medial side of the shaft than in other parts of the bone.

WET UNEMBALMED TIBIAL BONE
(Table LVIII)

Studies in this laboratory revealed that unembalmed wet tibial bone from adult men likewise exhibits topographic differences in its mechanical properties. Specimens from the middle third of the shaft had the highest mean tensile strength and modulus of elasticity while those from the distal third had the lowest. Mean tensile strain (% elongation) was greatest in specimens from the middle third and lowest in ones from the proximal third. As far as quadrants of the shaft were concerned, the highest and lowest tensile strength was found in specimens from the lateral and anterior quadrants, respectively. Specimens from the medial quadrant had the highest modulus of elasticity, and those from the anterior quadrants the low-

est. The greatest and the least percent elongation was found in specimens from the anterior and posterior quadrants, respectively.

The mean tensile strength of the specimens from the middle third of the shaft was significantly greater, at between the 0.05 and the 0.01 level, than that of the specimens from the distal third of the bone. No other significant differences were found between the mean tensile properties of specimens from various thirds and quadrants of the bone.

Compressive Properties (Table LIX)

Compressive properties, determined in this laboratory, of 118 specimens of wet cortical bone from unembalmed tibias of six adult men exhibited regional differences. Specimens from the middle third of the bone had the greatest average compressive strength, modulus of elasticity, and percent shortening (compressive strain). The lowest mean compressive strength and modulus of elasticity were found in the proximal third specimens while those from the distal third had the least percent shortening.

An evaluation of mechanical properties according to the quadrant of the shaft from which the specimens were obtained did not reveal that one quadrant was con-

TABLE LIX

TOPOGRAPHIC DIFFERENCES IN MEAN COMPRESSIVE PROPERTIES OF WET, UNEMBALMED
CORTICAL BONE FROM THE TIBIAS OF SIX ADULT MEN

Region	No.	Compressive Strength		No.	Modulus of Elasticity		No.	% Shortening
		lbf/in²	*kgf/mm²*		*× 10⁶ lbf/in²*	*kgf/mm²*		
Proximal third	19	12,935	9.09	19	2.56	1,800	15	0.95
Middle third	28	19,495	13.70	28	2.95	2,074	28	0.97
Distal third	12	13,090	9.20	12	2.71	1,905	9	0.64
Anterior quadrant	15	15,190	10.68	15	2.90	2,039	12	0.95
Lateral quadrant	15	16,140	11.35	14	2.77	1,947	14	0.74
Medial quadrant	16	17,568	12.35	16	2.79	1,961	13	0.87
Posterior quadrant	13	15,460	10.87	14	2.71	1,905	14	1.10

sistently dominant over the other quadrants. Specimens from the medial quadrant were the strongest and those from the anterior quadrant the weakest. Anterior quadrant specimens had the highest modulus of elasticity while posterior quadrant ones had the lowest. Compressive strain (percent shortening) was greatest in the posterior and least in the lateral quadrant specimens.

Compressive strength differences with respect to quadrant and shaft level were also found by Amtmann (1968) in 703 dry specimens of standardized size and shape obtained from embalmed femurs of six men and two women varying from 56 to 80 years of age. The specimens were taken from rings of bone, cut at various distances along the length of the femoral shaft, and their compressive strength in

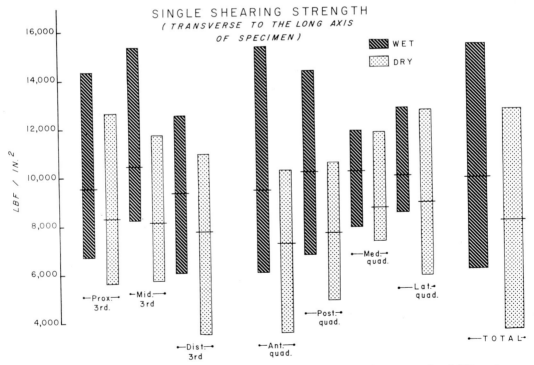

Figure 104. Average and range of variation in the single shearing strength of 121 wet- and 121 dry-tested specimens of cortical bone from different regions of embalmed femurs of 6 adult men. (Based on data from Evans and Lebow: *J Appl Physiol*, 1951)

the longitudinal direction, determined by loading them to failure at a rate of load increase of 50 kg/cm²/sec in a materials testing machine.

Examination of Amtmann's data showed that lateral quadrant specimens had the highest and posterior quadrant ones the lowest mean compressive strength at levels of 26%, 38%, and 50% of the shaft length. At 62% of the shaft length posterior quadrants were the strongest, and at 74% of the length the medial quadrant specimens were the strongest although the difference between them and the posterior quadrant specimens was slight. Anterior quadrant specimens were the weakest in both of these levels.

The mean compressive strength for all the specimens from each quadrant, regardless of the shaft level, was 1.97 for the posterior quadrant; 2.22 for the anterior quadrant; 2.36 for the medial quadrant; and 2.54 for the lateral quadrant. All possible differences between the means for the various quadrants were significant at the 1% level. The mean compressive strength for the three proximal-distal levels were 2.23, 2.31, and 2.30 × 10³ kg/cm², respectively, but the differences were not significant.

The significance of four variables—cross section (level), quadrant, body side, and individual—was also tested. Data obtained showed that all the main effects and the interactions level × quadrant, level × individual, quadrant × individual, and body side × individual were all significant.

Shearing Properties

WET EMBALMED FEMORAL BONE

Differences in the single shearing strength of wet specimens of cortical bone from various regions of adult human embalmed femurs were demonstrated first by Evans and Lebow (1951). A specially designed shearing tool was used (Fig. 10). A total of 242 specimens, half of them wet and half dry, were tested.

Evans and Lebow found that wet specimens from the middle third and dry ones from the proximal third of the bone had the highest mean shearing strength while the lowest strength occurred in specimens, wet as well as dry, from the distal third (Fig. 104). Medial and posterior quadrant wet specimens were the strongest and anterior quadrant ones the weakest. Among the dry specimens the ones from the lateral and anterior quadrants had the highest and lowest mean shearing strength, respectively. The mean shearing strength of all the wet specimens exceeded that of all the dry ones, just the reverse of what was found for the mean tensile strength of the two types of specimens. The data were not analyzed statistically.

A similar study made in this laboratory of 227 wet femoral specimens also showed that those from the middle third of the bone had the highest mean shearing strength. The lowest strength was found in specimens from the proximal, instead of the distal third of the shaft (Table LX) but the difference was slight. Specimens from the lateral quadrant were the strongest and those from the anterior quadrant the weakest.

An analysis of variance demonstrated that the mean shearing strength of the middle third specimens was significantly greater, at between the 0.05 and 0.01 level, than that of either the proximal or the distal third specimens. There was no significant difference between the shearing strength of the proximal and the distal third specimens. No significant differences were found in the mean single shearing strength of specimens from various quadrants of the shaft.

Wet Embalmed Tibial Bone (Table LX)

Determinations made in this laboratory of the single shearing strength of 116 wet specimens from embalmed tibias of adult men showed that the highest and lowest mean strength occurred in specimens from the middle and the proximal thirds of the bone, respectively. Medial quadrant specimens had the greatest and anterior quadrant ones the lowest mean strength. Thus, the tibia resembles the femur in having the greatest mean shearing strength in the middle third and the lowest in the proximal third and anterior quadrant of the bone. It differs from the femur in that its medial quadrant specimens, instead of the lateral quadrant ones, have the highest mean shearing strength.

From an analysis of variance it was found that the mean shearing strength of the middle third specimens was significantly greater, at better than the 0.01 level, than that of the proximal third specimens. The middle and distal third specimens showed no significant difference in their mean shearing strength.

Mean percent elongation of anterior quadrant specimens was greater, at the 0.01 or better significance level, than that of posterior quadrant specimens. Anterior quadrant specimens also had an ultimate tensile strength that was greater, at the 0.05 and the 0.01 significance level, than the strength of medial quadrant specimens. The modulus of elasticity of lateral quadrant specimens exceeded that of anterior quadrant specimens at a significance level of 0.05 to 0.01. The Rockwell superficial hardness of the posterior, the medial, and the lateral quadrant specimens was significantly greater at the 0.01 or better level, than the hardness of the anterior quadrant specimens. Lateral quadrant specimens were denser, at the 0.01 or better signifi-

TABLE LX

Topographic Differences in Mean Single (Punching) Shearing Strength Perpendicular to the Long Axis, in Wet Embalmed Adult Human Cortical Bone

	No.	lbf/in^2	kgf/mm^2
Femur			
Proximal third	76	$10,003 \pm 1,590$	7.03 ± 1.12
Middle third	76	$10,634 \pm 1,454$	7.48 ± 1.02
Distal third	75	$10,048 \pm 1,507$	7.06 ± 1.06
Anterior quadrant	58	$9,970 \pm 1,772$	7.01 ± 1.25
Lateral quadrant	60	$10,415 \pm 1,414$	7.32 ± 0.99
Medial quadrant	59	$10,283 \pm 1,360$	7.23 ± 0.96
Posterior quadrant	50	$10,243 \pm 1,593$	7.20 ± 1.12
Tibia			
Proximal third	37	$11,005 \pm 1,033$	7.74 ± 0.73
Middle third	40	$11,814 \pm 981$	8.31 ± 0.69
Distal third	39	$11,560 \pm 1,621$	8.13 ± 1.14
Anterior quadrant	30	$11,209 \pm 1,488$	7.88 ± 1.05
Lateral quadrant	29	$11,668 \pm 1,249$	8.20 ± 0.88
Medial quadrant	28	$11,731 \pm 1,057$	8.25 ± 0.74
Posterior quadrant	29	$11,293 \pm 1,263$	7.94 ± 0.89
Fibula			
Proximal third	8	$11,276 \pm 1,576$	7.93 ± 1.11
Middle third	10	$11,626 \pm 1,372$	8.17 ± 0.96
Distal third	8	$9,786 \pm 3,185$	6.88 ± 2.24

cance level, than those from the anterior quadrant. The density of the posterior and the medial quadrant specimens exceeded that of the anterior quadrant ones at between the 0.05 and the 0.01 significance level. No significant differences were found between the mechanical properties and density of specimens from the posterior, the lateral, and the medial quadrants.

WET EMBALMED FIBULAR BONE (Table LX)

Like the femur and the tibia, the specimens from the middle third of the bone had the greatest mean shearing strength. The distal third specimen had the lowest mean strength, as did the femoral specimens of Evans and Lebow. Because of its small size, only twenty-six fibular specimens were tested and no attempt was made to divide the bone into quadrants. The absence of significant differences in the mean shearing strength of specimens from various thirds of the shaft may be due to the small number of specimens tested.

WET UNEMBALMED TIBIAL BONE (Table LXI)

The mean single shearing strength of 1,126 wet specimens from unembalmed adult human tibias, was highest in specimens from the middle third and the posterior quadrant and lowest in those from the proximal third and anterior quadrant

of the bone. The unembalmed bones differed from the embalmed ones in having the greatest shearing strength in posterior, instead of medial quadrant specimens. However, comparison of the mean shearing strength of 116 embalmed and 126 unembalmed specimens from various regions of adult human tibias revealed no significant differences in mean shearing strength. Thus, if fresh specimens are unavailable, embalmed material may be used satisfactorily for studies on the single shearing strength of adult human cortical bone.

Our results differ somewhat from those of Ibuki who, according to Yamada (1970), reported that the ultimate shearing strength of formalin-fixed cortical bone was 1.05 times that of fresh bone.

Bending Properties

WET UNEMBALMED HUMAN BONE (Table LXII)

Variations in the breaking load (in bending) of standardized specimens of cortical bone from different quadrants of the middle of the shaft of the human humerus, ulna, femur, and tibia from forty subjects ranging from 5 to 90 years of age were reported by Maj (1942). Test specimens 1.2 mm thick, 3 mm wide, and 10-15 mm long, all oriented parallel with the shaft of the bone, were loaded to failure in a clasimeter, a jig especially devel-

TABLE LXI

TOPOGRAPHIC DIFFERENCES IN THE MEAN SINGLE (PUNCHING) SHEARING STRENGTH OF WET UNEMBALMED CORTICAL BONE FROM TIBIAS OF ADULT MEN

Region	No.	lbf/in^2	kgf/mm^2
Proximal third	27	10,903 ± 2,068	7.66 ± 1.45
Middle third	48	11,283 ± 2,366	7.93 ± 1.66
Distal third	51	11,106 ± 1,929	7.81 ± 1.36
Anterior quadrant	33	9,740 ± 2,509	6.85 ± 1.76
Lateral quadrant	33	11,393 ± 1,634	8.01 ± 1.15
Medial quadrant	30	11,707 ± 1,086	8.23 ± 0.76
Posterior quadrant	30	11,794 ± 2,294	8.29 ± 1.61

oped for the purpose. The clasimeter consisted of two knife blades, 7 mm apart, for supporting the specimen while it was loaded at the midpoint. The load was applied in the direction of the smallest dimension of the specimen and recorded in kilograms. The deflection occurring in the specimen was measured in millimeters per 5 kg load by a beam of reflected light magnified one hundred times.

Maj found that the relative strength of the various quadrants, arranged in order from highest to lowest breaking load, was anterior, posterior, lateral, and medial for the humerus; anterior, medial, and posterior (no data were obtained for the lateral) for the ulna; lateral, medial, anterior and posterior for the femur; and medial, lateral, anterior, and posterior for the tibia.

TABLE LXII

Topographic Differences in the Average Breaking Load (kg) in Bending of Unembalmed Human Cortical Bone (Data from Maj, 1942)

Bone	Anterior Quadrant	Medial Quadrant	Posterior Quadrant	Lateral Quadrant
Humerus ...	7.51	6.60	7.37	7.36
Ulna	9.39	8.87	7.17	—
Femur	6.92	6.94	6.02	7.10
Tibia	7.30	7.91	7.26	7.46

Hirsch and da Silva (1967) measured maximal deformation, residual deformation, and energy dissipated by 140 standardized autopsy specimens of femoral cortical bone from twelve subjects 30 to 74 years of age. The specimens were obtained from the lateral and medial aspects of the bone about 5 cm distal to the lesser trochanter. Test specimens were taken, at 10° intervals, at sites from 0° to 90° to the long axis of the shaft of the bone. The specimens were machined under dripping cold water and stored and subjected to bending tests in Ringer's solution.

Stiffness of the specimens progressively decreased as the orientation changed from 0° to 90° with a tendency toward a straight line relationship. An applied load of 0.100 Kp produced a negligible residual deformation. With a 0.250 Kp load, residual deformation was slight, up to a 60° orientation, after which it increased so that at a 90° orientation the load-deformation curve was almost horizontal. Increasing deformation was accompanied by greater energy dissipation. No statistically significant differences among the three variables were found in comparisons between specimens from the lateral and medial aspects nor from superior and inferior regions.

WET UNEMBALMED NONHUMAN BONE (Tables LXIII and LXIV)

Topographic variations in the mechanical properties of specimens from different regions of single nonhuman bones has not been investigated as thoroughly as those for human bones.

Olivo, Maj, and Toajari (1937) reported differences in the breaking load (in bending) and deflections (hundredths of a millimeter per 5 kg load) in small specimens of cortical bone from the same ring or cross section from the metacarpals and metatarsals of an ox and a mule as well as from the femurs of two women. A definite tendency was noted in some cases toward an increase in the breaking load at progressively greater depths within the cortex of the bone (Fig. 105). They also found an average breaking load of 8.0 kg for similar specimens from the anterior part of the femur of a 79-year-old man compared to an average of 8.4 kg for specimens from the posterior part of the same bone.

In a later study Maj (1938b) demonstrated that the breaking load (in bending) varied in different quadrants of ox metatarsal and metacarpal bones and at different levels along the bone (Table LXIII). In all quadrants of both bones

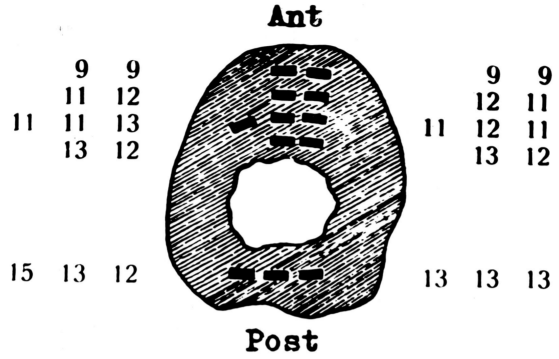

Figure 105. Variation in the breaking load (kg) in bending and deflection 0.01 mm/5 kg load (in parentheses) of specimens from different aspects and depths of the cortex of a mule metatarsal. (From Olivo, Maj, and Toajari, *Boll Sci Med (Bologna)*, 1937)

the breaking load was usually highest in the middle part of the shaft and decreased toward the ends, the decrease being greater at the distal than the proximal end. The relative strength of the various quadrants, in order from highest to lowest average breaking load, was medial, lateral, anterior, and posterior for the metatarsal, and medial, anterior, lateral, and posterior for the metacarpal. Thus, in the ox metatarsal and

TABLE LXIII

REGIONAL DIFFERENCES IN AVERAGE BREAKING LOAD (KG) UNDER
BENDING IN OX COMPACT BONE (Data from Maj, 1938b)

Bone	Distance (cm) from Proximal End of Intact Bone	Medial Quadrant	Lateral Quadrant	Anterior Quadrant	Posterior Quadrant
Metatarstal	7	7.50	9.50	7.25	5.00
	12	11.00	10.00	10.00	7.50
	17	11.20	11.00	10.30	10.00
	22	9.50	9.50	9.50	8.75
	27	6.00	4.00	6.50	4.50
Average		9.04	8.80	8.71	7.15
Metacarpal	5	10.50	9.50	9.00	6.00
	8	10.50	9.50	9.00	8.00
	10	10.50	11.00	10.00	9.00
	15	11.00	12.00	13.50	14.00
	20	4.00	3.00	4.75	3.50
Average		9.30	9.00	9.25	8.10

TABLE LXIV

Regional Differences in the Average Breaking Load (kg) Under Bending of Ox Compact Bone (Data from Maj, 1938)

Bone	Distance (cm) of Specimen from Proximal End	Anterior Quadrant Ext.	Mid.	Int.	Posterior Quadrant Ext.	Mid.	Int.	Lateral Quadrant Ext.	Mid.	Int.	Medial Quadrant Ext.	Mid.	Int.
Metatarsal	7	6		8.5	5			9		10	9		6
	12	10.5	11.5	8	8		7	13		7	13		9
	17	10.5	10.5	10.5	11.5	7	8	15	9	9	13	11.5	10
	22	10		9	10		7.5	9		10	8		11
	27	6.5			4.5			4			6		
Metacarpal	5	7		9.5	6			11		8	12		9
	8	6		10.5	7		9	12		7	12		9
	10	8.5		11.5	11		7	11	13	9	11	7	10
	15	12	14	15.5	16.5	12.6	13.5	14	14	8	10	11	12
	20	4.75			3.5			3			4		

Ext. = eternal; mid. = middle; Int. = internal.

TABLE LXV

Topographic Differences in Mean Torsional Properties of Wet Cortical Bone from Embalmed Femurs of Ten Adult Men

Region	Torsional Shearing Strength No.	lbf/in^2	kgf/mm^2	Shear Modulus No.	$\times 10^4\, lbf/in^2$	kgf/mm^2	Break Energy No.	$\dfrac{in\text{-}lb}{in^2}$	$\dfrac{kg\text{-}mm}{mm^2}$
Proximal third	172	6,429 ± 1,851	4.52 ± 1.30	172	83.8 ± 38.3	589 ± 269	172	1,984 ± 623	35.5 ± 11.1
Middle third	174	6,754 ± 1,979	4.75 ± 1.39	174	92.7 ± 45.9	652 ± 323	174	1,960 ± 587	35.1 ± 10.5
Distal third	69	5,894 ± 1,943	4.14 ± 1.37	69	79.8 ± 48.4	561 ± 340	69	1,821 ± 651	32.6 ± 11.7
Anterior quadrant	165	6,182 ± 1,784	4.35 ± 1.25	165	82.5 ± 38.7	580 ± 272	165	1,835 ± 582	32.8 ± 10.4
Lateral quadrant	82	6,524 ± 1,762	4.59 ± 1.24	82	86.8 ± 47.3	610 ± 333	82	2,055 ± 569	36.8 ± 10.2
Medial quadrant	82	7,194 ± 1,920	5.06 ± 1.35	82	99.5 ± 43.6	699 ± 307	82	2,136 ± 596	38.2 ± 10.7
Posterior quadrant	86	6,310 ± 2,238	4.44 ± 1.57	86	83.1 ± 46.7	584 ± 328	86	1,877 ± 678	33.6 ± 12.1

metacarpal the highest and lowest average breaking load occurred in specimens from the medial and posterior quadrants, respectively.

Even within individual quadrants topographic differences occurred in the breaking load. In the posterior, medial, and lateral quadrants of the metatarsal, the breaking load tended to decrease progressively from the periosteal surface toward the medullary cavity (Table LXIV). The opposite tendency was noted in specimens from the anterior quadrant of both bones.

A similar study was made by Toajari (1938) on specimens obtained from rings of bone from the radius, ulna, and olecranon process of oxen and the metacarpals and metatarsals of oxen, mules, and horses. These bones were chosen because of their peculiar position which, he assumed, made them continuously subjected to a particular stress. He also found that the breaking load (in bending) and the deflection varied with the depth within the cortex and the distance from the proximal end of the bone.

Torsion Properties

WET EMBALMED FEMORAL BONE

We have also found differences, according to the third and quadrant of the bone from which they were obtained, in torsional properties of 415 specimens of wet cortical bone from the embalmed femurs of ten adult men. Embalmed bones were used because intact unembalmed ones were not available.

Torsion specimens of standardized size and shape (Fig. 8E) were tested in a jig especially designed for that purpose (Fig. 16). A notch encircling the middle of the test section of the specimen reduced, if not entirely eliminated, the effects of tensile stresses and strains in the fracture mechanism. Thus, failure of the bone was primarily due to torsional shearing stress.

As mentioned previously, the shearing strength of a material is very difficult to determine because it is almost impossible to insure that the shearing force is uniformly distributed over the cross section of the specimen (Fig. 6). Torsional shear stress (strength) appears to be a function of the diameter of the cylinder tested. Therefore, if we had been able to obtain torsion specimens with a larger diameter than those used in the present study, the chance of having the shear stress more uniformly distributed over the cross section of the specimens would have been greater. Because of the marked effect of drying on the mechanical properties of bone, all specimens were tested wet. For further details of the torsion tests see Chapter 2.

Determination of shearing strength from torsion tests of cylindrical specimens with walls of uniform diameter, as in present studies, insures that the shearing force is more evenly distributed over the cross-sectional area of the specimen than was true for the punching shear tests of earlier experiments.

Maximum mean torsional shearing strength and shear modulus were found in specimens from the middle third of the shaft while those from the proximal third had the greatest mean break energy (Table LXV). Distal third specimens had the lowest mean value for all three mechanical properties. Specimens from the medial quadrant had the highest mean value for all three mechanical properties, followed in descending order by specimens from the lateral, posterior, and anterior quadrants.

The mean value for each of the mechanical properties of the middle third specimens was significantly greater, at better than the 0.01 level, than that of the distal third specimens. Middle third specimens also had a mean torsional shearing strength and shear modulus that was greater, at better than the 0.01 significance level, than those of proximal third specimens. Differences between the break energy of the proximal and middle third specimens and between the shear modulus of the proximal and distal third specimens were not significant.

Medial quadrant specimens had a mean torsional shearing strength, shear modulus, and break energy that were greater, at better than the 0.01 significance level, than those of posterior and anterior quadrant specimens. The difference between the mean shearing strength of the medial and lateral quadrant specimens was significant, at better than the 0.01 level. Lateral quadrant specimens had a mean shearing strength and break energy greater, at better than the 0.01 significance level, than those of the anterior quadrant specimens. Lateral quadrant specimens had a mean break energy greater at the same significance level than that of the posterior quadrant ones. No other significant differences were found.

Comparison of these results with other shear data shows that torsional shearing strength is considerably lower than single (punching) shearing strength although in both studies the shearing force acted on the cross section of the specimen in a direction transverse to its long axis. Rauber (1876) appears to be the only one who has compared the shearing strength of bone transverse to and parallel with the long axis. He reported that five fresh specimens of cortical bone from the femur of a 30-year-old man had an average shearing strength of 16,859 lbf/in² (11.85 kgf/mm²) when cut parallel with but loaded perpendicular to the long axis of the bone, compared to an average strength of only 7,152 lbf/in² (5.03 kgf/mm²) for five other specimens cut perpendicular to but

loaded parallel with the long axis. Rauber's value for shearing strength in the first series of tests is similar to those reported by Evans and Lebow (1951), while the results from the second series more nearly approach the value we found for torsional shearing strength.

In Rauber's tests the specimen was placed through coinciding holes in one center and two side plates. The side plates were fixed while the center plate was pulled from between them, thus shearing off the specimen like a rivet. In Rauber's experiments as well as those of Evans and Lebow the specimen was actually subjected to a double shearing action.

FRESH NONHUMAN BONE

The average maximum torsion strength of specimens from the distal part (the strongest region) of cattle femurs is, according to Yamada (1970), about 1.1 times greater than that of specimens from the middle part (the weakest region) of the bone.

Fatigue Life

WET UNEMBALMED TIBIAL BONE
(Table LXVI)

Regional differences also occur in the fatigue life of standardized specimens of wet unembalmed cortical bone from amputated tibias of adult men. The specimens (Fig. 8D) were tested in a Sonntag flexure fatigue machine at a constant stress of 5,000 lbf/in² (344.7 × 10⁶ dynes/cm²) at a rate of 1,800 cycles per minute. For further details of fatigue testing see Chapter 2.

Comparison of the mean fatigue life on the basis of the third of the shaft from which the specimens were taken showed that the longest and the shortest fatigue life were found in specimens from the middle and the proximal third, respective-

TABLE LXVI

<small>Regional Differences in the Mean Fatigue Life (No. of Cycles to Failure) of Wet Cortical Bone Specimens from Unembalmed Tibias of Adult Men Stress = 5,000 lbf/in² (344.7 × 10⁶ dynes/cm²) ; Rate = 1,800 cycles/minute</small>

Region of Bone	No. of Specimens	Mean	Standard Error
Proximal third	15	1,674,867	1,544,325
Middle third	20	2,792,050	1,941,915
Distal third	23	2,527,478	2,281,676
Anterior quadrant	13	1,765,692	1,747,064
Posterior quadrant	18	3,091,278	2,743,543
Lateral quadrant	14	2,642,214	2,176,670
Medial quadrant	13	1,808,308	1,887,778

ly. A similar comparison on the basis of quadrants of the bone revealed that the longest fatigue life occurred in specimens from the posterior quadrant, followed in descending order by those from the lateral, medial, and anterior quadrants.

None of the above differences between the means were statistically significant.

Impact Snapping Strength

WET UNEMBALMED HUMAN FEMORAL BONE

According to Yamada (1970) specimens from the anterior and the posterior sides of the adult human femur have a much greater impact snapping strength than specimens from the medial and the lateral sides. The impact snapping strength is also anisotropic being 0.26 ± 0.029 kg-cm/mm² (12.1 ± 1.35 ft-lb/in²) in the radial direction and 0.19 ± 0.21 kg-cm/mm² (8.87 ± 0.98 ft-lb/in²) in the tangential direction.

NONHUMAN FEMORAL BONE

It has been reported by Yamada (1970) that the impact snapping strength in the tangential direction of femoral bone of horses is a little greater on the anterior and lateral sides than on the posterior and medial sides. Femoral bone of cattle has an impact strength, in the radial direction, that is a little greater on the anterior than on the other sides. The impact strength in the tangential direction, in order from highest to lowest, is anterior, medial and lateral, and posterior sides.

Cleavage Properties

WET UNEMBALMED TIBIAL BONE

Yamada (1970) reported that the cleavage strength of tibial bone is highest on the lateral and medial sides, next on the posterior side, and least on the anterior side.

WET UNEMBALMED NONHUMAN BONE

Femoral bone from cattle has, according to Yamada (1970), the greatest cleavage strength in the middle and the least in the lower part of the bone.

Hardness

WET EMBALMED FEMORAL BONE
(Table LXVII)

Apparently the first to demonstrate regional differences in bone hardness were Evans and Lebow (1951) who performed Rockwell superficial hardness tests on 121 wet and the same number of air-dried specimens from embalmed femurs of six adult men. They reported that both wet and dry specimens from the middle third of the shaft were the hardest, while those from the proximal third were the softest (Fig. 106).

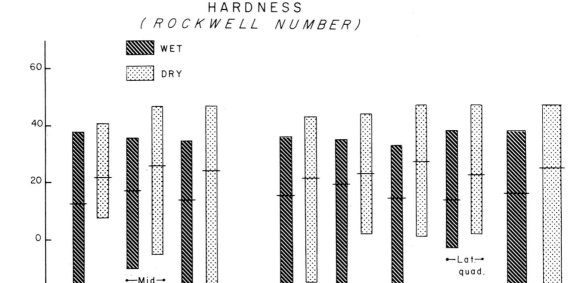

Figure 106. Average and range of variation in the superficial hardness of 121 wet- and 121 dry-tested specimens of cortical bone from different regions of embalmed femurs of 6 adult men. (Based on data from Evans and Lebow: *J Appl Physiol*, 1951)

Such uniformity was not found when the specimens were classified on the basis of the quadrant of the shaft from which they were obtained. Among the wet specimens those from the posterior quadrant were the hardest, followed in decreasing order of hardness by specimens from the anterior, lateral, and medial quadrants. Among the dry specimens the ones from the medial quadrant were the hardest, followed by posterior, lateral, and anterior quadrant specimens. However, the difference between the mean hardness for wet lateral and medial quadrant specimens was only 0.3. The mean hardness for all the dry specimens was greater than that for all the wet ones.

Rockwell superficial hardness tests of 285 wet specimens of embalmed femoral bones of adult humans made in this laboratory also showed that specimens from

the middle third of the bone were the hardest and those from the proximal third the softest (Table LXVII). Posterior quadrant specimens were the hardest, followed in order by medial, lateral, and anterior quadrant specimens. Thus, the order of hardness, according to quadrants, in this material was somewhat different than that of Evans and Lebow (1951). An analysis of variance in our data revealed that the differences between the mean hardness of the middle and proximal third specimens and the posterior and anterior quadrant specimens were significant at better than the 0.01 level. No other significant hardness differences were found.

WET UNEMBALMED FEMORAL BONE

According to Yamada (1970) Japanese investigators found that the hardness of the medial side of the femur exceeded that of the other sides by 1.2 times. It is also less in the distal than in the proximal and middle parts of the shaft.

Wet Embalmed Tibial Bone
(Table LXVII)

Regional differences were also evident in the Rockwell superficial hardness of 115 wet specimens from embalmed adult human tibias tested in this laboratory. Specimens from the middle third of the bone had the hardest and those from the proximal third the softest. When compared by quadrants the mean hardness values, from greatest to least, were found in specimens from the posterior, lateral, medial, and anterior quadrants of the bone. Thus, topographic differences in the mean hardness of wet embalmed tibial specimens are the same as those of femoral specimens when classified by thirds but not when classified by quadrants.

The mean hardness of the middle third specimens was significantly greater, at better than the 0.01 level, than that of the proximal third ones.

Wet Embalmed Fibular Bone
(Table LXVII)

The mean Rockwell superficial hardness of twenty-five wet specimens from embalmed adult human fibulas differed from that of similar femoral and tibial specimens in that distal third specimens were

the hardest and middle third ones the softest. An analysis of variance between the means revealed no significant differences. However, too few specimens were tested for definite conclusions.

Specimens from larger bones were usually harder than those from smaller bones, an observation previously reported by Yamada (1970).

Wet Unembalmed Tibial Bone
(Table LXVII)

Results obtained in this laboratory from tests of the Rockwell superficial hardness of 133 wet specimens from unembalmed tibias of adult humans agree with our results for wet embalmed femoral and tibial specimens, in that specimens from the middle and proximal thirds were the hardest and softest, respectively. They also agree in that the anterior quadrant specimens are the softest. However, they differ from the embalmed femur and tibia in having the medial quadrant specimens, instead of the posterior ones, the hardest. Thus, the differences in the relative hardness of various regions occurs primarily in the medial, lateral, and posterior quadrants of the bone.

There were no significant differences between the mean hardness of various thirds of the bone but the hardness of the posterior, lateral, and medial quadrant specimens was greater, at better than the 0.01

TABLE LXVII

Topographic Differences in Mean Superficial Rockwell Hardness of Wet Adult Human Cortical Bone

Region	No.	Embalmed Femur	No.	Embalmed Tibia	No.	Embalmed Fibula	No.	Unembalmed Tibia
Proximal third	98	11.17 ± 17.25	37	6.89 ± 14.24	8	7.50 ± 11.69	25	−5.80 ± 10.03
Middle third	93	17.01 ± 13.49	39	14.44 ± 6.65	9	5.00 ± 12.74	49	−1.59 ± 10.99
Distal third	94	13.69 ± 17.51	30	13.03 ± 6.96	8	10.63 ± 8.33	59	−3.53 ± 10.75
Anterior quadrant	70	9.70 ± 17.82	30	3.00 ± 10.47	—	—	29	−10.90 ± 11.33
Lateral quadrant	77	10.16 ± 17.75	29	14.31 ± 7.90	—	—	34	−0.65 ± 9.39
Medial quadrant	76	15.13 ± 16.78	28	14.25 ± 6.52	—	—	32	0.53 ± 6.94
Posterior quadrant	67	17.55 ± 16.26	28	15.07 ± 10.52	—	—	38	−2.90 ± 11.43

TABLE LXVIII

TOPOGRAPHIC DIFFERENCES IN THE MEAN VICKERS HARDNESS NUMBERS OF WET, NONHUMAN FEMORAL CORTICAL BONE

(Data from Yamada, 1970)

Layer	Horses	Cattle	Wild Boars	Pigs	Dogs	Cats	Rabbits	Guinea Pigs	Rats	Domestic Fowls
				(Transverse Cross Sections)						
Surface	27.0 ± 0.59	26.5 ± 0.70	25.9 ± 0.35	25.3 ± 0.22	—	—	—	—	—	—
Middle	34.6 ± 0.50	31.6 ± 0.70	31.1 ± 0.40	30.9 ± 0.23	30.6 ± 1.18	37.3 ± 1.51	41.3 ± 1.93	36.3 ± 0.50	38.8 ± 0.96	33.5 ± 2.12
				(Tangential Cross Sections)						
Surface	21.2 ± 0.54	21.6 ± 0.55	21.8 ± 0.70	20.5 ± 0.18	—	—	—	—	—	—
Middle	26.1 ± 0.50	25.8 ± 0.48	25.3 ± 0.46	24.5 ± 0.31	25.3 ± 0.58	30.4 ± 1.60	33.1 ± 1.78	29.5 ± 0.34	31.5 ± 0.77	27.5 ± 1.64

TABLE LXIX

SIGNIFICANT CORRELATION COEFFICIENTS FOR MECHANICAL PROPERTIES OF ADULT HUMAN CORTICAL BONE

Variables	Femur				Tibia				Fibula			
	No.	T	Coefficient	Sig.	No.	T	Coefficient	Sig.	No.	T	Coefficient	Sig.
Modulus vs tensile stress	44	5.701	0.661	>.001	77	3.237	0.350	>.001				
Modulus vs shear stress									43	2.570	0.373	>0.02
Modulus vs hardness	44	4.291	0.552	>.001	77	5.224	0.517	>.001				
Modulus vs density					76	3.609	0.387	>.001				
Tensile stress vs tensile strain	43	5.718	0.666	>.001	72	6.123	0.591	>.001				
Tensile stress vs hardness	45	5.435	0.638	>.001	79	4.409	0.449	>.001				
Tensile stress vs density					78	5.242	0.515	>.001				
Tensile strain vs density					79	3.091	0.332	>.01	25	-4.286	-0.666	>0.001
Shear stress vs hardness					78	2.265	0.251	>.05				
Shear stress vs density									28	5.132	0.709	>0.001
Hardness vs density	17	3.493	0.670	>.01	78	7.781	0.666	>.001	26	4.330	0.662	>0.001

significance level, than of the anterior quadrant specimens.

Wet Unembalmed Nonhuman Femoral Bone (Table LXVIII)

Hardness. Japanese investigators, cited by Yamada (1970), reported that in transverse and tangential cross sections of the femur of various animals, the Vickers hardness value of the surface layer was from 80% to 85% of that of the middle layer. The hardness of both layers (surface and middle) in all animals in the tangential cross sections was about 80% of that in the transverse cross sections.

Density (Table XLII). Differences have also been found in the density of specimens from various regions of adult human femurs, tibias, and fibulas. Femoral and tibial specimens from the middle third of the bone are the most dense and those from the proximal third are the least dense. Distal third fibular specimens are most dense and middle third ones the least dense. Femoral specimens from the posterior quadrant of the shaft are the most dense, followed, in decreasing order of density, by specimens from the medial, lateral, and anterior quadrants. Tibial specimens from the lateral quadrant are the most dense, those from the medial and posterior quadrants are next, and the anterior quadrant specimens are the least dense.

A statistical analysis of the data showed that the difference between the density of the posterior and anterior quadrant femoral specimens was significant at the 0.05 to 0.01 level. No other significant density differences were found for the femoral specimens.

In tibial bone, the difference between the density of the middle third and the proximal third specimens and the density of the lateral quadrant and anterior quadrant specimens in each case was significant at the 0.01 or better level. Density differences between specimens from the posterior and anterior quadrants, from the medial and anterior quadrants, and from the distal and proximal thirds were each significant at the 0.05 to the 0.01 level.

Differences between specimens from various thirds of the fibula were not significant. The fibula was not divided into quadrants because of its small size.

Because of the high correlations between density and mechanical properties of bone, the significant differences between the density of specimens from various regions of the femur and tibia may, in part, account for some of the significant topographic differences in their mechanical properties.

Correlations Between Mechanical Properties of Wet Embalmed Adult Human Cortical Bone

In addition to our investigations of topographic differences in mechanical properties of cortical bone, "t" values and coefficients of correlation were calculated in order to determine if there were any significant correlations between various mechanical properties of femoral, tibial, and fibular bone (Table LXIX).

Among the femoral specimens, significant correlations (> .01) were found between hardness and density, and highly significant ones (> .001) between modulus of elasticity and tensile stress, between modulus and hardness, between tensile stress and tensile strain, and between tensile stress and hardness.

Tibial specimens had a slightly significant correlation (> .05) between single shearing stress and density, a significant correlation between shear stress and hardness, and highly significant correlations between modulus and tensile stress, modulus and hardness, tensile stress and tensile strain, tensile stress and hardness, hardness and density, modulus and density, and tensile stress and density.

Significant correlations between modulus and shear stress, and highly significant ones between hardness and density, shear stress and density, and tensile strain and density were found among the fibular specimens.

CANCELLOUS (SPONGY) BONE

The mechanical properties of cancellous bone have been studied far less thoroughly than those of cortical bone. Cancellous bone is structurally an open cell foam, as a consequence of which it is much more difficult to prepare test specimens and determine their mechanical properties than it is for cortical bone. Most of the studies on mechanical properties of cancellous bone have been made on material obtained from the vertebrae, the femur, or the diploë.

Tensile Properties

Vertebrae. Sonoda (1962), who appears to be the only one who has determined the tensile properties of cancellous bone, reported that fresh moist specimens from thoracic and lumbar vertebrae of people 30 to 39 years of age had a tensile strength of 0.12 ± 0.01 kg/mm² (171 ± 14.22 lbf/ in²) and an ultimate elongation of 0.58 ± 0.03%.

Compressive Properties

Vertebrae (Table LXX). Compressive properties of cancellous bone were first investigated by Rauber (1876) who reported that four fresh cubes of spongy bone from the interior part of an adult human lumbar vertebra had an average compressive strength of 0.84 kgf/mm² (1,194 lbf/in²).

Messerer (1880) found that the mean compressive strength of fresh specimens of cancellous bone from thoracic and lumbar vertebrae of adult men was greater in specimens from the upper vertebrae of each region than in similar specimens from the lower vertebrae.

Intact vertebral bodies, because they consist almost entirely of cancellous bone, have also been used for determinations of its mechanical properties. One of the most thorough studies of this type was made by Göcke (1928) who tested vertebral bodies under static, impact, and rhythmic continuous (fatigue) loading. Specimens of standardized size and shape, taken from the interior of the vertebral bodies, were also tested.

Static loading tests were made with a five ton Amsler-Laffon press. Compressive strain (decrease in height of the body during a test) was measured by a precision gauge with a 0.01 mm scale division. For impact tests a 6.085 kg (13.4 lb) weight was dropped on the specimen through a distance of 2 m (6.6 ft). Rhythmic impact tests were made with a Krupp impact fatigue machine using a 4.185 kg (9.2 lb) weight and a drop height varying from 1 to 20 mm (0.039 to 0.78 in). A stamp mill with a 2 kg (4.4 lb) hammer was also used.

Göcke expressed the results of his experiments as load-deformation curves and usually reported the breaking load rather than the ultimate compressive strength. In some of the rhythmic (fatigue) loading tests, compressive strain (% shortening), elasticity curves, and energy (mkg) were also given.

A load-deformation curve, which Göcke states is typical for cancellous bone as a whole, shows that a cube of spongy bone from the second lumbar vertebra of a 29-

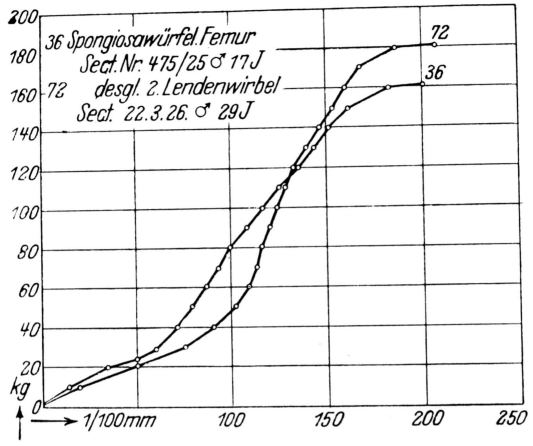

Figure 107. Compressive load-deformation curves for cubes of cancellous bone from the femur of a 17-year-old (curve 36) and the 2nd lumbar vertebrae of a 29-year-old man (curve 72). (From Göcke: *Bruns Beitr Klin Chir*, 1928)

year-old man (Fig. 107, curve 72) had a prominent elastic contraction of 1.0 mm (0.039 in) up to a load of 50 kg (132 lb), a proportional limit at a load of 170 kg (375 lb), and an ultimate compressive strength of 0.45 kg/mm² (640 lbf/in²). According to Göcke, the first part of the curve showing a gentle rise with small loads is unusual for most materials.

Göcke determined the compressive strength of some of his specimens by applying large static loads in the Amsler press. The first load was performed as a control in order to establish the dynamic characteristics for the particular specimen.

A neighboring vertebra was then subjected to repeated loading up to its proportional limit. In the 12th thoracic (control) vertebra of a 35-year-old man who died from appendicitis (Fig. 108, curve 7), the proportional limit was at 900 kg (1,985 lb) and failure at 1,050 kg (2,315 lb). When the second lumbar vertebral body of the same man was subjected to a prestress of 700 kg (1,544 lb) repeated three times, the curve became steeper and shorter indicating a reduction in plasticity and total endurance capacity (Fig. 108, curve 9). Although the structure of the specimen was more dense it was not improved from the technical standpoint. Prestressing the specimen beyond the proportional limit by application of a 900 kg (1,985 lb) load reinforced the condition. Similar but less extensive effects were produced in the first lumbar vertebral body of the same subject by a 500 kg (1,103 lb) load applied three times for forty-five seconds each time (Fig. 108, curve 8).

In static loading tests of the uninjured fifth thoracic vertebra of a 21-year-old man, who died as a result of a fall from a window, Göcke found a compressive strength of 0.485 kgf/mm² (690 lbf/in²) the first time the specimen was tested. Retesting the specimen four additional times with the same near failure load, showed that its deformation had increased from

330/100 mm (15%) to 395/100 mm (18.6%).

Variations in the dynamic behavior under impacts of the 11th thoracic through the 2nd lumbar vertebrae from a 51-year-old athletic man who died from cirrhosis of the liver were also investigated. In order to compare the results for different vertebrae, Göcke mathematically reduced all of them to the height of the 12th thoracic vertebra which was used as the control. The maximum load and contraction of this vertebra were 750 kg (1,654 lb) and 3.6 mm (12.8%), respectively (Fig. 109, curve 16). The other vertebrae were divided into two test groups. The vertebrae of the first group were subjected to nonfracturing impacts while the vertebrae in

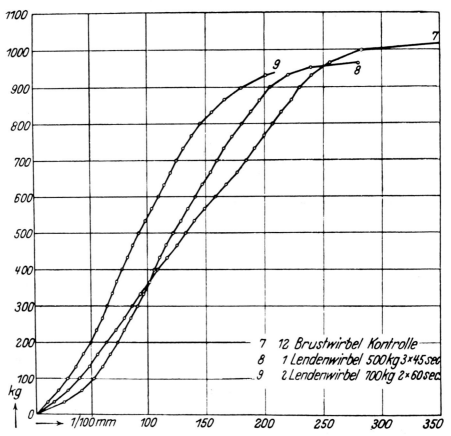

Figure 108. Compressive load-deformation curves for repetitive loading of vertebrae of a 35-year-old man. See text for explanation. (From Göcke: *Bruns Beitr Klin Chir,* 1928)

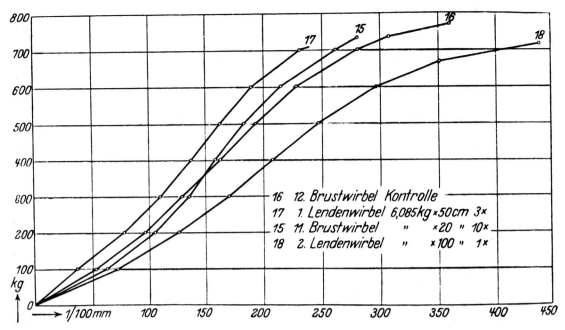

Figure 109. Compressive load-deformation curves for impact loading of the 11th thoracic through 2nd lumbar vertebrae of a 51-year-old man. See text for explanation. (From Göcke: *Bruns Beitr Klin Chir,* 1928)

the second group were tested with impacts exceeding those necessary for failure. Tests of the 11th thoracic vertebra with a nonfracturing impact or 1.217 mkg (8.802 ft-lb), repeated ten times at 0.25 minute intervals, produced a steeper load-deformation curve, indicating a reduced plasticity without any essential decrease in fracture strength (Fig. 109, curve 15). The first lumbar vertebral body was tested with three impacts of 3.04 mkg (21.99 ft-lb) each and the second lumbar vertebra with an impact of 6.085 mkg (44.02 ft-lb). In both of these the failure limit of the vertebrae was exceeded. Göcke found that the impacts applied to the first lumbar vertebra increased its stiffness (Fig. 109, curve 17) while the second lumbar vertebra suffered a typical strain fracture with a permanent deformation of 3.5 mm (Fig. 109, curve 18). In spite of the splintering of the vertebral margin the remaining un-

damaged part of the vertebra continued to support a surprisingly high load without failure.

For the rhythmic continuous loading (fatigue) tests, the body of the vertebrae was divided exactly in half along the midline—one half of it then being subjected to rhythmic repetitive impacts while the other half was tested under static loading in the Amsler press. In the repetitive loading tests, Göcke points out that it must be assumed that some of the impact energy was absorbed by the transverse elasticity of the 7 mm thick steel protective plate at the side of the specimen.

In fatigue studies of vertebrae from an 18-year-old man killed by a shot in the head, an impact of 0.027 mkg (0.196 ft-lb) was applied to half of the body of the fourth lumbar vertebra one thousand times, to the third lumbar vertebra two thousand times, and to the first lumbar vertebra four thousand times. The opposite halves of these vertebrae were the controls. In order to make the load-deformation curves comparable all the vertebrae were plotted to a uniform height of 30 mm (1.18 in).

Application of one thousand impacts with an energy of 27 mkg (1,000 × 0.027 mkg) to half the fourth lumbar vertebra, increased its density, reduced its plasticity, but did not change its failure limit (Fig. 110, curve 40). The two thousand impacts and 54 mkg of energy applied to half of the third lumbar vertebra enhanced these changes with a much reduced failure point (Fig. 110, curve 42). Still greater reduction in plasticity and ultimate limit occurred with four thousand impacts and an energy of 108 mkg (781 ft-lb) during the forty minutes of the test of half of the first

lumbar vertebra (Fig. 110, curve 44). Examination of the specimen with a magnifying glass disclosed fractures in the surface layer below the steel plate. However, the fractures did not extend into the specimen for a distance of more than 2 mm and no fracture was seen for 95% of the height of the vertebra although its strength characteristics and plasticity as a whole were modified. No new relationships were found for the control half specimens (Fig. 110, curves 41, 43, 45).

Not only did Göcke find differences in the compressive properties from one vertebral body to another but also in different regions of a single body. Thus, the center of the body of an externally normal appearing ninth thoracic vertebra of a 62-year-old man had a maximum compressive strength of 0.44 kg/mm² (626 lbf/in²)

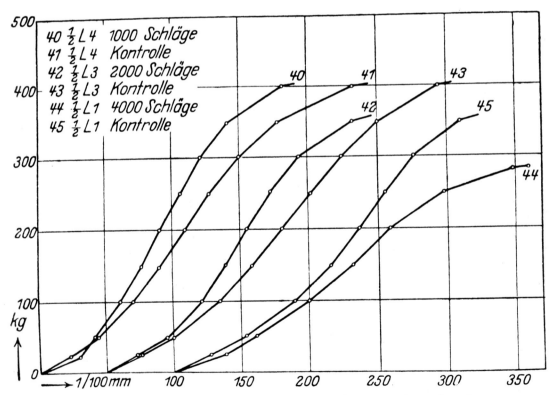

Figure 110. Compressive load-deformation curves for fatigue tests of vertebrae from an 18-year-old man. (From Göcke: *Bruns Beitr Klin Chir,* 1928)

compared to a maximum of 0.60 kg/mm² (853 lbf/in²) for a specimen from the anterior margin and 0.46 kg/mm² (654 lbf/in²) for a specimen from the posterior margin of the same vertebral body. Specimens from regions intermediate in position had intermediate values for compressive strength.

Yokoo (1952a) reported that the compressive stress (strength) and strain, of standardized specimens from lumbar vertebral bodies of people 40 to 49 years of age were greater than in similar specimens from people 60 to 69 years of age. However, the compressive strength of intact vertebral bodies exceeded that of the standardized specimens.

Sonoda (1962) demonstrated that the compressive strength and strain of intact vertebral bodies of people 20 to 39 years of age progressively decreased in a superior-inferior direction being greatest in cervical, next in thoracic, and least in lumbar vertebrae. Even within the thoracic region, the compressive strength and strain decreased from the upper, through the middle, to the lower vertebrae of the region.

Recently the compressive properties of 288 specimens of vertebral bone from seventy-two individuals, one month to 89 years of age, were determined by McElhaney et al. (1970b). The test specimens varied from intact vertebral bodies with the neural arches removed to 0.25 in³ (4.097 cm³) cubes of cancellous bone from within the bodies. All specimens were obtained at autopsy and usually tested within four days after death of the subject. Between time of removal of the specimens and testing they were stored in an isotonic saline solution buffered with calcium. All specimens were tested in the moist condition.

McElhaney et al. found a lower mean compressive strength than did Rauber, Messerer, Sonoda, Göcke, although it is higher than that reported by Yokoo and Galante et al. (Table LXX). The mean modulus of elasticity of the 288 specimens tested by McElhaney et al. was 220,000 ± 170,000 lbf/in² (154.7 ± 119.5 kgf/mm²) which is higher than that obtained by Yokoo (1952a) who gave an average modulus of 12,798 lbf/in² (9 kgf/mm²) for fresh cancellous bone from lumbar vertebrae of people 40 to 49 years of age and an average of 9,954 lbf/in² (7 kgf/mm²) for those 60 to 69 years of age.

In contrast to all the other investigators, McElhaney et al. determined Poisson's ratio for twenty-eight vertebral bodies from seven individuals varying from 45 to 79 years of age. They obtained an average value of 0.14 ± 0.09 which is higher than the Poisson's ratio they reported for cortical femoral bone, cranial bone alone, and full section cranial bone (*cf.* Table XLVI).

The higher values McElhaney et al. give for compressive strength and modulus of elasticity may be the results of (1) the wide age range (1 month to 89 years) in the subjects from whom their material was obtained and (2) the large number of specimens (288) tested. Because of the large number of specimens tested and the broad age range represented in their material, the mechanical property values obtained by McElhaney et al. are probably the most truly representative of the compressive strength and modulus of elasticity of cancellous bone in vertebral bodies.

McElhaney et al. account for their results on the basis of the structural arrangement of the trabeculae within the vertebral bodies. They consider compressive strength and modulus of elasticity as structural as well as mechanical properties. The large standard deviations they found in the values for these properties were attributed to variations in the porosity and in-

TABLE LXX

Mean Compressive Strength and Strain Under Static Loading in the Longitudinal Direction of Human Cancellous Vertebral Bone

Author	Vertebra	No. of Subjects	Age & Sex	No. of Spec.	Compressive Strength kgf/cm²	lbf/in²	Compressive Strain (%)
Rauber (1876)	lumbar	1	adult	4	84.0	1,194	
Messerer (1880)	T1	3	25-51 yrs	3	66.0	939	
	T6	4	25-56 yrs	4	67.0	953	
	T10	4	25-56 yrs	4	58.0	825	
	L1	5	25-81 yrs	4	52.0	739	
	L4	3	34-80 yrs	3	39.0	555	
	L5	4	25-56 yrs	4	59.0	839	
Göcke (1928)	T5	1	21, male	1	49.0	690	15
	L2	1	29, male	1	45.0	640	
	T9						
	center	1	62, male	1	44.0	626	
	anterior	1	62, male	1	60.0	853	
	posterior	1	62, male	1	46.0	654	
Yokoo (1952a)	L	5	40-49 yrs	—	19.0	270	2.5
			60-69 yrs	—	14.0	199	2.4
	vertebrae	—	—	—	61.0	867	5.8
Sonoda (1962)	cervical	—	20-39 yrs	—	127.0 ± 2.0	1,806 ± 28	8.1 ± 0.08
	upper thoracic	—	20-39 yrs	—	88.0 ± 0.02	1,251 ± 28	7.4 ± 0.15
	middle thoracic	—	20-39 yrs	—	78 ± 1.0	1,109 ± 14	6.6 ± 0.11
	lower thoracic	—	20-39 yrs	—	73 ± 1.0	1,038 ± 14	5.6 ± 0.08
	lumbar	—	20-39 yrs	—	64.0 ± 1.0	910 ± 14	5.6 ± 0.08
McElhaney, Alem & Roberts (1970)	vertebral bodies	72	1 mo-89 yrs	288	42.0 ± 35.0	600 ± 500	
Galante, Rostoker, & Ray (1970)	L3 or L4	23	Not stated	72	20.99 ± 2.57		

ternal arrangement of the trabeculae. To aid in explaining their results they developed a porous block model. Such a single material model was justified, on the basis of correlations reported in the literature, between mechanical properties and histological structure of cortical bone.

According to their model, the modulus of elasticity of bone is approximately proportional to the third power of the density which they found to be 0.017 ± 0.007 lbf/in³ (1.26 ± 0.52 kgf/mm²). Thus,

slight porosity changes in low relative density bone produces small strength and modulus of elasticity variations, while similar porosity changes in high relative density bone causes large variations in strength and modulus. Consequently, porosity distribution in a given bone specimen has more significant effects on strength and modulus in low than in high relative density bone.

Specimen size had no significant effect on the values for compressive strength and modulus of elasticity of intact vertebral bodies with the neural arches removed and of cubes of cancellous bone from within the bodies. This is contrary to data given by Yokoo (*cf.* Table LXX) and by Rockoff et al. (1969) who reported that usually 45% to 75% of the peak compressive load applied to an intact vertebral body with flat ends was supported by the cortical bone of the vertebra, regardless of the density or the percent ash of the cancellous bone within the specimen. However, Rockoff et al. used lumbar vertebrae only, which Sonoda (*cf.* Table LXX) reported were weaker than cervical and thoracic ones, and did not load their specimens to failure.

Recently, the relation of the compressive strength of human cancellous bone to its density was investigated by Galante et al. (1970). Cylindrical test specimens 10 mm long but of varying diameters were taken from the 3rd and the 4th lumbar vertebrae of twenty-three subjects within twenty-four hours after death. The experiments were divided into three series. In the first series, consisting of seventeen specimens, the relation between compressive strength and density was studied. In the second series of forty-six specimens, the effects of specimen orientation on compressive strength was investigated. In the third series the topic of study was the effect of deformation rate on compressive strength.

For these experiments, two types of density were calculated—real density and apparent density. Real density was calculated by dividing the wet weight by the volume of the bone matrix as determined by water displacement. Apparent density was computed by dividing the wet weight by the total specimen volume. The percent porosity of the specimens was obtained by dividing the apparent density by the real density and multiplying the quotient by 100. Ash weight per specimen volume was likewise computed.

In the first series of experiments, Galante et al. found a mean compressive strength of 20.99 ± 2.57 Kp/cm^2 for seventeen specimens, 10 mm $\times$ 10 mm, cut along the vertical axis of the vertebra and loaded at a rate of 0.1 cm/min. A kilopond (Kp) is the force that gives a mass of 1 kg an acceleration of 9.80665 m/s^2. Gravitational acceleration varies between 9.78 and 9.83 m/s^2. Thus, the value for force in kiloponds is approximately equivalent to the value for force in kilograms. For this reason and for the sake of uniformity, the value Galante et al. obtained for mean compressive strength is given in kg/cm^2 (Table LXX). Examination of the data in Table LXX shows that only Yokoo, for cancellous bone from lumbar vertebrae, found lower compressive strength values than Galante et al.

Some significant relations were found by Galante et al. between the compressive strength and density of their specimens. Compressive strength varied directly with apparent density and a straight line could be fitted, by the method of least squares, with a 0.01 significance. An equally significant regression was found between compressive strength and dry weight as well as ash weight per specimen volume. Compressive strength and real density had a negative regression at the same significance level, indicating that the denser the specimen, the lower its compressive strength. Negative regressions at the same significance level, were likewise found between compressive strength and dry weight per bone volume. In the other two series of experiments there were no significant negative regressions between compressive strength and real density.

In the second series of experiments, forty-six specimens, 7 mm $\times$ 10 mm, were cut along the anterior-posterior, the medial-lateral, and the superior-inferior axes of the vertebrae and tested at a deformation rate of 0.1 cm/min. In addition to their compressive strength, their real and apparent densities were determined.

In the superior-inferior direction, the mean compressive strength was 20.90 ± 1.61 kgf/cm² (297.20 ± 22.89 lbf/in²), in the anterior-posterior direction it was 8.51 ± 1.27 kgf/cm² (121.01 ± 18.06 lbf/in²), and in the bilateral direction it was 7.37 ± 1.05 kgf/cm² (104.80 ± 14.93 lbf/in²). Although the linear regressions relating compressive strength and apparent density were significantly different for each direction, the slopes of the lines were not. No correlations were found between compressive strength and real density.

The mean apparent density was 0.21 ± 0.001 g/cm³ for the specimens cut in the superior-inferior direction; 0.23 ± 0.02 g/cm³ for those cut in the anterior-posterior direction; and 0.23 ± 0.01 g/cm³ for the ones cut in the medial-lateral direction. Real density values for the three types of specimens were 1.83 ± 0.40 g/cm³, 1.79 ± 0.40 g/cm³, and 1.91 ± 0.10 g/cm³, respectively.

In the third series of experiments twenty-four specimens were loaded to failure at deformation rates of 0.01 and 1 cm/min. Specimens tested at a deformation rate of 1.00 cm/min had a mean compressive strength of 31.33 ± 3.75 kgf/cm², a mean apparent density of 0.22 ± 0.02 g/cm³, and a mean real density of 1.90 ± 0.01 g/cm³. Specimens loaded at a deformation rate of 0.01 cm/min had a mean compressive strength of 2.184 ± 3.83 kgf/cm², a mean apparent density of 0.20 ± 0.02 g/cm³, and a mean real density of 1.96 ± 0.01 g/cm³. The compressive strength of the two groups and the relation between strength and apparent den-

sity were significant at the 0.01 level but there was no correlation between compressive strength and real density.

Data obtained by Galante et al. suggests that apparent density is more important than real density in determining the compressive strength of trabecular bone. Thus, there is a direct linear relationship between compressive strength and apparent density —as one increases, so does the other. The same correlation was found between dry weight and ash weight as related to total specimen volume. However, apparent density was a more realistic entity and varied less around predicted regression lines. The key factor in causing apparent density changes is the volume of the void spaces, which is closely related to tissue strength. Major compressive strength changes are produced by minor porotic changes. The authors believe that the correlation between compressive strength and apparent density allows the investigation of more subtle biological variations influencing the compressive strength of trabecular bone.

Real density of trabecular bone, as pointed out by the authors, is a function of its composition—organic matrix, water, and mineral—and its increase is primarily the result of an increase in its relative mineral content. An increase in the real density was accompanied by a decrease in compressive strength, but the relation was not always statistically significant.

Orientational effects demonstrated in their experiments explain, in part, the anisotropy found in vertebral specimens. Regression equations excluded the possibility of variations induced by apparent density changes. Variations noted in the mean compressive strength of specimens tested at different strain rates suggested, in the author's opinion, indicate a complex rheological behavior.

Femur. Data on the mechanical properties of cancellous bone from long bones are not as abundant as those for vertebrae. Most of the data available pertain to femoral cancellous bone.

Examination of available literature revealed that the first investigation on mechanical properties of cancellous bone from human femurs was made by Rauber (1876) who reported that four fresh cubic specimens from the interior of a condyle of the femur of an adult man had an average compressive strength of 0.0625 kgf/mm² (88.88 lbf/in²).

Hardinge (1949) determined the force required to punch out little round pieces of cancellous bone from five cross sections

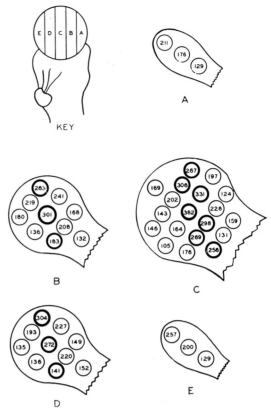

Figure 112. Average force (lbs) required to crush cancellous bone in cross sections of the femoral head and neck. (From Hardinge: *Surg Gynecol Obstet,* 1949)

of the head and neck of ninety-four femurs (sixty from men and thirty-four from women) from embalmed dissecting room cadavers (Figs. 111, 112). The data were reported as the average force (lbs) required to crush the specimens, not the strength (force per unit area) as suggested in the title of Hardinge's paper.

Although Hardinge demonstrated considerable topographic variation in crushing force from one cross section to another as well as in different parts of the same section (Figs. 111, 112), his data revealed a band, extending from the superior aspect of the head to the inferior aspect of the neck adjacent to the head (Fig. 113), in

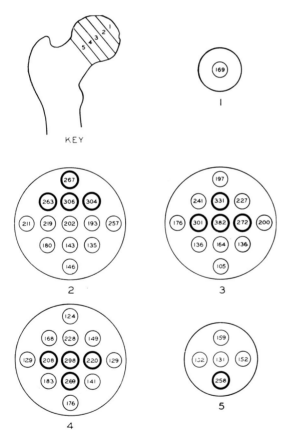

Figure 111. Average force (lbs) required to crush cancellous bone in cross sections of the femoral head and neck. (From Hardinge: *Surg Gynecol Obstet,* 1949)

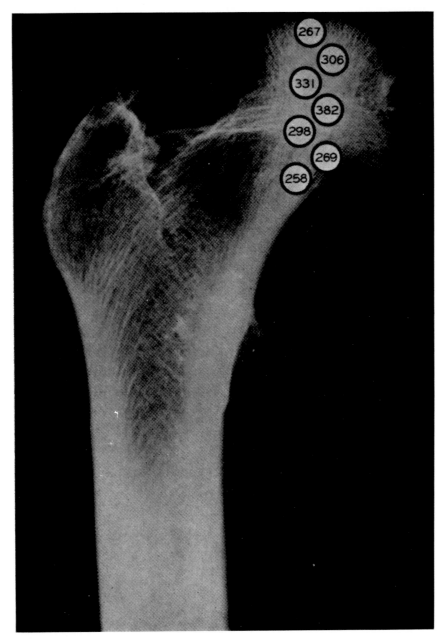

Figure 113. Areas of femoral head and neck requiring the largest average force to crush the cancellous bone. (From Hardinge: *Surg Gynecol Obstet,* 1949)

which the force was greater than in other adjacent regions.

Regional as well as directional differences in the compressive properties of cancellous bone from adult human long bones were shown by Knese (1958) who present-

ed his results as stress-strain curves. The shape of his curves are similar to those given by Göcke (1928). Thus, curves for a tibial condylar specimen loaded in a proximal-distal direction, and for fibular condylar specimens, one from the anterior and one from the posterior part—loaded in a transverse and a dorsal-ventral (front-to-back) direction, respectively, are all slightly s-shaped (Fig. 68). The first part of all three curves indicate a region of strengthening followed by a region of proportionality which, in the tibial condylar specimen loaded longitudinally, amounts to 90%, in the anterior fibular condylar specimen loaded transversely to 45.7%, and in the posterior fibular condylar cubes loaded dorsal-ventrally to 85.8% of the breaking load. The relative strain for the three specimens was 49.2%, 22.8%, and 60.5%, respectively. The modulus of elasticity of the tibial condylar cubes loaded longitudinally was 623 kg/cm²; of the anterior fibular condylar cube 518 kg/cm²; and of the posterior cube 1,565 kg/cm², respectively.

The head of the same femur was sectioned frontally and a cube from the anterior half was compressed in a dorsal-ventral direction. This cube had a compressive breaking strength of 116.5 kg/cm², and an elasticity modulus within the proportional limit of 580 kg/cm² (Fig. 114). A specimen from the posterior half, when compressed in the direction of the femoral neck, had a strength of 96.3 kg/cm² and an elastic modulus of 887 kg/cm². Thus, as Knese points out, specimens from the femoral head exhibit smaller directional differences in compressive strength than do specimens from the tibial and fibular condyles.

Differences in the compressive properties of standardized specimens of cancellous bone from various parts of the femur have been investigated most thoroughly by

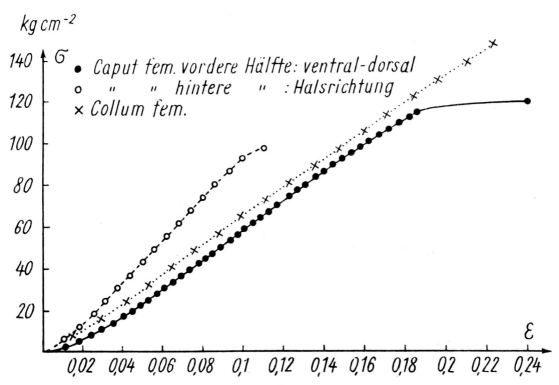

Figure 114. Compressive stress-strain curves for unembalmed femoral cubes of cancellous human bone. (From Knese: *Zwanglose Abhandlungen aus dem Gebiet der Normalen und Pathologischen Anatomie.* Courtesy of Georg Thieme)

TABLE LXXI

TOPOGRAPHIC DIFFERENCES IN MEAN COMPRESSIVE PROPERTIES OF WET CANCELLOUS BONE FROM
EMBALMED ADULT HUMAN FEMUR (Data from Evans and King, 1961)

Region	No.	Strength lbf/in	Strength kgf/mm²	No.	Modulus lbf/in²	Modulus kgf/mm²	No.	Failure Strain %	No.	Energy absorbed in-lb/in³	Energy absorbed kg-cm/cm³
Head	20	545 ± 161	77.5 ± 22.9	19	41,671 ± 1,270	5,926 ± 181	19	3.3 ± 1.6	19	8.00 ± 7.38	0.562 ± 0.519
Lateral condyle	16	362 ± 308	51.5 ± 43.8	13	40,395 ± 3,348	5,821 ± 476	15	2.7 ± 2.2	13	4.89 ± 2.05	0.344 ± 0.144
Medial condyle	4	333 ± 212	47.4 ± 30.1	23	29,947 ± 22,441	4,258 ± 3,191	23	2.2 ± 2.8		3.81 ± 2.37	0.268 ± 0.167
Greater trochanter	4	97 ± 47	13.8 ± 6.7	1	5,280	828	4	2.6 ± 0.4	3	2.79 ± 0.19	0.196 ± 0.013
Neck		627 ± 328	89.2 ± 46.6	5	55,960 ± 29,720	7,958 ± 4,226	5	2.0 ± 0.4	5	6.98 ± 3.72	0.491 ± 0.262

Evans and King (1961). Test specimens of two types—rectangular prisms 2.5 cm long and 0.79 cm on a side with a slenderness ratio of about 11:4, and 0.79 cm cubes—were taken from eleven embalmed dissecting room cadavers. The rectangular prisms (standard specimens), whose long axis was cut in various directions, were taken from different regions of the bone (Fig. 14), while the cubic specimens were obtained from the femoral head and condyles. A total of ninety-one rectangular and sixteen cubic specimens were tested. All specimens were kept in a physiological saline solution and tested wet in a 5,000-lb capacity Riehle materials testing machine calibrated to an accuracy of $\pm 1\%$.

Evans and King found that the prismatic (standard) specimens from the femoral head had the greatest mean compressive strength (Table LXXI) followed, in descending order, by specimens from the lateral condyle, medial condyle, neck, and greater trochanter. Mean modulus of elasticity was highest in the neck, followed, in order from highest to lowest, by specimens from the head, lateral condyle, medial condyle, and greater trochanter (one specimen only). Compressive strain was highest in specimens from the head, followed by those from the lateral condyle, greater trochanter, medial condyle, and neck. Specimens from the head also absorbed the most energy to failure, followed, in descending order, by specimens from the neck, lateral condyle, medial condyle, and greater trochanter. Thus, specimens from the head had the greatest compressive strength, strain, and absorbed the most energy. Greater trochanter specimens were the weakest and absorbed the least energy.

An analysis of variance between the means revealed that the difference between the compressive strain of the head specimens—the highest, and that of medial condylar specimens—the lowest, was significant at better than the 0.01 confidence level. The difference between the compressive strength of the neck specimens (highest) and that of the greater trochanteric specimens (lowest) was significant at the 0.02 confidence level. The same was true of the difference between the energy absorbing capacity of the head specimens (greatest) and that of the medial condylar specimens (least).

Comparison of the stress-strain curves for standard (prismatic) specimens and that for cubic specimens showed that the former were stiffer, i.e. had the higher modulus of elasticity (Fig. 71).

SUMMARY

Comparison of the mean values for mechanical properties of standardized specimens of wet, unembalmed adult human cortical bone showed that radial bone has the highest tensile and bending strength, and the greatest ultimate specific deflection in bending; fibular bone exhibits the greatest tensile and compressive strain, the longest fatigue life, and the highest modulus of elasticity; femoral bone has the greatest compressive and shearing strength (perpendicular to the long axis) and is the hardest.

Compressive strength, modulus of elasticity, and Poisson's ratio are highest in femoral bone, followed, in descending order, by cranial cortical bone, full section cranial bone when tested in the tangential direction, and full section cranial bone when tested in the radial direction. Full section cranial bone means the specimens tested consisted of the outer and inner tables of cortical bone separated by diploë. The only cortical bone for which Poisson's ratio has been determined was obtained from the femur and the skull.

Femoral bone has the lowest tensile and bending strength, tensile and compressive

strain, ultimate displacement in shear, ultimate specific deflection in bending, and the
shortest fatigue life. Radial bone has the
lowest compressive and shearing strength;
humeral bone has the lowest modulus of
elasticity; and ulnar bone is the softest.

Specimens from the middle third of the
shaft have the highest average tensile
strength (humerus, femur, tibia); compressive strength (tibia); single (punching) shear strength (femur, tibia, fibula);
torsion strength (femur); longest fatigue
life (femur); and are the hardest (femur, tibia). Fibular specimens from the
proximal third have the highest tensile
strength and those from the distal third
are the hardest.

Middle third specimens from the femur
and fibula have the highest modulus of
elasticity. Comparable specimens from the
humerus and tibia have the greatest percent elongation. Distal third humeral and
tibial specimens have the highest modulus
while proximal third femoral and fibular
specimens exhibit the most elongation.

Proximal third specimens have the lowest tensile strength (humerus, femur, tibia), compressive strength (tibia), single
shear strength (femur, tibia, fibula), shortest fatigue life (femur), and are the softest (femur, tibia). Femoral specimens
from the distal third have the lowest torsion strength, and fibular specimens from
the middle third are the softest. Specimens
from the proximal third have the lowest
modulus (humerus, femur, tibia, fibula)
and least elongation (humerus, tibia). Distal third femoral and fibular specimens
showed the least elongation.

Anterior quadrant specimens of femoral
and tibial bone have the minimum value
for mechanical properties more often
than specimens from other quadrants. No
such consistency is found with respect to
maximum mechanical property values.

Tensile property values for specimens
from the three major upper limb bones are
greater than those for comparable specimens from homologous lower limb bones.
Specimens from the proximal bones of the
limbs have tensile property values exceeding those of specimens from distal limb
bones. The mean value for the compressive properties of specimens from the
three major lower limb bones are greater
than those for similar specimens from
comparable upper limb bones. Specimens
from small bones usually have a higher
mean tensile strength and strain than those
from large bones. Large bone specimens
generally have a higher mean compressive
strength and hardness than small bone
specimens.

Many of the differences in mean mechanical property values for specimens
from different bones as well as those for
specimens from different regions of the
same bone are statistically significant (Table LXXII).

Cancellous bone from adult human femurs exhibits considerable regional variation in the mean values for its mechanical
properties. Compressive strength and modulus of elasticity are greater in the neck
while strain and energy absorbed at failure
are highest in the head of the bone. The
greater trochanter has the lowest compressive strength, modulus of elasticity, and
absorbs the least energy. The neck has the
lowest strain at failure.

The difference between the mean compressive strain of the head specimens and
that of the medial condyle specimens was
significant at the 0.01 confidence level. The
difference between the mean compressive
strength of the neck and that of the greater trochanter was significant at the 0.02
confidence level. The same was true for
the difference between the mean energy ab-

TABLE LXXII

STATISTICALLY SIGNIFICANT DIFFERENCES BETWEEN THE MEANS FOR MECHANICAL PROPERTIES OF
WET ADULT HUMAN CORTICAL BONE

Property	Embalmed		Unembalmed	
	1% or Better*	Between 5% and 1%*	1% or Better*	Between 5% and 1%*
Variation Among Bones				
Ult. tensile strength	Tibia > Femur Fibula > Femur		Tibia > Femur Fibula > Femur	Tibia > Fibula
Tensile strain (% elongation)	Tibia > Femur			
Modulus of elasticity (in tension)	Tibia > Femur Fibula > Femur	Fibula > Tibia	Tibia > Femur Fibula > Femur	
Single shear strength	Tibia > Femur	Fibula > Femur	Tibia > Femur Fibula > Femur	
Rockwell superficial hardness				Fibula > Femur Tibia > Fibula
Variation Within Bones				
Ult. tensile strength	Femur M/3 > P/3	Tibia AQ > MQ		Tibia M/3 > D/3
Tensile strain (% elongation)	Femur LQ > PQ Femur MQ > PQ Tibia AQ > PQ	Femur D/3 > P/3 Femur AQ > PQ Tibia M/3 > P/3 Tibia AQ > LQ Tibia AQ > MQ		
Modulus of elasticity (in tension)	Femur M/3 > P/3	Femur PQ > AQ Tibia AQ > MQ		
Single shear strength	Tibia M/3 > P/3	Femur M/3 > D/3	Tibia PQ > AQ Tibia LQ > AQ Tibia MQ > AQ	
Rockwell superficial hardness	Femur M/3 > P/3 Tibia M/3 > P/3 Tibia PQ > AQ Tibia LQ > AQ Tibia MQ > AQ	Femur PQ > LQ Tibia D/3 > P/3	Tibia PQ > AQ Tibia LQ > AQ Tibia MQ > AQ	

* Significance level.

AQ = anterior quadrant; LQ = lateral quadrant; MQ = medial quadrant; PQ = posterior quadrant. P/3 = proximal third; M/3 = middle third; D/3 = distal third.

sorbed to failure by the head specimens and the medial condyle specimens.

Specimens from the long bones of nonhuman animals also exhibit differences in their mechanical properties. However, the values for the properties of specimens from different limbs and limb segments do not show the rather consistent relationships seen in human material. There is also considerable species variation in the mechanical properties of homologous bones.

In all bones (human and nonhuman), compressive strength and strain are greater than tensile strength and strain. Values found for compressive modulus by various investigators are less than those for tensile modulus. However, in any given specimen, tensile and compressive modulus are probably the same.

Adult human cortical bone from the cranium has tensile properties, determined in a direction tangent to the skull surface, whose mean values are intermediate with those of similar specimens from long bones. Cranial bone is transversely isotropic whereas long bone specimens are highly anisotropic.

Full section cranial bone (outer and inner tables of cortical bone separated by diploë) has a mean compressive strength in the radial direction (perpendicular to the skull surface) that is less than that in the tangential direction with respect to the skull surface. Cranial cortical bone alone has a mean compressive strength greater than that of full section cranial bone. All three types of cranial bone specimens have a mean compressive strength greater than that of femoral cortical bone in the longitudinal direction but Poisson's ratio is less.

Mean compressive strength and strain of cancellous bone from human vertebral bodies as well as for intact vertebral bodies alone decreases in a superior-inferior direction. The mean compressive strength, modulus of elasticity, and Poisson's ratio of intact vertebral bodies are far less than the same properties for cortical femoral bone, when determined in the longitudinal direction, or any of the three types of cranial specimens.

CHAPTER 10

EFFECTS OF AGE, SEX, RACE AND SPECIES

AGE EFFECTS

Human Cortical Bone

LONG BONES

Tensile, Shearing and Hardness Properties. Although age differences in mechanical properties of bone would seem to be one of the most logical variables to study, data on it are not too plentiful in the available literature.

Wertheim (1847) found that four specimens of fresh cortical bone from the femur and the fibula of people less than 60 years of age had an average tensile strength of 10.67 kgf/mm² (15,173 lbf/in²) compared to an average of 5.34 kgf/mm² (7,593 lbf/in²) for four similar specimens from people over sixty.

A somewhat more extensive study was made by Rauber (1876). His data revealed that thirty-seven specimens from the fresh femur, tibia, and fibula of people less

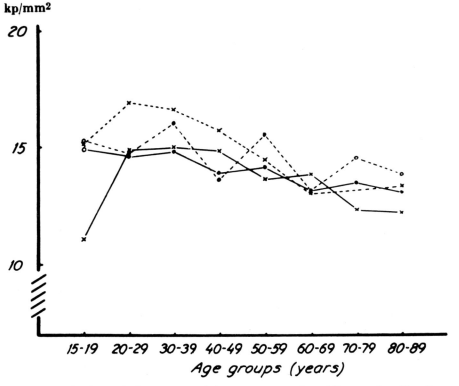

The variation of the mean ultimate strength with age for the femur and humerus, and for both sexes.

Men o. women x. femur ————, humerus – – – – –.

Figure 115. (From Lindahl and Lindgren: *Acta Orthop Scand,* 1967)

than 60 years of age had an average tensile strength of 10.08 kgf/mm² (14,334 lbf/in²) compared to a strength of 7.75 kgf/mm² (11,021 lbf/in²) for a single specimen from the femur of a 70-year-old man.

Age changes in the tensile strength of specimens of fresh moist cortical bone from tibias of twenty-eight subjects were investigated by Melick and Miller (1966). Specimens about 15 cm long and 2.5 cm wide were tested within three to five hours after removal from the body and within five minutes after preparation. The load was applied in the direction of the long axis of the specimens which coincided with that of the intact bone.

A mean strength of 20,050 ± 518 lbf/in² (14.10 ± 0.364 kgf/mm²) was found for specimens from adult people under 60 years of age compared to a mean of 17,197 ± 462 lbf/in² (12.09 ± 0.325 kgf/mm²) for people over 60. The difference between the means for the younger and older groups was significant. There were no significant changes in the amount of calcium, organic tissue or ash in the two groups.

Age and sexual variations in the tensile strength of fresh humeral and femoral cortical bone from sixty-four subjects were investigated by Lindahl and Lindgren (1967b). The specimens were obtained from four subjects of each sex in the 15 to 19 age group and thereafter in every decade up to 80 to 89 years of age. Most of

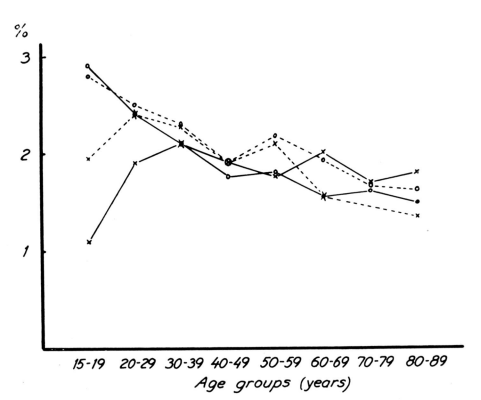

The variation of the mean deformation at failure with age for femur and humerus, and for both sexes.

Men o, women x, femur ———, humerus - - - - -.

Figure 116. (From Lindahl and Lindgren: *Acta Orthop Scand,* 1967)

the subjects were more than 40 years old and had died from cardiovascular disease, external violence, or poisoning. None died from tumors, had been bedridden for a long period of time, or had had fractures or bone diseases other than osteoporosis.

The tensile specimens, with a gauge length of 20 mm, were 6 to 8 cm long rods with a rectangular cross section 1.3 to 1.8 by 2.0 to 3.3 mm. Generally two or three specimens were obtained from each humerus and femur. The femoral test specimens were obtained from the anterior convex (tensile) side of the bone and the humeral ones from the thickest part of the circumference. The long axis of the specimen coincided with that of the bone. The specimens were prepared at a room temperature of 18° to 20° C and kept in air at 3° to 5° C until tested. Afterwards they were kept in a special test room.

Tensile tests were made in an Alwetron materials testing machine at a uniform deformation rate of 0.5 mm/min. The deformation was recorded continuously and from the curves obtained the ultimate tensile strength, elongation at rupture, proportional limit, and modulus of elasticity were calculated.

Data obtained from the tests (Fig. 115) showed that the mean tensile strength, except for women between 15 and 19 years of age, of both bones in both sexes significantly decreased (10%) with age.

The magnitude of the deformation (tensile strain) at failure, except for women between 15 and 19 years of age, also significantly decreased (about 35%) in both sexes (Fig. 116).

No significant age differences were found in the proportional limit and modulus of elasticity of specimens from both sexes.

Humeral specimens had a significantly greater tensile strength (about 10%) than femoral ones, but no other significant mechanical property differences were found between the two bones.

All mechanical properties had a very large intersubject range which was attributed to the great individual variation in the amount of bone present. This accounted for the great range of variation in the strength of individual bones.

Tensile properties of wet fresh cortical bone from Japanese subjects also vary with age (Yamada, 1970). In adult life mean tensile strength is greatest at 20 to 29 years of age, then progressively decreases in each successive decade to its minimum value at 60 years of age after which it does not change (Table LXXIII).

Although less than in the 20 to 39 age group, the mean tensile strength between 10 and 19 years of age exceeds that of people over 40 years of age. Tensile strain is maximum in the 10 to 19 age group after which it progressively decreases to a minimum in the 60 to 79 age group.

Weaver (1966) reported that the microhardness of normal cortical bone from adult human fibulas increases from childhood (two years) to a maximum about 30 years of age after which it remains about the same.

Rockwell hardness, according to Yamada (1970), likewise exhibits age differences, being greatest among adults in the 20 to 29 age group then steadily declining in each succeeding decade to a minimum value in the 70 to 79 age group (Table LXXIII).

Data obtained in this laboratory showed that the mean tensile strength of wet specimens of embalmed femoral cortical bone was lowest in the zero to 19 age group, rose to a maximum in the 20 to 39 age group, then gradually decreased in each older age group to a minimum between 80 and 99 years (Table LXXIV). However, the strength never again became as low as in the zero to 19 age group.

Tensile strain (% elongation) exhibited

TABLE LXXIII

MEAN MECHANICAL PROPERTY VALUES FOR WET FRESH CORTICAL BONE OF JAPANESE SUBJECTS OF DIFFERENT AGE GROUPS (Data from Yamada, 1970)

Property	10-19 yrs	20-29 yrs	30-39 yrs	40-49 yrs	50-59 yrs	60-69 yrs	70-79 yrs	Unit of Measurement
Tensile strength	11.6 ± 0.15 16,495 ± 213	12.5 ± 0.10 17,775 ± 142	12.2 ± 0.19 17,348 ± 270	11.4 ± 0.25 16,211 ± 356	9.5 ± 0.14 13,509 ± 199	8.8 ± 0.24 12,514 ± 341	8.8 ± 0.24 12,514 ± 341	kgf/mm² lbf/in²
Tensile strain	1.48	1.44 ± 0.007	1.38 ± 0.014	1.31 ± 0.027	1.28 ± 0.015	1.26 ± 0.005	1.26 ± 0.005	% elongation
Compressive strength	— —	17.0 ± 0.44 24,174 ± 626	17.0 ± 0.42 24,174 ± 597	16.4 ± 0.37 23,321 ± 526	15.8 ± 0.44 22,468 ± 626	14.8 ± 0.23 21,046 ± 327	— —	kgf/mm² lbf/in²
Compressive strain	—	1.9 ± 0.07	1.8 ± 0.02	1.8 ± 0.02	1.8 ± 0.02	1.8 ± 0.02	—	% contraction
Modulus of elasticity (torsion)	— —	350 497,700	350 497,700	320 455,040	320 455,040	300 426,600	300 426,600	kgf/mm² lbf/in²
Torsion strength	— —	5.82 ± 0.11 8,276 ± 156	5.82 ± 0.11 8,276 ± 156	5.37 ± 0.05 7,636 ± 71	5.37 ± 0.05 7,636 ± 71	4.96 ± 0.12 7,053 ± 171	4.96 ± 0.12 7,053 ± 171	kgf/mm² lbf/in²
Distortion (torsion)	0.028 ± 0.0009	0.028 ± 0.0009	0.025 ± 0.0005	0.025 ± 0.0005	0.027 ± 0.0010	0.027 ± 0.0010	0.027 ± 0.0010	mm
Bending strength	15.4 21,899	17.7 ± 1.1 25,169 ± 1,564	17.7 ± 1.1 25,169 ± 1,564	16.5 ± 2.1 23,463 ± 2,986	15.7 ± 2.0 22,325 ± 2,844	14.2 ± 2.9 20,192 ± 4,124	14.2 ± 2.9 20,192 ± 4,124	kgf/mm² lbf/in²
Specific deflection	0.086	0.075 ± 0.0041	0.066 ± 0.0054	0.062 ± 0.0070	0.062 ± 0.0070	0.053 ± 0.0045	0.053 ± 0.0045	mm
Cleavage strength	— —	9.0 (estimated) 12,798 (estimated)	8.8 ± 0.44 12,514 ± 626	8.6 ± 0.20 12,229 ± 284	— —	8.2 ± 0.10 11,660 ± 142	8.2 ± 0.13 11,660 ± 185	kgf/mm² lbf/in²
Rockwell hardness	—	49 ± 0.3	45 ± 0.5	43 ± 0.4	39 ± 0.8	34 ± 0.7	32 ± 1.0	

TABLE LXXIV

Mean Mechanical Property Values for Wet Embalmed Femoral Cortical Bone in Different 20-Year Age Groups

Property	No.	0-19 yrs	No.	20-39 yrs	No.	40-59 yrs	No.	60-79 yrs	No.	80-99 yrs	Unit of Measurement
Tensile strength*	6	7,237 ± 844	51	13,174 ± 2,518	87	12,411 ± 1,959	209	10,901 ± 2,554	47	10,341 ± 3,884	lbf/in²
		5.09 ± 0.59		9.26 ± 1.77		8.72 ± 1.38		7.66 ± 1.795		7.27 ± 2.73	kgf/mm²
% elongation*	6	1.66 ± 0.98	51	1.92 ± 0.80	83	1.48 ± 0.66	175	1.32 ± 0.57	47	1.39 ± 0.55	
Modulus of elasticity*			51	2.25 ± 0.45	87	2.16 ± 0.44	209	2.06 ± 0.45	47	1.88 ± 0.59	× 10⁶ lbf/in²
				1.58 ± 0.32		1.52 ± 0.31		1.45 ± 0.32		1.32 ± 0.41	× 10³ kgf/mm²
Single shearing strength†			51	9,226 ± 1,585	87	10,928 ± 1,340	209	9,729 ± 1,210	47	10,683 ± 1,974	lbf/in²
				6.49 ± 1.11		7.68 ± 0.94		6.84 ± 0.85		7.51 ± 1.39	kgf/mm²
Rockwell superficial hardness .	5	−34.4 ± 8.2	26	16.15 ± 15.37	87	15.72 ± 14.99	151	13.99 ± 17.34	24	4.21 ± 12.70	

*Parallel to long axis of bone.
† Perpendicular to long axis of bone.

a more erratic behavior, being highest between 20 and 39 years of age, second between zero and 19, third between 40 and 59, fourth between 80 and 99, and fifth between 60 and 79 years of age. Modulus of elasticity (in tension) decreased steadily with each older age group from a maximum at 20 to 39, to a minimum at 80 to 99 years of age.

The minimum mean value for single shearing strength, perpendicular to the long axis of the specimen, was found in the 20 to 39 age group with a subsequent decline in each succeeding age group from a maximum between 40 and 59 years. A slight increase in shear strength occurred in the 80 to 99 age group.

Rockwell superficial hardness was least in the zero to 19 year group in which a negative hardness value was found. However, only five specimens were tested. In specimens from adults, mean Rockwell hardness decreased from a maximum between 20 and 39 to a minimum between 80 and 99 years of age.

An analysis of variance in our data revealed that mean tensile strength in the 20 to 39 year group was significantly higher, at the 0.01 or better level, than in any other age group except the 40 to 59 age group for which the difference was significant at the 0.05 to 0.01 level (Table LXXV). Tensile strength of the 40 to 59 age group was also higher, at the 0.01 or better level, than that of all other groups except the 20 to 39 year group. Because of the small number of specimens, data from the zero to 19 age group were not included in the statistical analysis.

Tensile strain in the 20 to 39 age group was significantly greater, at the 0.01 or better level, than that in all other adult age groups. Specimens from the 40 to 59 age group had a tensile strain that was signifi-

TABLE LXXV

SIGNIFICANT AGE DIFFERENCES IN MEAN MECHANICAL PROPERTY VALUES OF
WET EMBALMED CORTICAL BONE OF ADULT HUMAN FEMURS

| | *Significance Level* | |
	0.01 or Better	Between 0.05 and 0.01
Tensile strength*	(51) 20-39 > 60-79 (209) (51) 20-39 > 80-99 (47) (87) 40-59 > 60-79 (209) (87) 40-59 > 80-99 (47)	(51) 20-39 > 40-59 (87)
Tensile strain*	(51) 20-39 > 40-59 (83) (51) 20-39 > 60-79 (209) (51) 20-39 > 80-99 (47)	(83) 40-59 > 60-79 (175)
Single shear strength†	(87) 40-59 > 20-39 (27) (87) 40-59 > 60-79 (89) (24) 80-99 > 20-39 (27) (24) 80-99 > 60-79 (89)	
Tensile modulus of elasticity* . .	(51) 20-39 > 80-99 (47) (86) 40-59 > 80-99 (47)	(51) 20-39 > 60-79 (195) (195) 60-79 > 80-99 (47)
Rockwell superficial hardness . .	(26) 20-39 > 80-99 (24) (87) 40-59 > 80-99 (24) (151) 60-79 > 80-99 (24)	

* Parallel to long axis of bone.
† Perpendicular to long axis of bone.
Figures in parentheses indicate the number of specimens in each age group.

cantly higher, at the 0.05 to 0.01 level, than that in the 60 to 79 age group.

Between 40 and 59 years of age, single shear strength was greater, at the 0.01 or better significance level, than that between 20 and 39 or between 60 and 79 years of age. Single shear strength was also greater, at the same significance level, in the 80 to 99 group than in either the 20 to 39 or the 60 to 79 age group.

Mean modulus of elasticity in the 20 to 39 and the 40 to 59 age groups was higher, at the 0.01 or better significance level, than in the 80 to 99 age group. In the 20 to 39 age group, the modulus was significantly greater, at the 0.05 to 0.01 level, than in the 60 to 79 age group. Between 60 and 79 years of age the modulus exceeded that of the 80 to 99 group at the 0.05 to 0.01 significance level.

In the 20 to 39, the 40 to 59, and the 60 to 79 age groups, the Rockwell superficial hardness was significantly greater, at the 0.01 or better level, than in the 80 to 99 age group.

Age differences were likewise evident in the mean values for mechanical properties of wet embalmed tibial cortical bone of adults studied in this laboratory (Table LXXVI). Mean tensile strength and percent elongation progressively decreased in each age group from a maximum between 20 to 39 to a minimum between 80 and 99 years of age. Modulus of elasticity was lower between 20 and 39, than the maximum between 40 and 59 after which it gradually decreased.

Single shearing strength and Rockwell superficial hardness were only determined in the 20 to 39, the 40 to 59, and the 60 to 79 year age groups. Shearing strength was greatest between 40 and 59 and least between 60 and 79 years of age. Hardness progressively decreased from a maximum

in the 20 to 39 to a minimum in the 60 to 79 age group.

Analysis of variance in the data revealed that tensile strength, strain, and modulus of elasticity in the 20 to 39 age group were each higher, at the 0.01 or better significance level, than in the 60 to 79 and the 80 to 99 age groups (Table LXXVII). The same was true for tensile strength and modulus of elasticity of the 40 to 59 age group. The 20 to 39 age group had a tensile strain and a Rockwell hardness that were greater, at the 0.01 or better significance level, than those of the 40 to 59 and the 60 to 79 age groups, respectively. Hardness of specimens from the 40 to 59 age group was also greater, at the same significance level, than that of the 60 to 79 age group.

Mean differences, significant at the 0.05 to the 0.01 level, between mechanical properties of various age groups were found for tensile strength (20 to 39 age group > 40 to 59); tensile strain (40 to 59 > 20 to 39); and single shearing strength (40 to 59 > 60 to 79).

Comparison of the data in Tables LXXV and LXXVII reveals that the mean ultimate tensile strength of wet cortical bone from embalmed femurs and tibias is greater, at the 0.01 significance level, in the 20 to 39 and the 40 to 59 age groups than in the 60 to 79 and the 80 to 99 age groups. In specimens from both bones the mean tensile strength in the 20 to 39 age group exceeded that in the 40 to 59 age group at the 0.05 significance level. Mean tensile strain (% elongation) in specimens from both bones in the 20 to 39 age group was greater, at the 0.01 significance level, than that in the 40 to 59, the 60 to 79, and the 80 to 99 age groups. In femoral specimens from the 40 to 59 age group, mean tensile strain exceeded, at the 0.05 signifi-

TABLE LXXVI

MEAN MECHANICAL PROPERTY VALUES FOR WET EMBALMED TIBIAL CORTICAL BONE IN DIFFERENT 20-YEAR AGE GROUPS

Property	No.	20-39 yrs	No.	40-59 yrs	No.	60-79 yrs	No.	80-99 yrs	Unit of Measurement
Tensile strength*	46	15,873 ± 2,568 11.16 ± 1.81	45	14,854 ± 2,201 10.44 ± 1.55	87	11,803 ± 2,041 8.30 ± 1.43	14	11,552 ± 2,578 8.12 ± 1.81	lbf/in^2 kgf/mm^2
% elongation*	45	2.29 ± 0.79	41	1.68 ± 0.81	75	1.53 ± 0.59	13	1.5 ± 0.73	
Modulus of elasticity*	46	2.46 ± 0.43 1.73 ± 0.30	45	2.68 ± 0.47 1.88 ± 0.33	84	2.08 ± 0.39 1.46 ± 0.27	13	1.91 ± 0.35 1.34 ± 0.25	$\times 10^6\ lbf/in^2$ $\times 10^3\ kgf/mm^6$
Single shear strength†	24	11,358 ± 2,321 7.98 ± 1.63	45	11,693 ± 737 8.22 ± 0.52	46	11,308 ± 904 7.95 ± 0.64			lbf/in^2 kgf/mm^2
Rockwell superficial hardness	24	15.2 ± 14.1	45	14.1 ± 8.3	46	7.1 ± 7.97			

* Parallel to long axis of bone.
† Perpendicular to long axis of bone.

TABLE LXXVII

SIGNIFICANT AGE DIFFERENCES IN MEAN MECHANICAL PROPERTY VALUES OF
WET EMBALMED CORTICAL BONE OF ADULT HUMAN TIBIA

Property	Significance Level	
	1% or Better	*Between 5% and 1%*
Tensile strength*	(46) 20-39 > 60-79 (87)	(46) 20-39 > 40-59 (45)
	(40) 20-39 > 80-99 (14)	
	(45) 40-59 > 60-79 (84)	
	(45) 40-59 > 80-99 (14)	
Tensile strain*	(45) 20-39 > 40-59 (44)	(45) 40-59 > 20-39 (46)
	(45) 20-39 > 60-79 (75)	
	(45) 20-39 > 80-99 (13)	
Single shear strength†		(46) 40-59 > 60-79 (46)
Tensile modulus of elasticity* ...	(46) 20-39 > 60-79 (84)	
	(46) 20-39 > 80-99 (13)	
	(45) 40-59 > 60-79 (84)	
	(45) 40-59 > 80-99 (13)	
Rockwell superficial hardness ...	(24) 20-39 > 60-79 (46)	
	(45) 40-59 > 60-79 (46)	

* Parallel to long axis of bone.
† Perpendicular to long axis of bone.
Figures in parentheses indicate the number of specimens in each age group.

cance level, that of specimens from the 60 to 79 age group. The same was true for tibial specimens of the 40 to 59 age group when compared to those from the 20 to 39 age group.

In both femoral and tibial specimens the mean modulus of elasticity in the 20 to 39 and the 40 to 59 age groups was higher, at the 0.01 significance level, than those from the 80 to 99 age group.

No other agreements were found between the femoral and tibial data with respect to significant differences in the mean values for mechanical properties of specimens from various age groups.

We have also investigated age differences in mechanical properties of wet unembalmed tibial specimens of adult cortical bone. Mean tensile strength, single shearing strength, and hardness were greatest in the 40 to 59 age group (Table LXXVIII). Percentage elongation and modulus of elasticity were highest in the 20 to 39 and the 60 to 79 age groups, respectively. Specimens from people between 20 and 39 years

of age had the lowest mean tensile strength, modulus of elasticity, and single shearing strength. The lowest percent elongation and hardness values were found in specimens from people in the 60 to 79 age group.

Fewer significant age differences were found for mechanical properties of unembalmed than for embalmed tibial specimens (Table LXXIX). However, the unembalmed specimens only covered a range from 20 to 69 years of age. Mean tensile strength in the 20 to 39 and in the 40 to 59 age groups was significantly greater, at better than the 0.01 level, than in the 60 to 79 age group. Modulus of elasticity between 40 and 59 and between 60 and 79 years of age was higher, at the 0.01 or better significance level, than that between 20 and 39 years of age. In the 40 to 59 age group, Rockwell superficial hardness was greater, at the 0.05 to 0.01 level, than in the 60 to 79 age group. No significant age differences were found for single shearing strength.

Although the total number of em-

TABLE LXXVIII

MEAN MECHANICAL PROPERTY VALUES FOR WET UNEMBALMED TIBIAL CORTICAL
BONE IN DIFFERENT 20-YEAR AGE GROUPS

Property	No.	20-39 yrs	No.	40-59 yrs	No.	60-79 yrs	Unit of Measurement
Tensile strength*	62	$12,524 \pm 3,956$	56	$12,813 \pm 2,603$	81	$12,605 \pm 2,116$	lbf/in²
		8.80 ± 2.78		9.01 ± 1.83		8.86 ± 1.49	kgf/mm²
% elongation*	56	2.06 ± 0.74	54	2.02 ± 0.87	74	1.20 ± 0.55	
Modulus of elasticity*	62	1.96 ± 0.48	55	2.41 ± 0.49	83	2.62 ± 0.70	$\times 10^6$ lbf/in²
		1.38 ± 0.34		1.69 ± 0.34		1.84 ± 0.49	$\times 10^3$ kgf/mm²
Single shear strength†	54	$11,038 \pm 2,664$	56	$11,243 \pm 1,607$	16	$11,049 \pm 1,711$	lbf/in²
		7.76 ± 1.87		7.90 ± 1.13		7.77 ± 1.20	kgf/mm²
Rockwell superficial hardness	53	-3.28 ± 12.48	51	-1.41 ± 8.34	29	-6.38 ± 10.65	

* Parallel to long axis of bone.
† Perpendicular to long axis of bone.

balmed and unembalmed tibial specimens was almost the same (192—embalmed; 194—unembalmed), the age range represented by the unembalmed material was smaller than that for the embalmed tibial and femoral specimens. This may account, in part, for the fewer significant age differences in the mechanical properties of the unembalmed tibial specimens.

Compressive Properties. The first to note age differences in compressive properties of fresh bone was Rauber (1876) who reported that forty-three femoral, tibial, and fibular specimens from people less than 60 years of age, had a mean compressive strength of 15.51 kgf/mm² (22,055 lbf/in²) compared to a strength of 13.21 kgf/

mm² (18,785 lbf/in²) for a single femoral specimen from a 70-year-old man.

Lindahl and Lindgren (1968) determined the compressive properties of humeral and femoral cortical bone specimens from the same sixty-four subjects used in their earlier study (1967b). Rods 2.1 to 3.8 mm long with a rectangular cross section of 1.3 to 2.0 by 2.7 to 3.3 mm were taken from the posterior (compressive) side of the femoral shaft and thickest part of the humerus. The test specimens were kept at a constant temperature of 28° C and a relative humidity of 65% until equilibrium, as previously described for their tensile specimens, was attained. The specimens were loaded to failure, at a constant rate

TABLE LXXIX

SIGNIFICANT AGE DIFFERENCES IN MEAN MECHANICAL PROPERTY VALUES OF WET
UNEMBALMED CORTICAL BONE OF ADULT HUMAN TIBIAS

Property	Significance Level	
	1% or Better	Between 5% and 1%
Tensile strain*	(56) 20-39 > 60-79 (74)	
	(54) 40-59 > 60-79 (74)	
Tensile modulus of elasticity*	(55) 40-59 > 20-39 (62)	
	(83) 60-79 > 20-39 (62)	
Rockwell superficial hardness		(51) 40-59 > 60-79 (29)

* In the long axis of bone.
Figures in parentheses indicate the number of specimens in each age group.

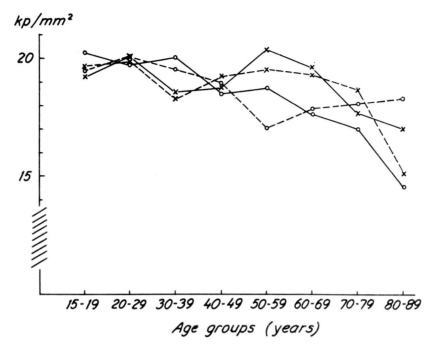

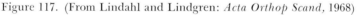

Mean compressive ultimate strength for the femur and humerus, both sexes and various age groups. Men ○, women ×, femur ———, humerus − − − −.

Figure 117. (From Lindahl and Lindgren: *Acta Orthop Scand,* 1968)

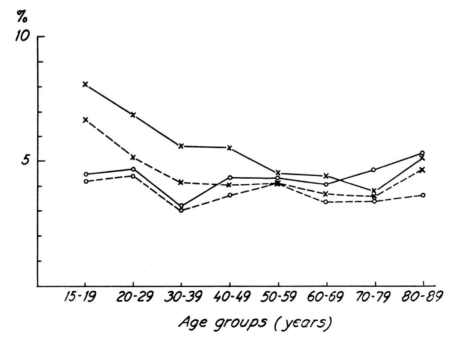

Mean compression at rupture for the femur and humerus, both sexes and various age groups. Men ○, women ×, femur ———, humerus − − − −.

Figure 118. (From Lindahl and Lindgren: *Acta Orthop Scand,* 1968)

of 0.05 mm/min, in an Alwetron testing machine.

Data obtained in their tests showed that from twenty years upward the mean ultimate compressive strength of humeral and femoral specimens from both sexes decreased about 15% with age, a reduction significant at the 1% level (Fig. 117). Mean compression (strain) from both bones of men less than 40 years of age declined about 40% with age, a decrease significant at the 1% level (Fig. 118). After 20 years of age, the proportional limit of both bones in both sexes declined about 15% with aging, a reduction that was not quite significant (Fig. 119). No significant variations were found in the modulus of elasticity (Fig. 120).

The authors compared their results for compression with those they previously found for tension (Lindahl and Lindgren, 1967b) and concluded that the higher tensile strength of the humeral specimens and compressive strength of the femoral specimens are the result of functional differences in the two bones.

Age, sex, and topographic differences in the compressive strength of 703 standardized dry specimens of cortical bone from the distal fourth of the proximal half of the femoral shaft of embalmed bodies of five men (56 to 64 years of age) and four women (62 to 81 years of age) were determined by Amtmann (1968). The test specimens were taken from rings from the five proximal sixths of the shaft. Each ring

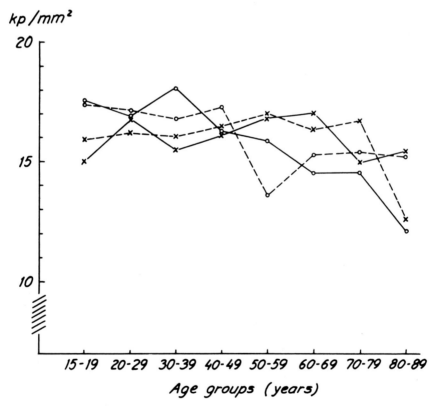

Mean limit of proportionality for the femur and humerus, both sexes and various age groups.   Men ○, women ✕, femur ———, humerus – – – –.

Figure 119. (From Lindahl and Lindgren: *Acta Orthop Scand*, 1968)

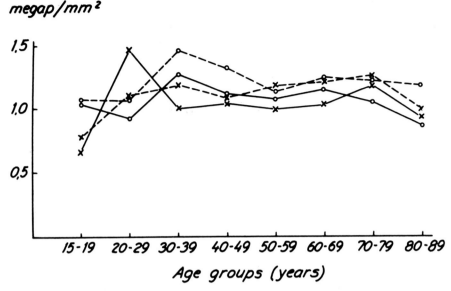

megap/mm²

Age groups (years)

Mean modulus of elasticity for the femur and humerus, both sexes and various age groups. Men ○, women ×, femur ———, humerus – – – –.

Figure 120. (From Lindahl and Lindgren: *Acta Orthop Scand*, 1968)

was subdivided into anterior, posterior, medial, and lateral quadrants. No known pathological bones were used. The specimens were loaded in a direction of the long axis of the shaft at a rate of load increase of 50 kg/cm²/sec.

In specimens from all quadrants of both right and left bones of men, the compressive strength fluctuated between 56 and 60 years of age after which it declined (Table LXXX). Although some fluctua-

tion also occurred in specimens from the women there was a more definite tendency for the strength of all quadrants to decrease from 62 to 81 years of age.

Amtmann and Schmitt (1968) related the compressive breaking strength and density of specimens from the anterior, posterior, medial, and lateral quadrants of cross sections of femurs of people less than and older than 67.8 years of age. They found that the mean breaking

TABLE LXXX

Average Compressive Strength ($\times 10^3$ kg/cm²) of Three Bone Samples of the Distal Quarter of the Proximal Half of the Femur (Data from Amtmann, 1968)

Body Side	Shaft Position	♂ 56	♂ 57	♂ 57	♂ 60	♂ 64	♀ 62	♀ 74	♀ 77	♀ 81
Left	posterior	1.32	2.54	1.93	2.45	1.83	2.42	1.79	1.29	1.20
	anterior	1.85	2.69	1.96	2.44	2.26	2.47	1.69	1.86	1.55
	medial	2.19	2.74	2.24	2.84	2.33	2.30	2.21	2.20	1.89
	lateral	2.31	2.92	2.42	2.84	2.80	2.46	2.27	2.35	2.28
Right	posterior	1.41	2.64	1.92	2.45	2.05	2.51	1.77	1.38	1.34
	anterior	2.29	2.72	2.28	2.59	2.59	2.53	2.01	1.94	1.69
	medial	2.23	2.69	2.35	2.70	2.48	2.69	2.11	2.26	1.71
	lateral	2.51	2.87	2.54	2.57	2.87	2.64	2.34	2.49	2.06

TABLE LXXXI

AGE DIFFERENCES IN MEAN COMPRESSIVE PROPERTIES, IN THE LONG AXIS OF THE BONE, OF
WET UNEMBALMED CORTICAL BONE FROM THE TIBIAS OF SIX CAUCASIAN MEN

Age (Yrs)	No.	Compressive Strength lbf/in²	kgf/mm²	No.	Modulus of Elasticity × 10⁶ lbf/in²	kgf/mm²	No.	% Shortening
26	14	10,413	7.32	14	3.24	2,278	10	0.68
31	12	20,440	14.37	12	2.70	1,898	11	1.36
54	13	20,624	14.50	13	2.53	1,779	13	1.91
61	12	17,148	12.06	12	2.70	1,898	12	0.66
66	15	14,755	10.37	15	2.29	1,610	11	0.86
75	12	16,823	11.83	12	2.63	1,849	11	1.33

strength of specimens from the older age group was significantly less than that of specimens from the younger age group.

Yamada (1970) cited data from Japanese investigators who found that maximum mean compressive strength of wet fresh cortical bone occurred between 20 and 39 years of age, after which it progressively declined to a minimum value in the 60 to 69 age group. Compressive strain also exhibited a gradual decrease with age, being maximum in the 20 to 29 and minimum in the 60 to 69 age groups, respectively.

Investigations made in this laboratory demonstrated that mean ultimate compressive strength of wet unembalmed tibial specimens, exclusive of those from a 26-year-old man whose leg was amputated for numerous nonunited fractures, is higher in men below than in those above 60 years of age (Table LXXXI). The same was true for modulus of elasticity and percent shortening (compressive strain) even when data from the 26-year-old man were included.

Bending Properties. Messerer (1880) reported that the bending strength of fresh cortical bone specimens from the humerus, femur, and tibia of nine male and seven female subjects increased to a maximum at 24 or 32 years of age after which it declined to a minimum in the seventies or eighties (Table LXXXII).

Modulus of elasticity was also determined for the humerus and femur of a 32-year-old man. The humerus had a modulus of 180,000 kgf/cm² and 152,000 kgf/cm² for the right and left bones, respectively. A modulus of 150,000 kgf/cm² and 153,600 kgf/cm² was found for the right and left femur.

Maj (1942) determined the breaking load (in bending), the standard deviation, and the coefficient of dispersion of dry specimens of cortical bone from the shaft of the humerus, ulna, femur, and tibia of forty people (twenty-four males, sixteen females) from 5 to 90 years of age. Test specimens 10 to 15 mm long, 3 mm wide and 1.2 mm thick were machined from 2 cm thick rings of bone from the middle of the shaft. Each specimen was oriented in the direction of the long axis of the shaft. From each person six test specimens were made from the humerus, three from the ulna, nine from the femur, and six from the tibia. The specimens were subjected to three-point bending in the same "clasimeter" used by Olivo, Maj and Toajari (1937).

Highest breaking loads, in the greatest statistical percentage, were found up to 35 years of age and during the fifties among the specimens from males (Table LXXXIII). Among specimens from females the highest fracture loads were found up to 27 years of age and during the forties. In both sexes lowest breaking loads occurred among specimens from people between 80 and 90 years of age.

Examination of Maj's data reveals that it falls into two groups with 60 years of age as the dividing line. Thus, the fourteen specimens from male subjects less than 60 years of age had an average breaking load of 8.05 kg compared to an average of only 6.52 kg for the ten specimens from subjects more than 60 years of age. The average age of the subjects in the younger and the older group was 42 and 69.7 years, respectively. Among female subjects the eight specimens from those less than 60 years of age had an average fracture load of 8.18 kg compared to an average of 6.22 kg for eight specimens from subjects more than 60 years of age. Subjects in the younger and the older group had an average age of 28.8 and 74.3 years, respectively.

Some interesting discrepancies were noted by Maj. Frequently low fracture loads occurred in periods of high resistance rather than the reverse. Between 25 and 35 years of age, the average resistance was approximately equal to that from 50 to 70 years of age. The coefficient of dispersion indicated that 76.5% of the determinations varied between 0.200 and 0.300.

Decrease in the bending properties of human cortical bone with advancing age was also noted by Sedlin (1965) who found that mean ultimate fiber stress, modulus of elasticity, and energy absorbed to failure all had a marked tendency to decrease with advancing age of the subject from whom the material was obtained (Table VII). Ultimate fiber stress decreased steadily with advancing age, but fluctuations occurred in the modulus of elasticity and the energy absorbed to failure.

According to data cited by Yamada (1970), wet fresh cortical bone from adult Japanese subjects has its maximum bend-

TABLE LXXXII

AGE AND SEXUAL DIFFERENCES IN BENDING STRENGTH OF FRESH HUMAN BONES
(*cf.* Table L) (Data from Messerer, 1880)

Age (Yrs)	Humerus kgf/cm²	Humerus lbf/in²	Femur kgf/cm²	Femur lbf/in²	Tibia kgf/cm²	Tibia lbf/in²
Male						
5.5	—	—	1,390	19,766	—	—
18	1,380	19,624	1,750	24,885	1,540	21,899
24	1,680	23,890	1,940	27,587	1,500	21,330
32 R	1,890	26,876	1,940	27,587	1,810	25,738
L	1,800	25,596	1,940	27,587	1,980	28,156
38	1,290	18,344	—	—	1,640	23,321
49	1,590	22,610	1,680	23,890	1,730	24,601
62 R	—	—	1,500	21,330	—	—
L	—	—	1,480	21,046	—	—
75	1,450	20,619	1,580	22,468	1,450	20,619
78	1,160	16,495	1,630	23,179	1,590	22,610
Female						
18 R	1,680	23,890	—	—	—	—
L	1,620	23,036	—	—	—	—
20	1,430	20,335	1,580	22,468	1,830	26,023
24	1,630	23,179	1,730	24,601	1,840	26,165
32	1,670	23,747	1,720	24,458	1,910	27,160
51	1,430	20,335	1,600	22,752	1,490	21,188
74	1,040	14,789	1,480	21,046	1,320	18,770
82	1,090	15,500	1,330	18,913	1,380	19,624

TABLE LXXXIII

FRACTURE LOAD IN BENDING OF HUMAN CORTICAL BONE (Data from Maj, 1942)

Yrs.	Male Average Fracture Load (kg)	S.D.*	C.D.*	Age (Yrs)	Female Average Fracture Load (kg)	S.D.*	C.D.*
10	6.26	2.15	0.344	5	8.80	3.24	0.360
23	12.27	1.66	0.135	22	10.81	2.13	0.197
29	7.91	1.66	0.209	27	7.50	1.60	0.212
31	8.82	2.23	0.253	28	6.50	1.54	0.236
32	6.53	1.64	0.252	30	6.78	2.89	0.426
35	7.53	1.64	0.217	32	6.44	1.65	0.256
46	7.40	1.59	0.215	42	9.84	2.82	0.287
47	8.78	1.70	0.194	45	8.77	2.36	0.269
50	7.95	1.90	0.239	65	7.52	1.70	0.226
54	6.78	2.22	0.327	66	7.25	2.10	0.290
57	9.43	2.02	0.214	69	5.86	1.54	0.263
57	7.42	2.23	0.301	72	5.35	1.45	0.271
59	7.34	1.60	1.218	74	6.08	2.11	0.247
59	8.31	1.74	0.209	77	5.81	1.32	0.227
60	6.95	1.24	0.178	82	6.27	1.48	0.236
63	6.43	1.63	0.253	90	5.62	1.09	0.194
64	6.21	2.18	0.351	—	—	—	—
67	7.09	1.67	0.236	—	—	—	—
67	6.55	1.93	0.295	—	—	—	—
69	8.55	2.06	0.241	—	—	—	—
71	5.27	1.19	0.226	—	—	—	—
77	4.77	1.06	0.222	—	—	—	—
79	6.50	1.54	0.237	—	—	—	—
80	6.91	2.63	0.381	—	—	—	—
Average 53.7	7.42	1.796	0.289	51.6	6.97	1.94	0.262

*S.D. = standard deviation; C.D. = coefficient of dispersion.

ing strength between 20 and 39 years of age and its minimum between 60 and 79 years of age (Table LXXIII). In the 10 to 19 age group the mean bending strength exceeds that of adults more than 60 years old. Ultimate specific deflection in bending is highest in the 10 to 19 age group after which it gradually decreases in each succeeding decade to a minimum after 60 years of age.

When considering values for bending strength it should be remembered that they are not directly comparable to those for tensile or compressive strength. In bending, the cross-sectional area of the specimen is subjected to a combination of tensile, compressive, and shearing forces none of which is uniformly distributed over the cross-sectional area. A similar situation exists for shearing strength, regardless of whether it is "punching" or torsional shearing strength, because in both types of tests the force is not uniformly distributed over the cross-sectional area of the specimen (*cf.* Figs. 1, 3, 4, 6, 7, and 10). This is in contrast to the conditions in pure tension or compression in which it can be assumed that the cross-sectional area of the specimen is subjected to a uniformly distributed pure tensile or compressive force.

Torsion Properties. Age variations in the torsion properties of fresh human cortical bone were first reported by Japanese investigators, cited by Yamada (1970), who found that the maximum torsion strength occurred between 20 and 39 years of age after which it declined in each successive 20 year age group to a minimum in the 60 to 79 age group (Table LXXIII). The magnitude of the distortion decreased from a maximum in the 10 to 29 age group to a minimum in the 30 to 49 group after which it slightly increased. Torsion modulus of elasticity was greatest between 20 and 39 years of age, thereafter declining to a minimum value in the 60 to 79 age group.

Torsional shearing strength, shear modulus, and energy absorbed to failure by standardized specimens (Fig. 8E) of wet cortical bone from embalmed femurs of adult human subjects have been determined in this laboratory. No consistent trend was noted with respect to aging. High values for torsional shearing strength were found in a 22-, a 58- and a 67-year-old subject while the lowest values occurred in a 44-year-old man (Table LXXXIV). Torsional shear modulus was highest in a 22-year-old subject, decreased during the forties and fifties, then rose again in the late fifties and the sixties. Energy absorbed to failure was greatest in the 22-year-old subject and least in the 55-year-old one. In the late fifties and during the sixties the energy absorbed to failure increased again.

Cleavage Properties. Yamada (1970) cites work of some Japanese investigators that showed a progressive decrease with advancing age in the mean cleavage strength which was greatest (estimate) in the 20 to 29 age group and least in the 60 to 79 age group (Table LXXIII).

Fatigue Life. Evans and Lebow (1957) found some age differences in the fatigue life of standardized specimens of wet unembalmed cortical bone from amputated tibias. The average number of cycles to failure was 2,229,999 for specimens from a 31-year-old man; 2,617,333 for specimens from a 53-year-old man; 2,469,999 for specimens from a 54-year-old man; and 2,029,999 for those from a 56-year-old man. However, the number of individuals used in their study was too small to draw definite conclusions regarding relations between age and fatigue life. One would expect that fatigue life would continue to decrease with advancing age because their specimens, which were tested in a flexure fatigue machine, probably failed in tension and, as previously discussed, the tensile strength of human cortical bone declines with advancing age.

Age and sexual differences in the fatigue properties of spindles of cortical bone from fresh femurs of twenty-two people have been investigated by Swanson et al. (1971). A total of sixty-eight specimens from men 37 to 92 years of age and thirty-

TABLE LXXXIV

AGE DIFFERENCES IN MEAN TORSIONAL PROPERTIES OF WET EMBALMED
CORTICAL BONE FROM CAUCASIAN MALE FEMURS

Age (Yrs.)	No.	Torsion Shear Strength		Torsion Shear Modulus		Energy Absorbed to Failure	
		lbf/in^2	kgf/mm^2	$\times 10^6\ lbf/in^2$	kgf/mm^2	$in\text{-}lb/in^2$	$kg\text{-}mm/mm^2$
22	3	8,147	5.73	1.486	1,045	27.46	0.489
44	15	3,857	2.71	0.292	205	17.68	0.315
55	16	4,060	2.85	0.362	254	15.01	0.267
56	17	4,715	3.31	0.432	304	16.59	0.295
58	10	8,433	5.93	1.360	956	24.68	0.439
60	31	6,766	4.76	1.042	733	21.03	0.374
67	27	7,466	5.25	1.235	868	20.62	0.367
68	26	6,876	4.83	1.145	805	20.10	0.358

nine specimens from women 35 to 98 years of age were tested. The specimens were loaded to failure, at a rate of 70 cycles/sec, in a Wöhler rotating fatigue machine. During preparation and testing the specimens were kept cool and wet with Ringer's solution. For more details of the testing procedure see Chapter 8.

When the data were analyzed, only a weak negative correlation was found when subject age was plotted against the number of cycles to failure for specimens tested at two different stress levels (Fig. 121). Furthermore, coefficients of correlation based on graphs with the best visual correlation were not significant for specimens

of male bone tested at a stress of 9,450 lbf/in² (65.1 MN/m²).

Density. Age variation in the density of 100 mm long cortical bone specimens from the middle half of the humerus and the femur of sixty-four subjects was investigated by Lindahl and Lindgren (1967a). Specimens were obtained from four subjects of each sex in the 15 to 19 age group and thereafter in each decade up to the 80 to 89 age group. In the interval between removal of the specimen and its density determination (usually less than fourteen days) the specimens were stored in air at a temperature of 3° to 5° C. Before the measurements were made, the specimens

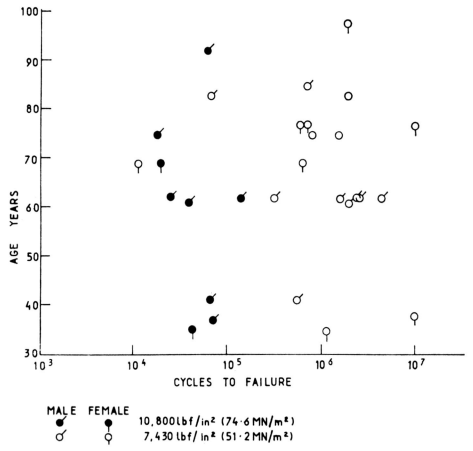

Figure 121. Age and sexual differences in fatigue life (cycles to failure) of human cortical bone. (From Swanson, Freeman, and Day: *Med Biol Engin,* 1971)

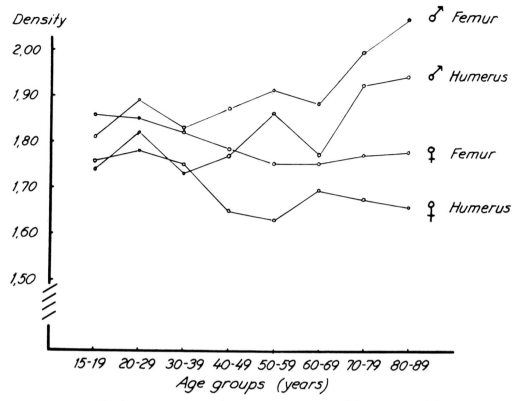

Variation of mean density of femur and humerus with age;
men and women.

Figure 122. (From Lindahl and Lindgren: *Acta Orthop Scand*, 1967)

were put into ordinary water for twenty-four hours and then wiped.

The two halves of the bones, each 100 mm long, were fitted together and the frontal diameters were measured to an accuracy of 0.1 mm with calipers at six equidistant sites. The means of the measurements were computed for each bone with allowance for the bone loss (1.5 mm) during sawing out of the specimen.

As soon as the specimens were removed from the water and wiped, they were weighed to an accuracy of 0.01 g. Their volume was then determined by water displacement to an accuracy of 0.01 mg and their density determined by dividing their weight by their volume.

Lindahl and Lindgren found that in men above 50 years of age the mean density of the femoral and humeral specimens increased significantly (1%) with age, but in women there was a slight, insignificant decrease with advancing age (Fig. 122). In both sexes the mean diameter of both bones increased significantly (0.1%) with age but there was a tendency for a decrease, after 30 to 39 years of age, in the mean cross-sectional area of the two bones. This decrease was significant (1%) in men but not in women.

Roentgenographic density determinations of the anterior, posterior, medial, and lateral quadrants of cross sections of the shaft of femurs of twelve men and twelve women, 56 to 87 years of age, were made by Amtmann and Schmitt (1968). They reported a negative correlation with a nonlinear regression between density and age for 398 specimens from men and 337 specimens from women. Significant differences between individuals were found in the mean density of the femoral shaft and the density spectra of the cross sections as well as between the density of right and left bones in individuals. The breaking strength of specimens of equal density was significantly lower in people more than 67.8 years of age than in those of individuals less than that age. However, this difference was equal in all density intervals. Amtmann and Schmitt attributed only 40% or 42% of strength variation to density differences.

Tensile Properties of Infant and Children's Bone. Practically all of the research on the mechanical properties of human bone has been based on material obtained from adults. One of the few exceptions is a study by Hirsch and Evans (1965) who determined the tensile properties of cortical bone from the femur of infants of both sexes, one day to six months of age, and from a 14-year-old boy.

The material was obtained from fresh autopsy limbs which were stored at $-20°$ C until the test specimens were made. Because of the small amount of cortical bone in the femur of infants, the test specimens were only 25 mm long, 1 mm thick, and 3 to 4 mm wide with a reduced middle region 5 mm long by 1.3 mm wide. An Instron materials testing machine was used to test the specimens which were loaded to failure at a constant rate of 0.1 cm/min, a room temperature of 20 to 22° C and a humidity of 65%. A pure tensile load in the direction of the long axis of the specimen was applied. All specimens were moist during a test.

Specially designed jaws were required to hold the specimens so they would not slip during a test. The jaws consisted of a pair of wedge-shaped chucks with rough surfaces and a thumb screw for exerting additional pressure on the expanded gripping ends of the specimens.

Tensile strain occurring in a specimen during a test was measured by a strain gauge mounted on the reduced area of the specimen with Eastman 910 cement. Budd Metafilm foil strain gauges (Type C12-LXL-M50A), 3 mm long with a gauge fac-

TABLE LXXXV

AVERAGE TENSILE PROPERTIES OF WET, UNEMBALMED CORTICAL BONE OF INFANT, CHILD, AND ADULT HUMAN FEMURS. LOADING SPEED FOR THE INFANT AND CHILD SPECIMENS = 0.1 CM/MIN

Property	Infant (newborn-6 mo) Hirsch and Evans (1965)	Child (14-yr-old boy) Hirsch and Evans (1965)	Wertheim (1847)	Rauber (1876)	Adult Hülsen (1896)	Yamada (1970)	Evans
Tensile strength							
kgf/mm²	10.0	17.63	7.77	9.74	10.58	12.4	6.51
lbf/in²	14,200	25,070	11,049	13,850	15,045	17,633	9,262
Tensile strain							
(% Elongation)	1.85	1.92	—	—	—	1.41	1.47
Modulus of elasticity							
kgf/mm²	1,012	2,245	2,264	2,246	1,735	1,760	1,195
× 10⁶ lbf/in²	1.40	3.19	3.20	3.19	2.47	2.50	1.699

TABLE LXXXVI

Age and Sex	Race	Maximum Stress (lbf/in²)	Modulus of Elasticity (lbf/in²)	Strain at Failure (%)	Energy Absorbed (in-lb/in³)	Density (dry specimen) (g/cm³)
45 M	N	409.8	35,384	2.5	4.86	0.659
53 M	N	859.7	74,211	2.4	11.08	0.713
58 M	N	292.0	25,665	2.9	—	0.667
69 M	W	629.3	48,800	2.1	—	0.988
70 M	W	455.5	51,444	2.2	—	0.824
72 M	W	437.2	47,650	2.2	5.07	0.694
77 F	W	185.0	15,577	3.6	4.34	0.588
78 M	W	241.4	20,087	3.1	3.53	0.694
80 M	W	340.7	32,340	1.9	3.07	0.561
88 F	W	137.6	10,523	3.2	3.07	0.345

tor of 2.01 ± 1% and a resistance of 120 ± 0.5 ohms were used. Strain was recorded with a Hottinger Strain Gauge Bridge (Model KWS/T = 5) and a Speedomax recorder using a paper speed of 30 cm/min.

Hirsch and Evans found that the mean tensile strength and strain of the specimens from infant femurs were within the same range of values which other investigators had reported for adult femoral bone, but the modulus of elasticity of the infant specimens was considerably lower (Table LXXXV). The average tensile strength and strain of the specimens from the femur of the 14-year-old boy were greater than similar values for adult femurs. Modulus of elasticity was about the same as that reported by some investigators for adult bone.

The data for tensile strength and strain of cortical bone from infant femurs strongly suggests that these two mechanical properties are not dependent upon mechanical stimuli of walking. However, the modulus of elasticity may not develop sufficiently until the infant tries to walk. That is to say, an infant cannot walk until the bones of the limbs are stiff enough, i.e. have a high enough modulus of elasticity to support the body weight.

Human Cancellous Bone

Age changes in the mechanical properties of cancellous bone have not been investigated as thoroughly as those for cortical bone. This is especially true for tensile properties of cancellous bone, probably because of the great difficulty of holding a specimen for testing.

Compressive Properties

Femur. Evans and King (1961) appear to be the only ones who have demonstrated age differences in some of the mechanical properties of cancellous bone from adult human femurs. They determined the compressive properties of ninety-one rectangular prisms (0.79 cm by 0.79 cm by 215 cm) of wet cancellous bone from the femurs of ten individuals varying from 45 to 88 years of age. Maximum compressive stress and strain, in the long axis of the specimen, were determined by loading the wet specimens to failure in a 5,000-lb capacity materials testing machine calibrated to an accuracy of ±1%. Modulus of elasticity and energy absorbed to failure were computed from the stress-strain curve for each specimen. Density was determined for dry specimens to avoid the effects of moisture in the interstices of the specimens.

TABLE LXXXVII

Mean Compressive Strength (lbf/in²) and Ash Weight (g/cc) of Moist Fresh Cubes of
Cancellous Bone from Adult Human 3rd Lumbar Vertebral Bodies and the Calcaneus.
Loading Speed Not Given (Data from *Chalmers and Weaver*, 1966)

Bone	All Cases	Male	Female	50 Years and Less	Over 50 Years
Vertebral strength	449.2	488.0	406.1	615.7	367.7
Calcaneal strength	532.7	578.7	472.9	566.8	514.2
Vertebral ash weight	0.128	0.136	0.120	0.153	0.116
Calcaneal ash weight	0.186	0.195	0.173	0.189	0.184

A definite tendency was noted toward a decrease in maximum compressive stress, modulus of elasticity, and energy absorbed to failure after 70 years of age, but strain at failure tended to increase. Density de-

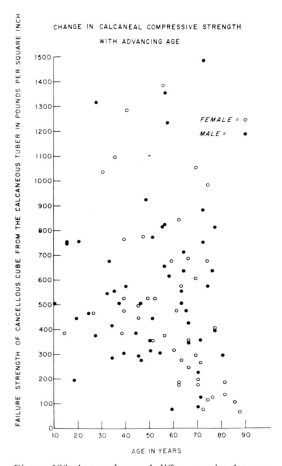

Figure 123. Age and sexual differences in the compressive strength of cancellous bone from the adult human calcaneus. (From Chalmers and Weaver: *J. Bone Joint Surg,* 1966)

clined after 70 years of age. Comparison of the mean values for these properties in individuals 45 to 70 with those of subjects 71 to 88 years of age showed that compressive strain was the only property greater in specimens from the older group (Table LXXXVI).

Calcaneus. Age differences in the compressive strength and ash weight of half-inch cubes of fresh cancellous bone from the calcaneus of ninety-nine subjects (fifty-five male, forty-four female) were studied by Chalmers and Weaver (1966). The bones were obtained at autopsies, usually a few hours after death, and stored at −20° C until used. No material was taken from patients with disease conditions affecting bone or who had been bedridden for more than three weeks. The volume of the test specimens was calculated from micrometer measurements and the results checked by water displacement measurements. Ash content (g/cm³ of fresh bone) was determined by incinerating the specimens at 700° C in a muffle furnace for ten hours. Since the volume of the specimens was known, the amount of actual bone in them could be determined by measuring their ash weight. Coefficients of correlation between compressive strength and ash weight were also computed. Test specimens were taken from the inferior part of the calcaneal tuberosity where the trabecular orientation was most uniform.

Chalmers and Weaver found that the

compressive strength of cancellous bone from the calcaneus decreased with advancing age (Table LXXXVII, Fig. 123), and that there was a close correlation between mineral content and compressive strength (Table LXXXVII). However, this relationship was less predictable for calcaneal than for vertebral specimens (*cf.* Figs. 124 and 125).

Vertebrae. Tensile Properties. Because of the great technical difficulty of holding specimens for testing, Sonoda (1962) appears to be the only person who has determined the tensile properties of cancellous bone. For this purpose fresh vertebral bodies, supplemented with specimens of cancellous bone from within the bodies, from twenty-six subjects (22 to 76 years of age) were used.

Sonoda found that the ultimate tensile strength and strain (% elongation) of wet cancellous bone from thoracic and lumbar vertebral bodies of people between 20 and 39 years of age was 0.12 ± 0.01 kgf/mm² and $0.58 \pm 0.03\%$, respectively. Between 40 and 70 years of age the ultimate tensile strength was 90% and the percent elongation 84% of those in people 20 to 39 years of age.

Compressive Properties. Messerer (1880) noted a marked tendency toward a decrease in the ultimate compressive strength of thoracic and lumbar vertebral bodies with advancing age (Table LXXXVIII).

A similar tendency was found by Yokoo (1952a) who determined the compressive properties of cancellous bone from lumbar vertebrae of five people. He reported a mean ultimate compressive strength of 0.19 kgf/mm², an ultimate contraction of 2.5% and a modulus of elasticity of 9 kgf/mm² in specimens from people 40 to 49 years of age. Specimens from people 60 to 69 years of age had a compressive strength of 0.14 kgf/mm², a contraction of 2.4% and a modulus of elasticity of 7 kgf/mm².

A more recent study of age changes in the compressive properties of vertebral bodies and cancellous vertebral bone was

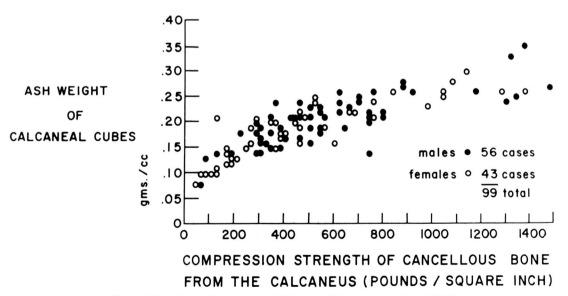

RELATIONSHIP BETWEEN THE STRENGTH AND THE ASH WEIGHT OF CANCELLOUS BONE FROM THE CALCANEUS

ASH WEIGHT OF CALCANEAL CUBES

gms./cc

males ● 56 cases
females ○ 43 cases
99 total

COMPRESSION STRENGTH OF CANCELLOUS BONE FROM THE CALCANEUS (POUNDS / SQUARE INCH)

Figure 124. (From Chalmers and Weaver: *J Bone Joint Surg,* 1966)

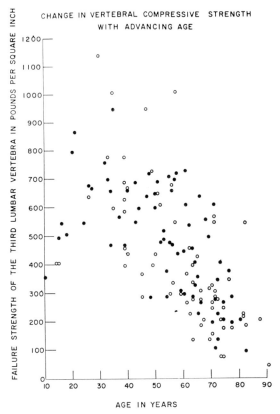

CHANGE IN VERTEBRAL COMPRESSIVE STRENGTH
WITH ADVANCING AGE

Figure 125. (From Chalmers and Weaver: *J Bone
Joint Surg*, 1966)

specimens were taken at random from the general hospital population which, unfortunately, had few patients between 15 and 25 years of age. After removal from the body, the 3rd and 4th lumbar vertebral bodies were radiographed to determine their uniformity. Afterwards, the 3rd and 4th bodies were separated from the others, saran-wrapped as were the unseparated vertebrae, and frozen until needed.

In addition to the mechanical properties of the specimens, the amount of bone present was determined by finding the grams of ash per cubic centimeter of hydrated medullary tissue. For this purpose vertebral bodies had all the soft tissue, cartilage and cortical bone removed, after which the external surfaces of the prepared sample was waxed with paraffin. The volume of the cube of bone thus obtained was determined by water displacement. Ashing of the sample was performed at 580° C for forty-eight hours in a muffle furnace. Ash weight was determined with a Mettler microanalytical balance. Ash weight divided by volume of bone yielded ash content per unit volume. This value was then compared to the stress values obtained in adjacent vertebral bodies after examination to be certain that the two vertebrae were radiographically uniform.

The compressive strength of the specimens was determined by loading them to

made by Bartley et al. (1966). In this study, both whole vertebral bodies as well as specimens of trabecular bone from within the vertebral body were tested. The material was obtained at autopsy from lumbar bodies of forty patients who died from various disease processes. The bone

TABLE LXXXVIII

Age and Sex Differences in the Ultimate Compressive Strength (kgf/cm²), in the Longitudinal Direction, of Fresh Human Vertebrae (Data from Messerer, 1880)

| | Thoracic Vertebrae | | | Lumbar Vertebrae | | | Average—All Vertebrae | |
Subject	1st	6th	10th	1st	4th	5th	kgf/cm²	lbf/in²
25-year-old woman	52	63	51	56	—	64	57	810.54
30-year-old man	92	92	80	78	—	78	84	1,194.48
34-year-old woman	—	—	—	—	62	—	62	881.64
51-year-old woman	55	67	57	67	—	60	61	867.42
56-year-old man	—	44	45	32	32	34	38	540.36
80-year-old woman	—	—	—	—	22	—	22	312.84
81-year-old woman	—	—	—	27	—	—	27	383.94

failure at a constant rate of one-half inch per minute in an Instron testing machine. Before testing, the circumference of the vertebral bodies was measured with a planimeter, after which the bodies were saran-wrapped and frozen until tested. Before testing the vertebrae were thawed for four hours so they were moist when tested.

Differences between the compressive strength of whole vertebral bodies and samples of trabecular bone from within the vertebral body were also investigated. For this purpose, two adjacent vertebrae from five representative male subjects, selected on the basis of the median value for ash/cc content, were used. One vertebral body was crushed whole while the adjacent one was compressed after the cortical bone and soft tissue were trimmed away. Crushing strength and the characteristic curves between the two specimens were then compared.

Bartley et al. found a striking similarity between the distribution of the ash/cc vs age and crushing strength vs age, as well as a high correlation (0.88) between the crushing strength of a vertebra and the ash content of adjacent vertebral bodies. The greatest crushing strength before maximum deformation occurred was 582 lbf/in² in specimens from a 30-year-old man while the lowest was 89 lbf/in² in those from a 57-year-old woman who had scleroderma and a clinical diagnosis of osteoporosis. These same specimens also had the highest and the lowest ash weight/cc values of 0.23 GN and 0.06 GN, respectively. The average force required for crushing was 916 lb.

Chalmers and Weaver (1966) also investigated the relation between compressive strength and age (Fig. 125) and between compressive strength and ash weight (Fig. 126) in specimens from vertebral bodies of 137 cadavers. Although relatively few subjects were less than 30, compressive strength seemed to increase up to that age. Afterwards both strength and ash weight decreased and were considerably less in people over 50 than in those under 50 years of age (Table LXXXVII). Vertebral specimens showed a significantly greater decrease in both properties than did calcaneal specimens. Separation of the specimens according to age and sex revealed that this relationship was maintained except in individuals less than 50 years of age in whom the compressive strength of calcaneal bone was less than that of vertebral bone although ash weight was higher. In the opinion of the authors, this indicated that bone strength is not a simple function of mineral content. A high coefficient of correlation was found between the compressive strength and the mineral content of both the vertebral and the calcaneal specimens.

Chalmers and Weaver think that the activity and occupation of the individual may influence the bone strength, as evidenced by the broad normal range seen in the middle age group when compared to those below and above 30 and 60 years of age, respectively. Thus, increased activity may influence bone strength via the trabecular structure independent of its mineral content. The authors noted that the mean vertebral ash content is much less than the mean calcaneal content in all groups and that the differences are proportional to the differences in compressive strength. Trabecular structure in the vertebrae primarily parallels the compressive force whereas in the calcaneal tuberosity a more complex trabecular orientation is found. They believe that these variations in trabecular orientation account for differences in bone strength occurring independently of its mineral content.

McElhaney et al. (1970b) found that the mean compressive strength of human

RELATIONSHIP OF ASH WEIGHT TO COMPRESSIVE STRENGTH OF L$_3$

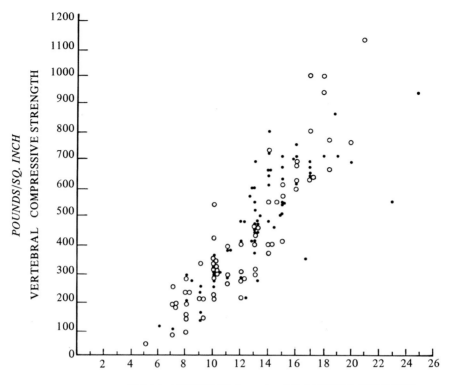

Figure 126. (From Chalmers and Weaver: *J Bone Joint Surg,* 1966)

vertebral bodies was greatest between 10 and 20 years of age, after which it steadily declined to a minimum value at 80 to 90 years of age. In the first decade of life the mean compressive strength was intermediate between the mean value in the fourth and fifth decades.

Torsion Properties. Apparently Sonoda (1962) is the only one who has determined the torsion properties of cancellous bone. According to him the breaking torsion moment of vertebral bodies in people 20 to 39 years of age is 60 ± 5.4 kg-cm for the upper thoracic, 108 ± 7.3 kg-cm for the middle thoracic, 165 ± 10.2 kg-cm for the lower thoracic, and 255 ± 18.4 kg-cm for the lumbar vertebral bodies. The estimated breaking torsion moment between 40 and

59 years of age is 83% and between 60 and 79 years of age—68% of that in the 20 to 39 age group.

Torsion strength in the 20 to 39 age group is 0.37 ± 0.04 kgf/mm^2 in the upper thoracic, 0.35 ± 0.01 kgf/mm^2 in the middle thoracic, 0.34 ± 0.02 kgf/mm^2 in the lower thoracic and 0.32 ± 0.02 kgf/mm^2 in the lumbar vertebral bodies. The estimated strength in the 40 to 59 age group is a little less but in the 60 to 79 group is only 80% of that between 20 and 39 years of age.

The ultimate angle of torsion between 20 and 39 years of age is 13 ± 0.7° for the upper thoracic, 10 ± 0.8° for the middle thoracic, 8 ± 0.4° for the lower thoracic and 5 ± 0.6° for the lumbar vertebral bodies. Between 40 and 59 years of age the estimated torsion angle is 89% and between 60 and 79 years of age, 63% of that in the 20 to 39 age group.

When using data on mechanical properties of cancellous bone one should remember that the values obtained represent those for the specimen tested more than those of the bone itself. Cancellous bone has many relatively large spaces within it and the methods usually used for determination of the cross-sectional area of the test specimens generally do not allow for these spaces or irregularities in the margins of the specimen. Consequently, the cross-sectional area upon which the ultimate strength of the specimen is based is actually the area of the whole specimen rather than that of the bone within it. The same is true, but to a lesser extent, for most property values given for cortical bone. However, these values may be closer to the true values for bone because there is much more bone present in a cortical specimen than in a cancellous one.

SEX EFFECTS

Human Cortical Bone

TENSILE PROPERTIES

Effects of sex on mechanical properties of bone do not seem to have been investigated as thoroughly as those for age. Wertheim (1847) and Rauber (1876) both reported that bone from men had a greater tensile strength than that from women. However, only a few specimens were tested by each investigator.

A more complete study of tensile properties of cortical bone from the humerus and femur of adult men and women was recently made by Lindahl and Lindgren (1967). No significant sexual difference was found in ultimate tensile strength (Table LXXXIX, Fig. 115) although the strength of the humeral specimens was higher, at the 0.001 significance level, than that of the femoral specimens. There were no significant sexual or bone differences in mean deformation at failure (Fig. 116), the limit of proportionality, or the modulus of elasticity.

Japanese investigators, according to Yamada (1970), also found no significant differences in tensile strength and percent elongation in cortical bone from Japanese subjects.

The above results differ from those obtained in this laboratory. An analysis of variance of our data for tensile properties of wet embalmed tibial specimens of American Caucasians revealed that the percent elongation of specimens from women (1.94%) was greater, at the 0.01 or better significance level, than that of specimens from men (1.54%). However, the modulus of elasticity of the male specimens (2.65 × 10^6 lbf/in^2) was higher, at the same significance level, than the modulus of female specimens (2.03 × 10^6 lbf/in^2).

A similar analysis of tensile properties of embalmed wet femoral specimens for American Caucasians revealed even more significant sexual differences in mechanical property values. Thus, mean ultimate tensile strength (11,794 lbf/in^2) and modulus of elasticity (2.14 × 10^6 lbf/in^2) of the male specimens were greater, at the 0.01 or better significance level, than the strength (10,508 lbf/in^2) and modulus of elasticity (1.89 × 10^6 lbf/in^2) of the female specimens. Tensile strain (percent elongation) was higher, at the 0.01 or better significance level, in the female (1.74%) than in the male (1.36%) specimens.

Mean ultimate tensile strength of wet

TABLE LXXXIX

SEXUAL DIFFERENCES IN TENSILE AND COMPRESSIVE PROPERTIES OF FRESH, MOIST HUMAN CORTICAL BONE. LOADING
SPEED = 0.5 MM/MIN (Data from Lindahl and Lindgren, 1967 & 1968)

In Tension

| | Men | | Women | |
| | Femur (n = 29) | Humerus (n = 27) | Femur (n = 30) | Humerus (n = 16) |
Property				
Ultimate tensile strength (kp/mm²) *	14.1 ± 0.2	14.9 ± 0.2	13.4 ± 0.3	15.1 ± 0.5
	(12.2-16.1)	(12.0-17.5)	(8.5-16.7)	(11.9-18.1)
Deformation at failure (%)	2.0 ± 0.1	2.2 ± 0.1	1.8 ± 0.1	1.9 ± 0.1
	(1.4-3.1)	(1.5-3.3)	(0.5-2.4)	(1.0-2.6)
Limit of proportionality (kp/mm²) *	4.4 ± 0.1	4.3 ± 0.1	4.2 ± 0.1	4.3 ± 0.2
	(3.1-5.7)	(3.2-5.4)	(2.6-5.7)	(2.9-5.3)
Modulus of elasticity (megap/mm²)	1.52 ± 0.03	1.56 ± 0.03	1.50 ± 0.04	1.61 ± 0.08
	(1.19-1.88)	(1.16-1.89)	(1.08-2.02)	(0.72-2.08)

In Compression

| | Men | | Women | |
	Femur (n = 30)	Humerus (n = 30)	Femur (n = 30)	Humerus (n = 30)
Ultimate strength (kp/mm²) *	19.7 ± 0.3	18.8 ± 0.4	18.3 ± 0.4	19.1 ± 0.3
	(14.8-22.2)	(13.3-21.4)	(12.7-22.4)	(16.4-21.7)
Compression at rupture (%)	5.3 ± 0.5	4.5 ± 0.3	4.3 ± 0.2	3.9 ± 0.2
	(3.5-14.8)	(2.8-9.6)	(2.8-7.7)	(2.3-6.4)
Limit of proportionality (kp/mm²) *	15.8 ± 0.4	16.1 ± 0.4	15.7 ± 0.4	16.7 ± 0.3
	(10.1-18.3)	(10.6-19.1)	(9.3-20.5)	(13.6-19.2)
Modulus of elasticity (megap/mm²)	1.05 ± 0.06	1.10 ± 0.05	1.07 ± 0.05	1.20 ± 0.07
	(0.30-1.76)	(0.45-1.58)	(0.46-1.55)	(0.71-1.85)

* 1 kp/mm² = 1,422 lbf/in²
1 megap = 1,000 kp, 1 kp (kgf) = 9.80665 newtons = 2.2046 lbf
1 megap = 1,422,000 lbf/in²

embalmed tibial specimens from American Negro women (14,422 lbf/in²) was greater, at the 0.01 or better significance level, than the strength (12,109 lbf/in²) of similar specimens from American Negro men. The modulus of elasticity (2.71 × 10⁶ lbf/in²) of the female specimens was significantly higher, at the 0.05 to 0.01 level, than that (2.42 × 10⁶ lbf/in²) of the male specimens.

COMPRESSIVE PROPERTIES

Wet unembalmed cortical bone from women has, according to Rauber (1876) and Calabrisi and Smith (1951), a lower compressive strength than that of men. However, relatively few specimens were tested and no statistical analysis was made of the data.

The compressive properties of fresh

moist cortical bone from the humerus and femur of adult men and women were recently determined by Lindahl and Lindgren (1968). They reported that femoral specimens from men had a compressive strength that was significantly greater (at the 0.01 level) than that of similar specimens from women with a mean difference of 8% (Table LXXXIX). No sexual differences were noted in compression at rupture, limit proportionality, or modulus of elasticity.

Yamada (1970) reported that no significant sexual differences were found in compressive properties of Japanese cortical bone.

BENDING AND TORSION PROPERTIES

Japanese investigators, cited by Yamada (1970), found no significant sexual differences in bending properties of Japanese cortical bone, but specimens from females had a lower torsion strength than those from males.

DENSITY

Because the mechanical properties of bone are also a function of the amount of bone present, sexual differences in density must be considered, too. Thus, Lindahl and Lindgren (1967) have shown that the density of cortical bone specimens from the humerus and femur of men gradually increases with advancing age while that of comparable specimens from women decreases (Fig. 122).

Human Cancellous Bone

Sexual differences in mechanical properties of cancellous bone have been most thoroughly documented for material from human vertebral bodies. Messerer (1880) reported that the compressive strength of various vertebral bodies of a 25-year-old woman was less than that of comparable specimens from a 30-year-old man (Table LXXXVIII). However, specimens from a 51-year-old woman had a higher compressive strength than those from a 56-year-old man.

The most research in this area was done by Sonoda (1962) who determined the tensile, compressive, and torsional properties of fresh vertebral bodies of twenty-six subjects varying from 22 to 76 years of age. No significant sexual differences were found in tensile, compressive, and torsional strength nor in tensile and compressive strain. However, the breaking torsional moment in specimens from females was only 80% of that in males. Also, the ultimate torsion angle in females was slightly smaller than in males.

According to data given by Chalmers and Weaver (1966) the mean compressive strength and ash weight of fresh vertebral and calcaneal cancellous bone is less in females than in males (Table LXXXVII).

Specimens of cancellous femoral bone from two females in a study by Evans and King (1961) had a lower mean ultimate compressive stress than any of the specimens from males, a lower modulus of elasticity than all but one of the males, absorbed less energy to failure than most of the males, had a higher maximum compressive strain than all males but one, and were less dense than any of the male specimens. These differences are probably related to the fact that the women were 77 and 88 years of age and undoubtedly osteoporotic.

RACIAL DIFFERENCES

Very little data are available on racial differences in the mechanical properties of human bone. Most of the early investigators did not give the race of the subjects from whom their material was obtained but they were very likely European Caucasians.

All of the data reviewed by Yamada (1970) were obtained from Japanese subjects. The average value given by Yamada for ultimate tensile strength in the longitudinal direction of fresh cortical bone from the adult human humerus, femur, tibia, and fibula, in all cases, is higher than that reported by other investigators for material from non-Japanese subjects (Table XXXVIII). Wertheim, Rauber, and Hülsen undoubtedly used material from European Caucasians while my material was obtained from American Caucasians. However, since Wertheim and Hülsen each tested only four specimens, their data may not be typical. Average compressive strength values given by Yamada (Table XXXVIII) are within the same range of variation reported by other investigators

TABLE XC

RACIAL DIFFERENCES IN MEAN MECHANICAL PROPERTY VALUES FOR WET AND DENSITY VALUES FOR DRY ADULT HUMAN CORTICAL BONE

Race and Bone	No.	Ultimate Tensile Strength (lbf/in²)	No.	Single Shearing Strength (lbf/in²)	No.	% Elongation	No.	Elastic Modulus (lbf/in² × 10⁶)	No.	Rockwell Hardness	No.	Density (g/cm³)
American Caucasian men, emb. tibia	108	14,100 ± 2,228	108	11,578 ± 1,475	99	1.54 ± 0.76	107	2.65 ± 0.599	108	14.46 ± 10.63	108	1.96 ± 0.07
American Caucasian women, emb. tibia ...	61	13,248 ± 3,949	—	—	52	1.94 ± 0.96	60	2.03 ± 0.476	—	—	—	—
American Negro men, emb. tibia	58	12,109 ± 1,261	58	11,308 ± 904	55	1.43 ± 0.58	56	2.42 ± 0.398	58	7.13 ± 7.97	58	1.83 ± 0.10
American Negro women, emb. tibia	15	14,423 ± 1,214	—	—	12	1.16 ± 0.28	17	2.71 ± 0.474	—	—	—	—
Japanese* (Yamada, 1970) unemb. tibia .	—	20,335 ± 171	—	11,660 ± 270	—	1.50	—	2.61	—	—	—	—

* All specimens from subjects 20-39 years of age.

for specimens from comparable bones of Caucasians.

Mean tensile strain of wet unembalmed cortical bone from Japanese subjects is less than we found for Caucasian material but the compressive strain is greater (Table XXXIX). Mean modulus of elasticity in tension is higher in Japanese bone than we found in Caucasian bone (Table XL).

The mean tensile strength we found for wet cortical bone from embalmed tibias of adult American Negro men is considerably less than that reported for Japanese subjects (Table XC). This is true in spite of the fact that embalming significantly increases the tensile strength of bone (Table XI). Tensile strain and modulus of elasticity in American Negro men are also

less than in Japanese subjects.

Comparison of the mechanical properties of wet cortical bone for embalmed tibias of adult American Caucasian and Negro men revealed that ultimate tensile strength, strain, modulus of elasticity, single shearing strength, and density were each greater in the Caucasian than in the Negro men. Opposite results were found from comparison of the mechanical properties of American Caucasian and Negro women, bone from Negro women having a higher ultimate tensile strength and modulus of elasticity than that from the Caucasians. No data were available on single shearing strength and density in the two groups of women.

Whether or not the above racial differ-

SPECIES DIFFERENCES IN MEAN TENSILE STRENGTH OF WET UNEMBALMED CORTICAL BONE IN THE LONGITUDINAL DIRECTION
(Data from Hulsen, 1896 and Yamada, 1970)

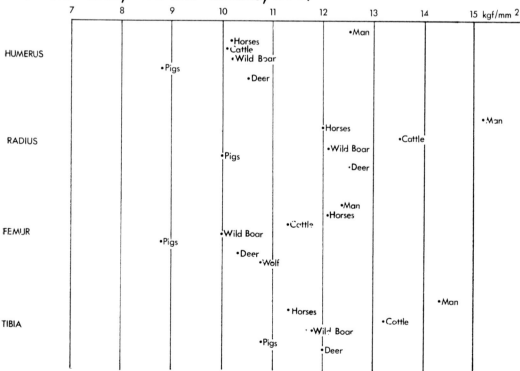

Figure 127

SPECIES DIFFERENCES IN MEAN TENSILE STRAIN IN LONG AXIS OF WET UNEMBALMED CORTICAL BONE (Data from Yamada, 1970)

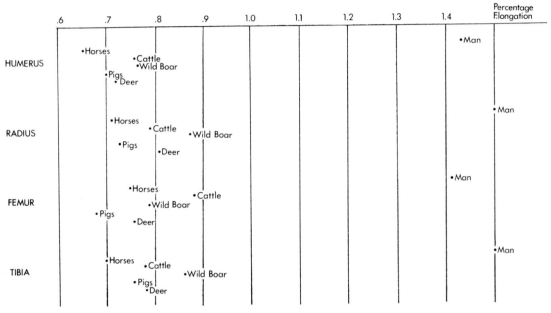

Figure 128

TENSION

SPECIES DIFFERENCES IN MEAN MODULUS OF ELASTICITY* OF WET UNEMBALMED CORTICAL BONE (Data from Yamada, 1970)

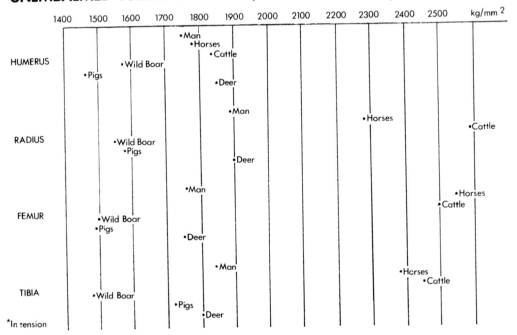

Figure 129

ences are statistically significant cannot be determined from the available data, because the number of specimens used to determine the various mechanical properties of each race is not large enough for statistical evaluation or not known.

SPECIES EFFECTS

Aside from man, relatively few data are available on mechanical properties of mammalian cortical bone. Most of the data that are available were obtained, almost exclusively, from the long bones of domestic animals. Comparison of the mechanical property values for humeral, radial, femoral and tibial bone of animals with those of man reveals rather unexpected differences.

The mean ultimate tensile strength of human bone exceeds that of other mammals (Fig. 127) while the mean tensile strain is very much greater (Fig. 128).

Mean compressive strength of femoral bone of other mammals is considerably less than that for man (Fig. 130). However, the mean modulus of elasticity (Fig. 129) and compressive strain (Fig. 131) of human bone are intermediate with respect to the values obtained from bones of other mammals. Dempster and Liddicoat (1952) reported a mean modulus of elasticity of $1,450 \pm 820$ kgf/mm² for wet human cortical bone in compression which is much higher than that given for other mammalian bone (Fig. 132).

Modulus of elasticity in tension is high-

SPECIES DIFFERENCES IN MEAN COMPRESSIVE STRENGTH OF WET UNEMBALMED CORTICAL BONE IN THE LONGITUDINAL DIRECTION (Data from Yamada, 1970)

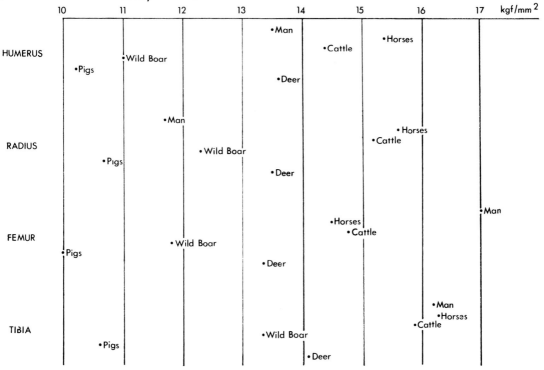

Figure 130

est in horse or cattle bone (Fig. 129), and the same is true for compressive strength of humeral, radial, and tibial bone in horses (Fig. 130). Specimens from horses also have the highest compressive strain for each bone (Fig. 131).

Pig bone has the lowest mean tensile and compressive strength (Figs. 127 and 130),

and the lowest modulus of elasticity in tension is found in specimens from pigs or wild boars (Fig. 129). Compressive strain is lowest in deer or cattle bone (Fig. 131). Among nonhuman mammals, horse bone has the highest and pig bone the lowest mean modulus of elasticity in compression (Fig. 132).

SUMMARY

Ultimate tensile, compressive, shearing, bending, torsion, and cleavage strength of cortical bone decrease with advancing age. The same is true for percent deformation and hardness. Most of the changes between the maximum value, usually between 20 and 39 years of age, and those found in old age groups are statistically significant at the 5% to 1% or the 1% or better levels. There is no significant age difference in the proportional limit (in tension) or the modulus of elasticity. Fatigue life (strength) has only a weak negative correlation with age. Above 50 years of age, density in male bone increases significantly but in female bone it decreases.

No significant sexual differences in ultimate tensile strength, deformation at failure, and proportional limit have been found in cortical bone specimens from

SPECIES DIFFERENCES IN MEAN COMPRESSIVE STRAIN IN LONG AXIS OF WET UNEMBALMED CORTICAL BONE (Data from Yamada, 1970)

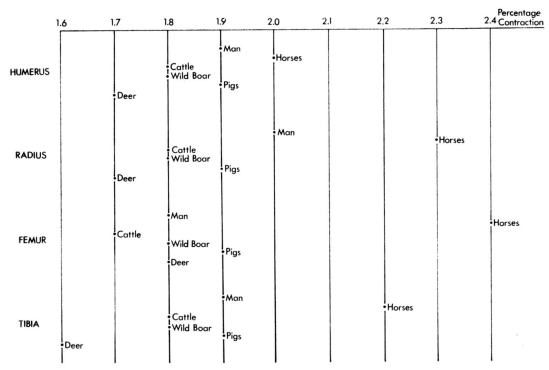

Figure 131

COMPRESSION

SPECIES DIFFERENCES IN MEAN MODULUS OF ELASTICITY OF WET UNEMBALMED CORTICAL BONE (Data from Yamada, 1970)

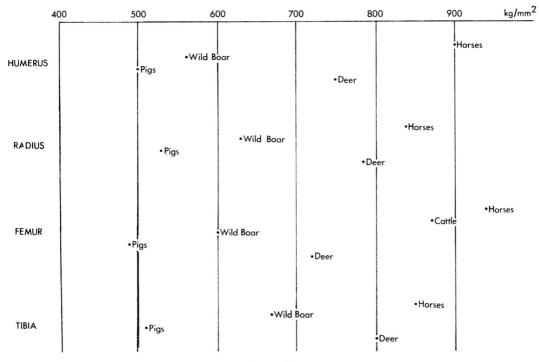

Figure 132

Swedish people. The same is true for tensile strength and strain in material from Japanese subjects. However, tensile strength and modulus of elasticity of wet embalmed femoral bone from American Caucasians are significantly higher in male than in female bone. Tensile strain is significantly greater in female than in male bone. Ultimate tensile strength and modulus of elasticity of wet embalmed tibial bone of American Negroes are significantly greater in females than in males. Wet cortical bone from embalmed femurs of American Caucasians has a significantly greater compressive strength in men than in women, but there is no sexual difference in compressive strain, proportional limit, and modulus of elasticity. No significant

sexual differences have been found in the compressive properties of cortical bone of Japanese subjects. The same is true for bending properties of Japanese bone, although the torsional strength of male bone exceeds that of female bone. Density of male bone increases with advancing age while that of female bone decreases.

Among Japanese subjects there are no significant sexual differences in the tensile, compressive, and torsional strength or in tensile and compressive strain of cancellous vertebral bone. However, male cancellous bone from vertebrae has a greater torsional breaking moment and ultimate torsion angle than female bone. Compressive strength and ash weight in vertebral and calcaneal cancellous bone of Swedish people are higher in men than in women. Wet femoral cancellous bone of American Caucasian men has a greater compressive strength, modulus of elasticity, energy absorbing capacity, and density than similar bone from American Caucasian women. Compressive strain is higher in specimens from the women than in those from the men.

Ultimate tensile strength, in order from highest to lowest, is American Negro women, American Caucasian men, American Caucasian women, Japanese and American Negro men. Tensile strain (percent elongation), in order of decreasing value, is highest in American Caucasian women, American Negro men, American Caucasian men, Japanese and American Negro women. Modulus of elasticity is highest in American Negro women, followed by American Caucasian men, Japanese, American Negro men, and American Caucasian women.

Single shearing strength, in descending order, is American Caucasian men, American Negro men, and Japanese, while the order for Rockwell hardness is Japanese, American Caucasian men, and American Negro men. No data are available on shearing strength and Rockwell hardness for American Caucasian and Negro women.

Bone from American Caucasian men is more dense than that of American Negro men.

The data for American Caucasian and Negro subjects were obtained from wet embalmed tibial specimens, that for Japanese subjects from wet unembalmed cortical bone.

There appears to be no data on racial differences in mechanical properties of cancellous bone.

Most of the data on mechanical properties of mammalian cortical bone, aside from man, were obtained from domestic animals. Mean tensile strength of human bone is somewhat greater and tensile strain very much greater than in other mammals. Modulus of elasticity of human bone in compression is much higher than that of other mammals but compressive strain and modulus in tension are intermediate with respect to those of other mammals. Modulus of elasticity in tension is higher in horse or cattle bone. Horse bone (humerus, radius, tibia) also has the greatest compressive strength and strain. Pig or wild boar bone has the lowest tensile and compressive strength and modulus of elasticity. Deer or cattle bone has the lowest compressive strain.

CHAPTER 11

VISCOELASTIC AND PLASTIC PROPERTIES OF BONE

THE MECHANICAL BEHAVIOR of bone, as the result of the application of a force, is influenced by the fact that bone is a viscoelastic material. Consequently, when a force is applied to bone it tends to undergo creep or plastic flow. As long as the force does not cause deformation of the bone beyond its elastic limit, practically all of the deformation is recovered as soon as the load or force is removed. If the yield point of the bone is exceeded, most of the deformation is recovered immediately or soon after removal of the force, and with sufficient time almost all of the remaining deformation is finally recovered. This recovery with extended time is called the elastic aftereffect. The portion of the deformation that is never recovered remains as a permanent set.

Viscoelastic properties of bone were first recorded by Rauber (1876) who studied the effects of prolonged loading on bone. The details of this work were discussed in Chapter 8.

The effect of *in vitro* loading on plastic flow of fresh wet specimens of cortical bone from human femurs and tibias was investigated by Roth et al. (1961a) in specimens from amputated limbs of an 18-year-old and a 63-year-old patient. One amputation resulted from a soft tissue neoplasm and the other from vascular insufficiency.

Test specimens, about 10 by 5 by 5 mm, were cut so that one of the surfaces of the specimen was parallel with one of the major axes of the intact bone. Thus, the specimen could be loaded in the longitudinal, radial, or tangential axis of the shaft of the bone. During preparation and testing, the specimens were kept moist with tap water.

Nonfracturing loads were applied to the specimens by two methods. In the first method, specimens were compressed between a ram and an anvil of mild steel which were positioned in a vise. When the jaws of the vise were closed the 3 mm wide ram was forced into a slightly wider slot in the anvil. In the second method, a dissecting needle was laid on the surface of the specimen which was then compressed between the jaws of the vise. During the compression the needle was pushed into the surface of the specimen, thus creating a complex force system between them.

Lightly loading a specimen produced a visible indentation which disappeared completely on removal of the load. Heavy loads caused a permanent indentation or set in the form of a mirror image of the ram. If a too heavy load was applied, a shear failure occurred as a piece of the specimen was punched out by the ram. This shear failure was in contrast to the tension failure produced by forcing the specimen apart as the needle was pushed into its substance.

A permanent set could be produced by loading the specimen in any direction. When a nonfracturing load or a load smaller than that required to cause a permanent set was applied for longer periods of time the specimen would fail suddenly with a loud snap.

Although a permanent set arose from plastic flow, the authors do not think that plastic flow is a normal physiological problem in bone, because the load required to produce it is almost as large as the fracture load. The results obtained by Roth et al. are difficult to evaluate because neither the magnitude nor the duration of the loads applied to the specimens are given.

In a second paper based on material from the same two patients, Roth and his colleagues (1961b) demonstrated biphasic elastic behavior in fresh human bone. Test specimens of the same dimensions used in their earlier study were loaded as before until a permanent set was produced.

The surfaces of the specimens were then ground under running water until all evidence of the indentations was removed and the surface appeared perfectly flat when examined with optical aid in oblique light. Afterwards the specimens were immersed in: (1) 95% ethanol for ten minutes, (2) pure dioxane for ten minutes, and (3) 2% nitric acid for four minutes, after which they were boiled in water for ten minutes.

When the first two procedures were completed a hump, which was a negative image of the original indentation and a positive image of the ram producing it, was found on the surface of the specimens. The hump was considerably shallower than the original permanent set and disappeared completely after boiling the specimen. This behavior was easiest to elicit by loading the specimen parallel with the long axis of the intact bone.

The results were explained on the basis of two elastic components—mineral and matrix—which have additive effects under normal loads. With abnormal loads the authors believe that the mineral component

is loaded into the region of plastic flow and given a permanent set at slightly lower loads than those needed to cause the same behavior in the matrix component. Thus, the permanent set in the mineral component "locks in" elastic strain from the matrix component. If the effect of the bonds holding the permanent set can be eliminated, the elastic strain of the matrix corrects itself, producing the original shape or hump.

The mineral phase is weaker than the matrix and takes a permanent set before the matrix does. Decalcification removes the mineral phase, while dehydration in some way cancels the intercrystalline bond holding the permanent set of the mineral phase against the tendency of the elastically strained matrix to return to its original shape and dimensions. In the specimens not developing humps after ethanolization, it was possible that the matrix was also given a permanent set.

According to the authors, there are two theories to explain plastic flow in bone. One theory is that it is a sort of cog-wheel phenomenon, the cogs interlocking with each other after plastic flow. Shrinking the specimen with alcohol disengages the cogs.

The second theory is that alcohol, because of its polar nature, attaches to and blocks certain bonds holding adjoining crystal masses together so that the elastic strain in the matrix is released. If such a situation occurs, the strength of bone may be affected considerably by the type and number of hydroxyapatite ions in it.

If the shrinkage explanation is correct, the strength and rigidity of bone should vary with the amount of water in it. The marked effects of moisture on the mechanical properties of bone (see Chapter 4) seem to support the shrinkage theory.

Currey's studies (1965) of the effects of prolonged loading on anelasticity of wet and dry specimens of cortical bone tested at various temperatures have already been discussed (see Chapter 8).

Dynamic measurements of the viscoelastic properties of bone were made by Smith and Keiper (1965) with an electromechanical transducer especially developed for the purpose. With this instrument dynamic, nondestructive tests were successfully made of small specimens of human and dog cortical bone. Cylindrical specimens about 2 by 2 by 12 mm, with a uniform diameter of 1.00 to 1.03 mm, were cut from the subperiosteal cortex of the ribs and long bones. The long axis of the specimen usually coincided with that of the intact bone. Similar specimens were taken from the inner cortex of the ilium just below and roughly parallel to the crest. The specimens, which were obtained at operation or autopsy, were stored in 50% alcohol and then immersed in Ringer's solution for at least twenty-four hours before testing. After brief blotting they were weighed to the nearest 0.10 milligram on a micro-balance.

Storage of the specimens in 50% alcohol did not change their elastic modulus although their viscous modulus was uniformly increased with a mean change of 13%. This effect was reversed by immersing the specimens in Ringer's solution for twenty-four hours. Apparently alcohol had a dehydrating action.

In rib specimens from patients with diseases not apt to affect the bone, the elastic/viscous stiffness ratio tended to decline with age (Table XCI). However, the small number of specimens and the effect of alcohol on viscous stiffness, which was not realized at first, prevented analysis of cor-

TABLE XCI

ELASTICITY, VISCOSITY, AND DENSITY MEASUREMENTS OF HUMAN RIB BONE (Data from Smith and Keiper, 1965)

Age	Primary Diagnosis	Elastic Modulus* $\times 10^{11}$ dynes/cm²	Viscous Modulus† $\times 10^{9}$ dynes/cm²	Stiffness Ratio elastic/viscous	Bone Density (mg/mm³)
Males					
13	Coarctation Aorta	1.41	3.02	46.6	1.74
19	Subaortic Stenosis	1.96	2.95	66.4	1.90
33	Diabetes Mellitus	2.03	3.00	67.7	1.80
49	Carcinoma, Kidney	1.72	3.02	56.9	1.97
54	Diabetes Mellitus	2.10	4.58	45.8	1.80
60	Chronic Nephritis	1.92	3.72	51.6	1.81
62	Pneumonia	1.67	3.67	45.5	1.78
		(1.86) ‡	(3.60)	(53.5)	(1.83)
72	Lymphoma, Colon	1.82	3.49	52.2	1.83
73	Gout; Arteriosclerosis	1.97	3.49	56.4	1.81
Females					
50	Carcinoma, Ovary	1.91	3.48	54.9	1.77
51	Cerebral Thrombosis	1.89	3.72	50.8	1.86
51	Lymphoma, Neck	2.17	3.05	71.2	1.90
52	Carcinoma, Breast	1.66	3.18	52.2	1.79
58	Mitral Insufficiency	1.74	4.55	38.2	1.84
63	Carcinoma, Breast	1.93	4.87	37.6	1.88
		(1.88)	(3.81)	(51.1)	(1.83)

* Elastic stiffness $\times \dfrac{\text{length}}{\text{cross-sectional area}}$ (cylinder).

† Viscous stiffness $\times \dfrac{\text{length}}{\text{cross-sectional area}}$ (cylinder).

‡ Figures in parentheses are mean values for the last five entries in the group.

relation. Apparently the viscous modulus was not influenced by bone density or the sex of the subject.

Two iliac specimens (Table XCII) had an elastic modulus comparable to those of specimens from adult ribs but the elastic moduli of the rest of the iliac specimens were considerably lower. Mean values of iliac specimens from adult men and women were considerably less than those for the rib specimens. However, the number of specimens tested was too small for statistical evaluation of sexual difference. The rib specimens from the 19-year-old male had the lowest viscous modulus but it was also low in the iliac specimens.

Density was usually less in iliac than in rib specimens but the difference was not as great as that between the elastic moduli of the two types of specimens. Iliac specimens in males had a higher average viscous modulus than rib specimens but in females it was lower.

Specimens from the long bones (Table

XCIII) had elastic moduli similar to those of the rib specimens. The elastic modulus of one tibial and two femoral specimens were 20% to 40% less in the transverse than in the longitudinal direction. The elastic/viscous ratio, transverse to the long axis of the bone, approached the lowest values for the iliac specimens from the male individuals. No differences were found between the specimens from Michigan patients and those from Texas patients where the water had a high fluoride content.

Sexual differences were not found in the elasticity of rib specimens, but iliac specimens from females had higher elastic moduli despite comparable densities. The low elastic modulus and density of the rib specimen from the 13-year-old boy may have been the result of submaximal mineralization.

Femoral specimens from adult male beagle dogs had a substantially higher elastic modulus than specimens from female dogs, although the viscous moduli were

TABLE XCII

Elasticity, Viscosity, and Density Measurements of the Human Iliac Crest
(Data from Smith and Keiper, 1965)

Age	Primary Diagnosis	Elastic Modulus* $\times 10^{11}$ dynes/cm²	Viscous Modulus† $\times 10^{9}$ dynes/cm²	Stiffness Ratio elastic/viscous	Density (mg/mm³)
Males					
19	Subaortic Stenosis	1.19	3.59	33.2	1.62
42	Cerebral Thrombosis	1.51	3.88	38.9	1.75
45	Carcinoma, Pancreas	1.18	3.71	31.8	1.82
63	Myocardial Infarction	1.48	4.97	29.8	1.71
66	Myocardial Infraction	1.42	3.59	39.6	1.88
		(1.39) ‡	(4.04)	(35.0)	(1.79)
Females					
39	Carcinoma, Breast	1.90	3.93	48.4	1.93
71	Carcinoma, Stomach	1.42	3.01	47.2	1.77
80	General Arteriosclerosis	1.22	2.78	43.8	1.62
83	Myocardial Infarction	1.75	3.82	45.9	1.77
		(1.57)	(3.39)	(46.3)	(1.77)

* Elastic stiffness $\times \dfrac{\text{length}}{\text{cross-sectional area}}$ (cylinder).

† Viscous stiffness $\times \dfrac{\text{length}}{\text{cross-sectional area}}$ (cylinder).

‡ Figures in parentheses are mean values for the preceding entries.

TABLE XCIII

ELASTICITY, VISCOSITY, AND DENSITY MEASUREMENTS OF HUMAN LONG BONES (Data from Smith and Keiper, 1965)

Bone and Age	Primary Diagnosis		Elastic Modulus* $\times 10^{11}$ dynes/cm²	Viscous Modulus† $\times 10^{9}$ dynes/cm²	Stiffness Ratio elastic/viscous	Bone Density (mg/mm³)
Tibia						
Male—70	Arteriosclerosis	(a)	1.67	3.25	51.4	1.78
		(b)	0.97	2.96	32.8	1.85
Clavicle‡						
Male						
20	Trauma		1.64	3.55	46.2	1.84
64	Sarcoma		1.89	3.26	58.0	1.85
Femur						
Male						
70	Arteriosclerosis	(a)	1.62	3.10	52.3	1.67
		(b)	1.23	3.81	32.3	1.73
Female						
35	Trauma	(a)	1.96	4.80	40.8	1.19
		(b)	1.55	3.57	43.4	—

* Elastic stiffness $\times \dfrac{\text{length}}{\text{cross-sectional area}}$ (cylinder).

† Viscous stiffness $\times \dfrac{\text{length}}{\text{cross-sectional area}}$ (cylinder).

‡ High fluoride area of Texas.

(a) = Specimen cut parallel to longitudinal bone axis.

(b) = Specimen cut across longitudinal bone axis.

comparable and the density was essentially constant. Specimens from the control and the fluoride-treated dogs had similar moduli.

In discussing the results of their studies, Smith and Keiper point out that the small size of their specimens (the cross-sectional area of the cylinders being equivalent to that of approximately eleven osteons) is a disadvantage because too little of the atomic unit is present. The advantage was that several specimens could be machined from a single bone section.

The studies by Bonfield and Li (1966, 1967) on elastic and plastic deformation as well as the anisotropy of nonelastic flow in cortical bone were discussed in Chapters 6 and 7.

Viscoelastic properties of wet specimens of unembalmed cortical bone of adult human femurs have also been investigated by

Sedlin (1965). He tested standardized specimens under a constant deformation, under different rates of deformation up to a constant load, during loading and unloading at different constant rates, and finally under a constant load.

The material used in the constant deformation experiments consisted of twelve groups of ten specimens each. The specimens, cross sections of the middle femoral shaft, were obtained from ten subjects, 19 to 64 years of age. One group of specimens was tested as cantilevers, sixteen specimens from sixteen subjects were tested in tension, and twenty-five from fourteen subjects were tested as end-supported beams. Five complete cross sections from five subjects were tested in longitudinal compression while compression tests were also made of fifteen blocks from the same subjects.

A constant deformation rate of 0.2 cm/ min to 1.0 cm/min varying in accordance with specimen size and type of loading was used. Progressive loading was stopped at an estimated 25% of the failure load and the resultant deformation maintained. By keeping the recorder running, stress as a function of time with a constant deformation was recorded. Recording time varied among the tests and recording was stopped when no further deformation occurred. The predominant recording time was thirty seconds to two minutes but in some instances was extended to ten to fifteen minute periods to verify that no additional changes were occurring.

All specimens from all subjects gave identical qualitative results. When deformation became constant, i.e. when loading was stopped, a stress decrease occurred with 50% to 60% of it being evident in thirty seconds. Depending upon the direction of loading there were quantitative differences in the amount of stress decrease with time. This behavior was attributed to the natural heterogeneity of bone. These data demonstrated that stress relaxation and relaxation time are material properties of bone.

Deformation at different deformation rates up to a constant load was investigated in twelve cantilever specimens from a 68-year-old woman and five tension specimens from five subjects. Cantilever specimens were loaded to 100 grams at a rate of 0.1 cm/min, then at 1.0 cm/min with two minutes between loads. After overnight refrigeration they were retested first at 1.0 cm/min, then at 0.1 cm/min with two minutes for recovery between tests. Larger specimens from the 68-year-old woman were loaded to 250 grams but otherwise the procedure was not changed. Tension specimens were loaded to 10 kg at a rate of 0.1 cm/min then at a rate of 0.2 cm/min.

Unit stress was about 3.5 kp/mm² and 0.8 kp/mm² in the cantilever and tension specimens, respectively. Average deformation in the twelve cantilever specimens was 0.86 mm when loaded at a speed of 0.1 cm/min and 0.82 mm when loaded at a rate of 1.0 cm/min. When tested the following day, average deformations of 0.85 mm and 0.87 mm were found with loading rates of 1.0 cm/min and 0.1 cm/min, respectively. In both cases the individual differences were highly significant. Consistent and highly significant differences were likewise found in the cantilever tests of the larger specimens. Similar results were obtained in the tensile tests.

These tests showed that bone deforms less with rapid than with slower loading and agree with data obtained by McElhaney and Byars (1965) from compression tests.

In another series of experiments Sedlin studied the behavior of bone during loading and unloading at constant rates. Test material consisted of five compression specimens from three subjects, fifteen simple beam specimens from two subjects, and ten tensile specimens from five subjects. The testing machine was cycled between zero load and 50% of full scale with smaller loads of 100 or 250 grams for the cantilever tests and 100 kg for the compression tests. Each specimen was tested twice, first at a rate of 0.1 or 0.2 cm/min and second at a rate of 1.0 cm/min.

Although the general shape of the hysteresis loop obtained in the experiments varied with the direction of loading, the results were similar in all tests and demonstrated that the amount of residual deformation varied with the deformation rate. Residual deformation was greater at zero stress at the slower rate than at the faster rate, indicating that with this type of testing more energy was dissipated at a slower than at a faster rate.

Sedlin also investigated creep phenomena in bone in a three-part study. In a preliminary study (Part 1), four tensile specimens from a 69-year-old man were tested first at 5 kg, then at 10 kg with approximate stresses of 0.85 and 1.7 kp/mm², respectively. The constant load was maintained for thirty minutes while deformation readings were taken at 1, 2, 3, 4, 5, 15 and 30 minutes, respectively. At thirty minutes the load was released and the specimen allowed to recover for half an hour before the second load was applied.

With 5 kg load the final deformation was reached almost immediately and remained unchanged. After application of a 10 kg load, deformation increased for about ten minutes, then seemed to remain constant. These results suggested that total deformation with a constant stress is approached asymptotically and that deformation is a function of stress duration.

In Part 2 of his studies, two tensile speci-

mens were successively subjected to 5, 10, 20, and 30 kg loads in order to determine if they returned to their original length after removal of the load. Then three other specimens were tested with successive loads of 10, 20, and 30 kg. Loads were applied for thirty minutes and then released. Deformation was recorded constantly and numerically with a voltmeter printing readout. A test was considered complete if the specimen returned to its original length. Tests were performed at ten minute intervals.

With a constant 5 kg load, two specimens reached maximal deformation almost immediately with no further increase for the rest of the experiment (Table XCIV). They also returned to their original length with release of the load, most of the recovery occurring immediately and the remainder within a few minutes.

With a 10 kg load some specimens had a definite delay in reaching total deforma-

TABLE XCIV

CHANGES IN DEFORMATION OVER TIME UNDER DIFFERING CONSTANT LOADS*
(Data from Sedlin, 1965)

Subject	Load Kg	Loaded				Unloaded			
		Initial Deformation	Seconds 5	15	30	Initial Recovery	Seconds 5	15	30
1	5	24.0	24.5	24.5	24.5	0	0	0	0
	10	26.4	31.8	32.3	32.7	3.8	1.8	1.1	.7
	20	82.1	89.4	91.3	92.7	13.6	7.0	5.4	4.7
	30	154.2	182.6	192.5	198.9	42.4	26.9	24.1	23.2
2	10	55.0	59.8	60.5	60.6	5.1	3.5	2.6	0
	20	71.0	74.6	76.0	78.0	2.6	0	0	0
	30	98.7	104.1	106.3	108.2	11.8	3.9	2.5	2.2
3	10	83.3	86.3	86.9	87.4	3.4	0	0	0
	20	146.3	170.2	173.1	175.3	20.1	9.9	8.1	6.9
	30	207.4	231.9	247.4	261.4	51.8	29.6	26.1	24.7
7	5	11.5	11.9	12.0	12.0	.6	0	0	0
	10	14.6	14.7	14.8	14.8	1.2	0	0	0
	20	54.0	62.9	63.8	64.3	14.9	12.8	12.3	12.3
	30	92.7	99.2	101.0	102.0	18.7	14.5	14.5	13.4
19	10	28.8	30.3	30.9	—	2.0	0	0	0
	20	94.8	103.3	105.7	107.5	17.7	4.8	0	0
	30	146.0	187.4	210.3	232.3	90.0	64.0	60.1	58.3

* Deformation units are in micra, and are the difference between a recorded value and original length.

tion. Of the five specimens tested, four regained their original length and one did not. A 20 kg load caused a progressive deformation up to thirty minutes. After removal of the load only one specimen returned to its original length after half an hour. Similar but greater deformation occurred with 30 kg load and none of the specimens returned to its original length after half an hour. In all tests initial deformation occurred as rapidly as the specimen could be loaded and initial recovery length as fast as it could be unloaded. From this it was concluded that bone has both instantaneous and retarded elasticity.

These experiments demonstrated that under certain constant loads, bone will gradually yield and that larger loads produce larger yields. However, the latter characteristic varies from one subject to another.

In a third part of Sedlin's study, five additional specimens from the 69-year-old man were subjected to a 30 kg load for twenty-five hours before it was removed. The recovery period was then recorded for an additional twenty-four hours.

Data obtained showed that two specimens reached a constant deformation within twenty-four hours, two continued to deform for the entire time, and one failed after one hour (Table XCV). All three

specimens for which a record of unloading was obtained showed persistent deformation after a 24-hour recovery period. Data from the two specimens with continuing deformation for twenty-four hours indicated that eventually a constant deformation would have been reached. The recovery records showed that a decrease in deformation would have occurred although the specimen would not have returned to its original length.

Quantitative data on viscoelastic properties of fresh wet cortical bone of Japanese subjects have been cited by Yamada (1970), who gives values for the elastic limit (percent of ultimate stress), percentage of recovery with and without the elastic aftereffect, creep limit (percent of ultimate stress), maximum creeping time, and a comparison of the deformation at creeping rupture with that of a normal test. Values were obtained for tensile, compression, shearing, bending, and torsion tests.

Examination of these data (Table XCVI) reveals that the elastic limit is highest in tension and torsion and lowest in shearing. Maximum and minimum values for percentage of recovery without the elastic aftereffect were found in bending and in shearing, respectively. The greatest percentage of recovery with the elastic aftereffect was seen in compression and

TABLE XCV

DEFORMATION AND RECOVERY FROM A 24-HOUR CONSTANT LOAD* (Data from Sedlin, 1965)

Subject	Initial Deformation	Loaded Time in Hours						Initial Recovery	Unloaded Time in Hours					
		1	5	10	15	20	24		1	5	10	15	20	24
1	109.0	137.7	143.9	144.4	146.3	147.1	147.1	†						
2	103.9	135.1	157.5	171.6	178.5	184.8	190.6	61.1	29.3	20.8	16.6	15.2	13.9	11.9
3	113.8	178.1	187.6	194.7	199.3	203.0	205.3	83.0	59.4	54.3	52.3	51.6	50.0	49.0
7	103.6	128.9	140.7	142.1	143.7	144.2	144.2	37.8	18.2	15.0	12.9	12.5	11.3	11.2
19	198.8	341.9	—	Fracture										

* Deformation is recorded in micra. In the unloaded half of the table, the deformations are to be interpreted as the remaining deformation at the time cited.

† This test had to be discontinued at this time to permit electrical work in other parts of the laboratory.

TABLE XCVI

VISCOELASTIC PROPERTIES OF FRESH, WET COMPACT BONE OF ADULT JAPANESE
(Data from Yamada, 1970)

Test	Elastic Limit (% of Ult. Stress)	% Recovery (Without Elastic Aftereffect)	% Recovery (With Elastic Aftereffect)	Creep Limit (% of Ult. Stress)	Maximum Creep Time (hrs)	Deformation at Creeping Rupture Compared with Ult. Deformation in a Normal Test
Tensile (femur)	80	84	92	65	24	1.6 times
Compressive (femur)	75	88	93	70	15	1.2 times
Shear	25	63	—	75	48	1.6 times
Bending	70	89	92	60	80	no change
Torsion	80	85	93	70	36	1.6 times

Ult. = ultimate.

shearing while the least (1% lower) occurred in tension and bending. No values were reported for shearing.

Shear produced the maximum value for creep limit while bending resulted in the minimum value. Creeping time was maximum in bending and minimum in compression.

Deformation at creeping rupture was 1.6 times the ultimate deformation of a normal test for tension, shearing, and torsion but only 1.2 times the normal deformation in compression. Bending caused no change in the rupture deformation in comparison with that of a normal test.

Sonoda (1962) is apparently the only one who has investigated viscoelastic properties of cancellous bone. For this purpose he used fresh wet vertebral bodies from Japanese subjects. He reported that the elastic limit in compression exceeded that in tension but the reverse was true for percentage of recovery with and without the elastic aftereffect (Table XCVII). Lumbar and cervical vertebrae in compression provided the maximum and minimum values for creep limit, respectively. Maximum creeping time was greatest in lumbar vertebrae in compression and lowest in vertebral bodies (region not given) in torsion. No torsion values were given for elastic limit, percentage of recovery without the elastic aftereffect, and percentage of recovery with the elastic aftereffect.

Because of its viscoelastic nature, attempts have been made to explain the mechanical behavior of bone under load by means of rheological models. Rheology,

TABLE XCVII

VISCOELASTIC PROPERTIES OF FRESH, MOIST HUMAN VERTEBRAL BODIES
(Data from Sonoda, 1962)

Test	Elastic Limit (% of Ult. Stress)	% Recovery Without Elastic Aftereffect	% Recovery With Elastic Aftereffect	Creep Limit (% of Ult. Stress)	Maximum Creeping Time (hours)
Tension	15	11	12	40	15
Compression	25	7	11	30 cervical & upper thoracic 35 lower thoracic 50 lumbar	24 cervical & upper thoracic 48 lumbar
Torsion				40	10

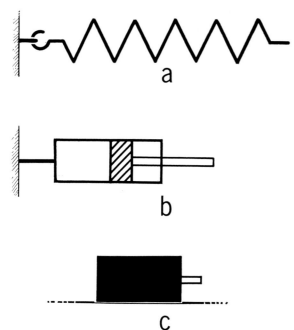

Figure 133. Rheological models: a—The Hooke Body, b—The Newton Body or dashpot, c—The Saint-Venant Body.

released the spring returns to its original length. The amount the spring is pulled out depends upon the magnitude of the force applied to it.

Pure viscous flow is represented by the Newton body or "dashpot" (Fig. 133b) which is an oil-filled tube with a loose stopper which acts like a piston. Application of a tensile or a compressive force to the stopper makes it move through the oil at a rate proportional to the magnitude of the force. As soon as the force is removed motion ceases and the stopper remains where it is at that time.

The Saint-Venant body is simply a weight on a horizontal surface (Fig. 133c). The weight can only be moved by a force

the science dealing with deformation and flow of matter, is commonly thought of as being concerned only with fluids although flow also occurs in solids. In fluids the rate of flow is directly proportional to the applied force and inversely proportional to the viscosity of the material. The problem in solids is not that large forces make them flow but that small forces do not.

Although rheological laws are primarily mathematical they are often represented graphically by simple mechanical models— the Hooke body, the Newton body or "dashpot," and the Saint-Venant body— based on three elementary principles (Reiner, 1959, 1960).

Elastic behavior of matter is represented by the Hooke body (Fig. 133a) which is a coiled spring firmly supported at one end. Application of a force to the free end of the spring pulls it out but if the force is

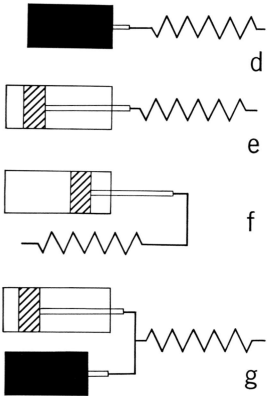

Figure 134. Rheological models: d—The Prandtl Body, e—The Maxwell Body, f—The Kelvin Body, g—The Bingham Body.

large enough to overcome the friction between the weight and the surface. On removal of the force the weight stays in its new position. While accurately representing yield stress, the Saint-Venant body is a defective model since it does not represent the motion after the yield point is exceeded. A steady force large enough to move the body will make it move faster and faster after movement is initiated. Once movement is started a steady force will cause a constant rate of flow. In this respect plastic and viscous flow are similar.

Correction of the defects of the Saint-Venant body can be attained by combining a weight and a "dashpot" in parallel to form a Bingham body (Fig. 134g) which represents the similarities and differences between various materials.

Elastic deformation of a material below the yield point is represented by the Prandtl body consisting of a weight in series with a spring (Fig. 134d). A small force stretches the spring while a large force also moves the weight.

A third combination of the three primary rheological models is the Kelvin body which consists of a dashpot in parallel with a spring (Fig. 134f). A perfectly elastic sponge whose holes are filled with a viscous liquid represents a Kelvin body. Under a steady static load the sponge elongates in proportion to the load and returns to its original length upon removal of the load. If the load is rapidly applied energy is absorbed by the viscous flow of the liquid in the sponge so that it behaves like rubber or jelly.

A fourth combination of the primary models is the Maxwell body which is composed of a dashpot and a spring in series (Fig. 134e). The Maxwell body demonstrates that fluids, even ideal gases, may have both elastic and viscous properties.

Thus, a tensile force applied to the spring immediately stretches it and causes the piston to begin to move behind the spring. If the model is kept stretched to a certain length the piston will continue to move until the elastic strain disappears. The disappearance of the strain indicates that the elastic forces in the liquid have "relaxed" by the time the piston has completed its movement.

The Maxwell body can also be considered in another way. Suppose the spring is rather weak and the dashpot is filled with a very viscous oil. If the spring is pulled out and quickly released it returns almost exactly to its original position with hardly any movement of the piston. The body now looks like an elastic solid and, depending upon the viscosity of the dashpot, it might be hours or centuries before the fluid properties are apparent. Thus, the everyday qualitative differences between a solid and a liquid become only quantitative differences, dependent upon the relation between the time of relaxation and of observation.

Sedlin used the data obtained from his experiments, already discussed in this chapter, as the basis for the development of a rheological model to account for the observed behavior of cortical bone.

The fact that the load-deformation curves obtained in the tests had no straight line eliminated the perfectly elastic body. Perfectly plastic and rigid bodies were eliminated by the fact that stress progressively increased until failure. The cycle and creep studies demonstrated that elastic behavior is a feature of bone.

Some type of viscous damping in bone was deduced from the following facts: (1) deformation up to some constant load is a function of the deformation rate, (2)

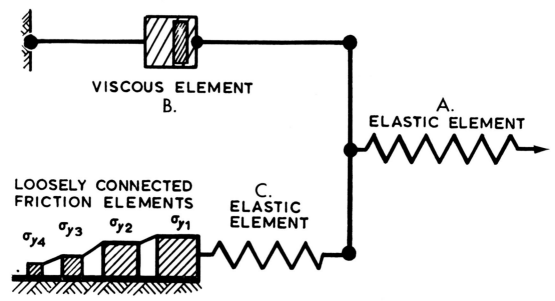

Figure 135. Sedlin's rheological model for bone. (Slightly modified from Kenedi: Courtesy of Proceedings of the Institution of Mechanical Engineers, 1966-67)

total deformation under a constant stress was not attained instantaneously, i.e. there is a retardation time, (3) there is relaxation time, and (4) the presence of a hysteresis on load-unload cycle testing.

The *generic* model he finally developed (Fig. 135) consists of a Hooke body linked in series to a unit composed of a Newton body (dashpot) in parallel with a modified Prandtl body. Unfortunately, Sedlin did not attempt to equate the various components of his model with specific anatomical features of bone. The number and relative size of the friction elements are arbitrary.

The Hooke body (Fig. 135*A*) shows that bone undergoes instantaneous deformation proportional to the load applied to it. If the load is maintained, the Newton body (Fig. 135*B*) alters the shape and puts a constantly increasing load on the Prandtl body (Fig. 135*C*) as they are both stretched. This, in turn, decreases the rate of stretching of the dashpot or Newton body. These parts of the model show that

bone, after its original deformation, continues to exhibit some extra deformation which appears at an ever increasing rate and approaches the same asymptotic value as Smith and Walmsley (1959) and Currey (1965) previously showed.

During unloading the reverse behavior occurs. The friction elements explain the irreversible deformation that appears with time above some load. The value depends upon the condition of loading. Irreversible deformation does not appear at low loads, no matter how long the time, because the friction of the first element (σ_{y1}) cannot be overcome by the load. If the load is large enough to make the friction element (σ_{y1}) move, it does so immediately, because originally before the dashpot (B) has stretched much, the spring C will not have transmitted much of the force to σ_{y1}. Because of frictional losses under it, friction element σ_{y1} does not have to move at all. This results in less load being transferred to the other friction elements than that transferred from the spring C to σ_{y1}.

SUMMARY

Bone, both cortical and cancellous, is a viscoelastic material that exhibits the phenomena of creep, plastic flow, permanent set, stress relaxation, hysteresis, elastic recovery, and the elastic aftereffect.

Attempts have been made to explain the viscoelastic behavior of bone by means of rheological models. However, the various elements of the model have not been equated with specific anatomical elements of bone.

CHAPTER 12

EFFECTS OF REDUCED FORCES, RADIOACTIVE ISOTOPES AND PIEZOELECTRICITY

REDUCED FORCES

THUS FAR WE HAVE been concerned with data obtained from experiments in which standardized specimens of bone were subjected to some kind of force. The question now arises as to how mechanical properties of bone are affected by reduced forces or absence of forces to which bone is normally subjected during life. It is already known from data collected during space flights up to fourteen days duration that measurable changes occur in the chemistry and density of the calcaneus and metacarpal bones of pilots and crews of space vehicles (Kazarian and Von Gierke, 1969). With increasing advances in space age technology, which may permit man to stay on the moon or in outer space for extended periods of time, the effect of reduced or zero gravitational forces on the mechanical properties of human bone becomes a problem of extreme practical importance. Unfortunately, there are little experimental data on this problem.

Kazarian and Von Gierke (1969) investigated the effects of immobilization on bone loss, chelation, and mechanical properties of bones of thirty-two male Rhesus monkeys. The monkeys, varying from 7 to 10 kg in weight, were clinically screened and surveyed radiographically to insure, by epiphyseal closure, that they were skeletally mature. They were then divided into sixteen control and sixteen experimental animals. For seven days preceding the experiments the animals were conditioned in metabolic cages.

The experimental animals were anesthetized and then immobilized in a fast-setting full body plaster of Paris cast. Twice daily the animals were hand fed and sixteen times daily, at regular intervals, given distilled water to drink. At two week intervals the animals were anesthetized, removed from the casts, weighed, radiographed, and examined for complications. After a sixty day period they were killed. Rigid immobilization was assumed to simulate weightlessness.

Bones of interest were dissected out, the soft tissue removed, and midsagittal sections made so that the trabecular orientation could be examined. Comparable specimens from control animals were compared with those from the demineralized and immobilized animals. Demineralization was obtained by a 0.04% solution of Na_2EDTA, diluted with 250 ml of 0.9% NaCl solution which was infused intravenously every Monday, Wednesday, and Friday for a three-month period.

In twelve specimens (six immobilized and six controls) lumbar vertebrae five through seven were removed, stripped of their articulations as well as ligamentous and tendinous attachments, and prepared for immediate compression testing. The vertebral bodies and the intervening discs were then loaded to failure at a constant rate in an Instron materials testing machine with an automatic recorder. The rate of loading was 10×10^{-3} sec^{-1}.

Load-deformation curves (Fig. 136) showed that the compressive strength of

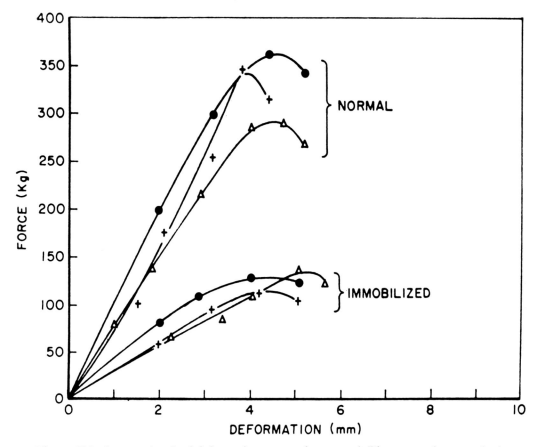

Figure 136. Compressive load-deformation curves for normal Rhesus monkey vertebral segments and after 60 days of immobilization. (From Kazarian and Von Gierke: *Clin Orthop*, 1969)

the vertebrae from the immobilized animals was two or three times less than that of similar vertebrae from the control animals. Similar curves for tension tests at points of muscle insertion on the bones showed that the force required to pull these attachments away was 30% less in the specimens from the immobilized animals than in those from the control animals (Fig. 137).

Fresh femurs from chelated animals had a considerably lower compressive strength than those from the control animals (Fig. 138). The reduced compressive strength in the chelated animals was attributed to extensive thinning of the femoral cortex and

loss of secondary trabeculae with thickening of the principal trabeculae.

Effects of forced immobilization by a pelvic cast on mechanical, chemical, and anatomical features of growing hind limb bones of guinea pigs were recently investigated by Eichler (1970). The hind legs were immobilized in the frog position in which there is 90° flexion and abduction of the hips, 90° flexion of the knee and mid-position of the ankle. Food intake was reduced the first two days of the experiments but by the fourth week, average food intake was about the same as that in the control animals. Food intake decreased somewhat later but not enough so that

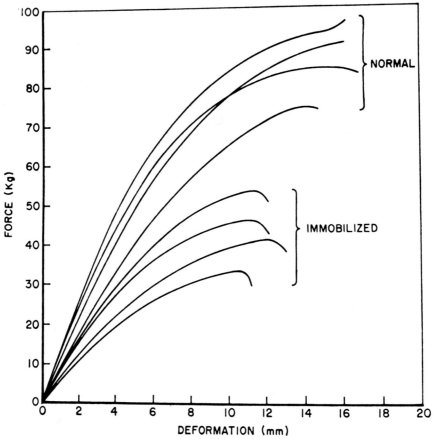

Figure 137. Tensile load-deformation curves for points of muscle attachment in normal and immobilized Rhesus monkeys. (From Kazarian and Von Gierke: *Clin Orthop,* 1969)

changes due to immobilization were the result of malnutrition.

Newborn as well as young animals weighing 150, 250, 350, and 500 g in addition to adults (800 to 1,000 g) were used to provide sufficient comparative material. To avoid errors due to fluctuations in estrus, only male animals were used. Initially mixed breeds were employed to eliminate genetic effects but this was later abandoned because of difficulty in obtaining them; only white purebred Pirbright strain animals were used.

The "physiological breaking strength" was determined for the humerus and femur of 285, mostly male, guinea pigs. "Physiological breaking strength" is not equivalent to "ultimate stress" used in materials testing science but is, in the author's opinion, more appropriate for growing bone. The bones were tested under static compression-bending loads in an apparatus constructed for that purpose, with which a maximum load of 25 kp (55 to 125 lb) could be applied. Energy for fracture was produced by a pendulum with a locking device so that the specimen could be loaded in 100 p increments. By use of a size dependent support, the bending loads acted on the epiphysis while the dynamic load was applied to the middle of the shaft. Collapse of the cortex of the bone was avoided by a relatively large surface for support. The loading apparatus was adjustable in order to accommodate bones of various sizes. All bones were positioned so that the dorsolateral surface rested on two arms while the entire shaft was loaded.

A water level was used to insure that the instrument was not tilted. Load was increased in increments of 10 p/sec. By manually turning a knob an almost constant rate of loading could be obtained. In the beginning of an experiment, torsion of the bone occurred. Later, torsion was prevented by the clamps. Before testing, the bones were stored in physiological saline solution. The unfixed bones were tested on the day of autopsy.

In the normal animals the physiological breaking strength of the humerus and the femur increased markedly during the growing period. Femoral strength during this period was 30% to 40% and in adult life 17% to 30% greater than humeral strength. In 350 g animals, femoral breaking strength of females exceeded that of males by 4.1%. At the time of the tests the

Weight class (g)	Time of fixation (weeks)					
	1	2	3	4	5	6
150 (10-5) kp		7,6 / 3,4		7,0 / 3,1		
Loss %		54,47		55,93		
250 (10-5)	5,3 / 5,6	9,3 / 5,7	9,7 / 4,2	10,5 / 4,1	11,7 / 3,9	11,7 / 3,8
Loss %	−5,9	37,7	56,3	60,6	66,2	67,0
350 (15-10-5)			11,7 / 7,1			
Loss %			39,5			
500 (15-10-5)			16,8 / 10,9			
Loss %			35,0			
800 – 1000 (20-15-10-5)			20,3 / 15,5	20,8 / 14,7		
Loss %			23,6	29,5		

■ Experimental animals   □ Controls

Reduction of the physiological breaking strength of femora by pelvic-plaster immobilization (guinea pigs)

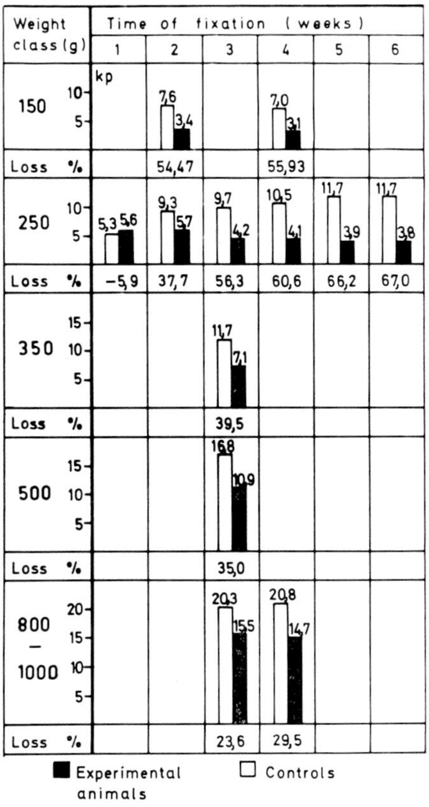

Figure 139. Effects of immobilization on physiological breaking strength of guinea pig femurs. (From Eichler: *Aktuelle Orthopädie*, 1970)

animals were at the age of puberty so it can be assumed that females of this age and weight class were skeletally more mature than comparable male animals. Femoral breaking strength of adult male animals (800 to 1,000 g) was 15% greater than in females of the same weight. Similar sexual differences were found for the breaking strength of the humerus.

Immobilization reduced the breaking strength of the femur as a function of immobilization time, sex, and age—the greatest reductions occurring in the youngest animals (Fig. 139). One week after immobilization the femoral breaking strength

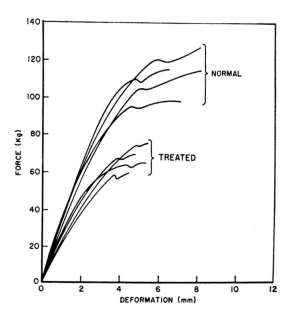

Figure 138. Compressive load-deformation curves for fresh normal and chelated monkey femurs. (From Kazarian and Von Gierke: *Clin Orthop,* 1969)

of somewhat older animals (250 g starting weight) was reduced 24%. Additional strength reductions of 21% occurred after two weeks, of 8% after three weeks, and of 4% between the fourth and sixth weeks of immobilization (Fig. 140). After six weeks in the cast, the breaking strength was only 38% of its original value—a 62% loss compared with the strength of bones from the control group! Femoral tensile strength losses in younger animals were based on a logarithmic decrement.

Femoral strength of animals in the 400 g group also underwent a loss of 25% after three weeks in the cast. This loss was equivalent to about 8% loss in one week. Femoral tensile strength declined another 17% after four weeks of immobilization. Although six week comparisons were unavailable, the evidence seemed to justify the assumption that loss rate has a logarithmic increment with immobilization period.

Femurs of adult animals lost 28% of their original strength after three weeks and 33% after eight weeks of immobilization. A linear decrease in breaking strength with immobilization was assumed.

Among the experimental animals, humeral breaking strength increased about 20% in young animals of both sexes. This was attributed to the greater strength of the forelegs, due to muscle training, since they were the only legs that could be used for pulling the animal around.

Calculations of the specific breaking strength, based on the pipe formula and the cross-sectional area of the bones at the fracture region, were also made. It was found that after three weeks in the cast the specific breaking strength of the femur of 400 g female guinea pigs declined 33% and that of male animals in the same weight group by 40%. These values are somewhat higher than those for physiological breaking strength.

Three weeks in a cast reduced the specific breaking strength of adult femurs by 29%. This reduction is particularly large compared to physiological breaking strength and is nearly equal to the decrease in tensile strength of femurs of young animals.

Specific breaking strength of the humerus of young growing experimental animals increased 20% to 30%, which is the reverse of the condition for physiological breaking strength which increased only in adult animals. The author explains this difference partially on the basis of age dependent differences in the cross-sectional shape of the femur in young and mature animals. Femurs of young animals have a tubular cross section shape while in adult animals it is triangular. A bone with a tubular cross section shape has a considerably lower tensile strength than one with a triangular cross section. Consequently, specific breaking strength values can only be correlated within identical age and weight groups when the strength calculations are based on the simplified formula for a tubular pipe.

Effects of immobilization on microhardness of guinea pig bone were also investigated by Eichler. Femoral microhardness of growing experimental animals weighing 250 g increased after one week of immobilization. However, animals of 500 g weight required three weeks of immobilization for surface strengthening of the bone. In young animals an initial increase in microhardness was followed by a decrease of up to 60% compared with that of control animals (Fig. 141). Hardness losses were greatest in animals between birth and puberty (350 g). After four weeks of immobilization the Vickers hardness number for the femurs decreased from 61 to 25. The tests were made with a Durimet (Leitz) microhardness tester and a Vickers diamond cone.

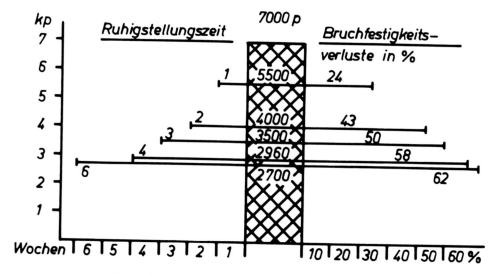

Bruchfestigkeit der Femora 200g schwerer
Meerschweinchen nach Ruhigstellung im
Beckengips
Startfestigkeit 7000 p

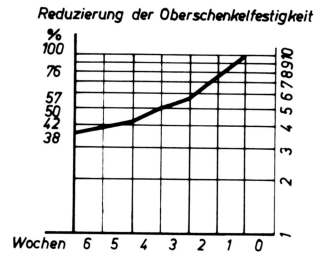

Knochenfestigkeitsverluste der Jungtiere
folgen einer einfachen logarithmischen
Funktion

Figure 140. Effects of immobilization on breaking strength of guinea pigs. (From Eichler: *Aktuelle Orthopädie*, 1970)

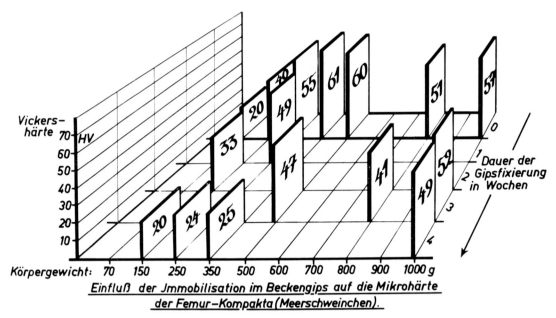

Figure 141. Effects of immobilization on microhardness of cortical bone of guinea pig femurs. (From Eichler: *Aktuelle Orthopädie*, 1970)

In a few cases, hardness of adult guinea pig bone was increased by immobilization. In most of the animals femoral surface microhardness was decreased by 8.8% after three weeks and by 13.6% after four weeks of immobilization. Humeral microhardness of immobilized animals was 5% less than that of control animals. The author interpreted this decrease as the result of fewer movements as the animal dragged itself and the cast around the cage. Thus, reduction of movement frequency causes a smaller bone, i.e. the humerus to undergo a decrease in its microhardness in spite of increased strength requirements for movement.

RADIOACTIVE ISOTOPES

A problem of major importance in the atomic age is the effect of radioisotopes on bone as a result of above-ground testing of atomic bombs. Much attention has been given to dangers from absorption by bone of radioactive isotopes, especially strontium, but there has been little attention paid to the way in which such isotopes might affect the mechanical properties of bone.

Apparently the only studies on the effects of radioactive isotopes on mechanical properties of bone have been made at the Radiobiology Laboratory of the University of Utah, Salt Lake City, Utah, by Hollingshaus and Mays (1958) and Taysum et al. (1962). Hollingshaus and Mays investigated the bending properties of intact tibias of purebred Beagle dogs who had been given different bone-seeking radioisotopes. The isotopes used were plutonium, radium, mesothorium, radiothorium, and strontium. In each case the dosage (rad) and length of time the isotope was in the animal were known. Taysum et al. obtained their material from the same source but used standardized specimens instead of whole bones. For this reason the following discussion will be limited to results of their experiments.

Taysum and colleagues used cylindrical test specimens with a reduced central region which were machined to a standardized size from various parts of the cortex of fresh, unembalmed dog tibias. Specimens from "hot" bones were prepared inside a glove box so that none of the bone dust was inhaled by the technician. The tibias were kept at $-20°$ C until the test specimens were made. The specimens were then returned to the freezer and not removed until a short time before testing to allow thawing. Specimens were moist when tested.

Jaws were especially designed to hold the specimens so that they could be loaded to failure under pure tension. The specimens were tested in a standard 120,000-lb capacity Baldwin testing machine equipped with a Tate-Emery load cell with an accuracy of ±0.5 lb in the range used in the tests. Strain was measured with a flexible leaf cantilever extensometer to which an SR4 electric strain gauge was cemented. Strain was measured by a conventional strain gauge bridge and amplifier. In order to monitor drift the equipment was calibrated with a micrometer repeatedly during each test.

A loading rate of approximately 15 lb/min was used with stress and strain readings being taken at 2 lb increments. All tests were made at room temperature. Stress-strain data for each specimen were plotted against each other and the proportional limit determined by the 25% offset method. This was later found to provide no advantage so values determined by eye were subsequently used.

In order to increase the number of control animals, animals with less than 200 rad were also considered as controls. This was considered to be acceptable because of the small effect of dosages of thousands of rad.

The parameters primarily investigated and reported were age and radiation dosage versus stress and energy absorbed to the proportional limit. Values for strain and the modulus of elasticity, also obtained during the experiments, were not discussed although they were included in the tables.

In the first experiment mechanical property data for specimens from tibias of male and female aging control dogs were compared with those from dogs of both sexes that had received various dosage levels of radium and plutonium. Dogs given the isotopes varied from 348 to 2,726 days in age and the average skeleton dose (rad) from 170 to 11,200. Aging control dogs were from 529 to 4,089 days of age. In specimens from the radioactive dogs tensile stress varied from 7.1 to 16.5×10^3 lbf/in^2; strain from 2.20 to 6.40 in/in $\times 10^{-2}$; modulus of elasticity from 1.54 to 4.74×10^5 lbf/in^2; and energy absorbed from 0.715 to 4.05 ft-lb/in^3. No consistent trends were evident when data from dogs given different isotope dosages were compared. Specimens from the aging control dogs had an ultimate stress varying from 9.18 to 22.0×10^3 lbf/in^2, a strain from 2.40 to 6.72, a modulus of elasticity from 2.24 to 5.80×10^5 lbf/in^2, and absorbed from 1.10 to 5.01 ft-lb/in^2 energy.

In the second experiment, data from dogs given radium, plutonium, strontium, and mesothorium were compared with those of aging control dogs. Data from both sexes were given. The radioactive dogs ranged from 539 to 2,032 days of age and had dosages varying from 107 to 6,670 rad. Stress varied from 9.04 to 22.89×10^3 lbf/in^2; strain from 0.88 to 3.14; modulus from 7.050 to 23.03×10^5 lbf/in^2; and energy from 0.30 to 2.89 ft-lb/in^2. In the aging control dogs stress ranged from 11.27 to 24.56; strain from 0.73 to 2.10; modulus from 9.056 to 23.03; and energy absorbed from 0.342 to 1.71. Again no consistent trends were observed in any of the data.

Data from dogs given thorium, strontium, plutonium, and mesothorium were compared with those from normal dogs in the third experiment. The radioactive dogs varied from 455 to 1,832 days of age and received from 10 to 1,680 rads as an average dose. Specimens from these dogs had a stress ranging from 9.131 to 23.5; strain from 0.362 to 1.46; modulus from 9.05 to 47.0; and absorbed from 0.20 to 1.30 ft-lb/in³ of energy. No definitive tendencies were noted. The normal dogs were 275 days old and had a stress ranging from 12.9 to 23.5, strain from 0.432 to 2.01, modulus from 10.2 to 37.7, and an energy absorption from 0.293 to 3.94.

Taysum and his colleagues were primarily interested in age and radiation dosage vs stress to the proportional limit and energy absorbed to the proportional limit, so they were the only parameters discussed or analyzed for statistical significance. Data from each of the above-mentioned three experiments were plotted as stress vs age, energy absorbed vs age, stress vs dose, and energy absorbed vs dose. Regression analyses and tests of the significance of the regression coefficients were then made.

The results of these analyses, in view of the ranges of variation found for the values of the various mechanical properties determined, showed no significant correlations at the 0.05 confidence level in changes of stress or of energy with increased age or dosage! Thus, at least in purebred Beagle dogs, bone-seeking radioisotopes do not significantly alter tensile properties or the energy absorbing capacity of tibial cortical bone.

PIEZOELECTRICITY

Piezoelectricity, i.e. the electricity or electric polarity due to pressure, has also been found in bone. The phenomenon is especially prominent in crystalline substances and its presence in bone is the result of the apatite crystals which give an electric response when they are deformed by a force. The strength of the electric current (microvoltage) depends upon the type of crystal being deformed and the direction of the current on the axes of the crystal.

The "piezoelectric effect" in bone was first measured by Fukada and Yasuda (1957) and has since been studied by Bassett and Becker (1962), Shamos et al. (1963), Shamos and Lavine (1964), Becker et al. (1964), Bassett et al. (1964), McElhaney (1967), and Cochran et al. (1968).

Piezoelectricity in quartz and other materials results from the fact that pressure deforming the crystal lattice also separates the centers of gravity of the positive and negative which generates a diploë moment in each molecule. The diploë moment is the product of the values for the charges times the amount of their separation.

Fukada and Yasuda used 2,000 cycles per second and recorded both direct and indirect piezoelectrical effects. The same effect was found in both whole and demineralized bone so they concluded that it was related to the organization of the collagen molecules into a quasi-crystalline matrix instead of to the bone mineral content.

Similar observations for whole bones tested in compression and bending were made by Shamos et al. (1963). The bones were mechanically cleaned and the potential differences recorded from ring electrodes around the shaft of the bone. The potential decayed at a rate of 0.5 seconds and removal of the stress caused another potential surge of equal magnitude but opposite polarity. In this respect the results approximated those obtained from a classic piezoelectrical device of multicrystalline nature instead of from a single crystal.

In the experiments of Bassett, Becker and their associates, stress generated electrical phenomena were measured from the tibia-fibula complex of amphibians as well as standardized specimens of cortical bone taken from various bones of man and other mammals. The test specimens had all soft tissue and blood removed and care was taken to prevent heating them during preparation. All specimens were kept "dry" at all times. Specimens were tested immediately or stored at 20° C and 60% relative humidity. Stress potential was measured on fresh specimens. Various degrees of dehydration were produced by controlling the relative humidity, drying in ovens at different temperatures, or by lyophilization. Demineralization was obtained by constant agitation of the specimens in 5% formic acid solution until they were flexible. Refluxing the specimens with ethylenediamine for 30 to 40 cycles removed the organic matrix. The demineralized and anorganic specimens were then washed in running tap water for twenty-four hours followed by the same procedure in distilled water.

One end of the bone was fixed in a polyethylene clamp while it was loaded like a cantilever beam by applying a series of calibrated weights to the free end of the bone. Electrical current generated in the middle third of the shaft of the bone by the applied force was detected by "painted on" silver electrodes with pressure contacts of fine platinum wire. A 10^{11}-ohm resistor was then put into the circuit and the voltage generated across it by the current flow was measured with an electrometer and recorded on a galvanometer recorder. With this apparatus a record of 100 cps could be recorded with distortion or damping.

Becker et al. (1964) found that the initial current surge produced by the stress decayed to a steady output in a few seconds which lasted as long as the load was applied. Because of technical difficulties their observations were limited to sixty seconds but during this time no measurable decay occurred in the current. Removal of the stress produced current in the opposite direction but the amount was considerably less than when bone was loaded.

According to Shamos and Lavine (1964) the ordinary electrical properties of hard tissues are intermediate between those of good insulators and poor semiconductors. At room temperature the energy gaps are about 2.5 electron volts. They believe that the dielectric constant measurements indicate a highly ordered structure of hard tissues and that the semiconductor-rectifier theory is unnecessarily elaborate to account for piezoelectric phenomena in bone.

Piezoelectric phenomena occurring under load were investigated by McElhaney (1967) in the dry intact right femur of a 38-year-old white man who died from trauma sustained in an automobile accident. The repeatability of the results obtained were verified in specimens from fifty-two other adult human femurs. Effects of embalming were studied in three bovine femurs tested first in the fresh and then in the embalmed condition. After embalming, the bones were baked for two weeks at 105° C by which time their weights were stabilized. Baking decreased the dissipation of the electric charge which was measured at more than 600 silver epoxy quarter-inch squares cemented on the surface of the femur.

The bone was eccentrically loaded, in a vertical direction, through the head of the bone in a closed loop hydraulic testing machine. Charge amplitude, with respect to the ground, was measured with a spring-loaded contracter against the silver squares while a triangular load-time function of 50 lb amplitude was applied to the bone at a rate of one cycle per second. A 100 lb preload was applied first to stabilize the loading procedure. Load-charge relationships were not influenced by varying the preload-force amplitude combination. Repeated testing for three months verified reproducibility.

In other experiments, sections of the shaft of the same bone were tested in direct compression. Small right parallelepipeds, $0.25 \times 0.125 \times 1.00$ in, from the cor-

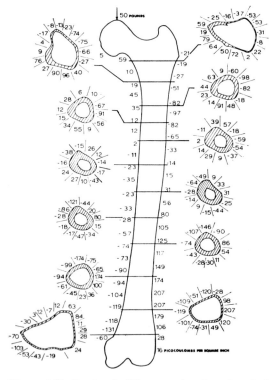

Figure 142. Regional differences in piezoelectrical properties of an adult human femur under a 50-lb compressive load. (From McElhaney: *J Bone Joint Surg*, 1967)

tex of the shaft of this and fifty-two other femurs were also tested for load-charge relationships.

The advantages of this experimental design are that the amplitude and frequency of the loads can be precisely controlled and that the charge amplifier and frequency have very high input impedances. Precise control of amplitude and frequency are important because even in well-dried bone the charge dissipates exponentially with time thus requiring dynamic measurements. High input impedance insures that charge leakage does not occur via the measuring-recording system. Load-time and charge-time histories were recorded by oscilloscopes during cycle loading of the femur in the testing machine.

A load and charge out of phase, e.g. in the compression direction, produced a positive charge indicated by a minus sign $(-)$, while a load and charge in phase, e.g. in the tensile direction, also produced a positive charge which, in this case, was indicated by a positive sign $(+)$. These were the only two-phase relationships clearly found and most regions of the femur were strongly positive or negative. Some non-linearities and phase lags were found in regions of the bone where the charge was very weak. The charge in picocoulombs divided by the area (in²) of the silver plates gave the number of picocoulombs/in² (Fig. 142). A coulomb is the standard unit of electrical charge.

The number of picocoulombs/in², some positive and some negative, varied continually but inconsistently along the length of and around the periphery of the femoral shaft. No correlations were found between charge distribution with Koch's data on stress distribution, with wall thickness, curvature, or other topographic features of the bone. This lack of correlation is attributed to the markedly different directions over the bone surface in the ordered ultra-structure necessary for the piezoelectric effect.

Similar measurements were obtained from one-inch high right cylinders from the proximal end of the femoral shaft when tested under cyclic compression loading. Sections of the intact bone which gave a positive charge and those with a negative charge gave similar results when sections of the bone were cut away and tested. In order to insure that these small specimens had only compressive strain when tested, resistance-wire strain gauges cemented adjacent to the silver squares on the bone surface recorded the strain produced in a test.

Undecalcified sections, cut parallel with and perpendicular to the long axis of the bone, revealed some histological differences in bone from areas that were strongly positive or negative. In bone from negative areas the periosteal region had significantly fewer haversian canals, more unorganized haversian bone, and more subperiosteal circumferential lamellae than sections from a comparable region that tested positively. Also, in negative bone the osteocytes and surrounding lacunae had a more random and less organized pattern than in positive bone which usually had many more young developing osteons.

In contrast to all the previous studies in which piezoelectrical phenomena were studied in dry bone, Cochran et al. (1968) investigated electromechanical properties of physiologically moist bone. For this purpose 160 thin strips of cortical bone, cut longitudinally from the middle third of the linear aspect of fifty pairs of dog femurs, were used. The bone strips were classified as Control, Standard, and Assorted Specimens, the latter including bone and calcified tissues of diverse origins.

Hand-prepared control specimens were kept moist with Hanks' Balanced Saline and tested immediately after removal.

Standard specimens were 30 mm long, 2 mm wide, and 0.6, 1.2 or 2.4 mm thick, and were stored in a 0.9% saline solution for periods of not more than seventy-two hours before testing. The majority of specimens tested were of this type.

Assorted specimens included sections of all quadrants from other long bones of adult, immature, and senile dogs. Sections of Squibb Boplant, human tibia from a bone bank, bovine mandibles, and ossified turkey tendons were also included.

Whole rat, cat, and dog femurs and tibias were tested *in vitro* with the surface fat removed by chloroform methanol if necessary.

In the *in vivo* experiments with fifteen adult cats under Nembutal anesthesia, the middle region of the right tibia or fibula was denuded—care being taken to preserve the blood supply, washed, and kept moist with Ringer's solution until tested.

An apparatus was especially designed so that the specimens could be loaded like a cantilever beam. The force was applied to the free end of the specimen by a plunger with a load cell attached to the end in contact with the specimen. A pneumatically operated piston moved the plunger whose rate of onset and velocity were controlled. In most cases the rate of deformation was 25 cm/min although a maximum rate of 30 cm/min could be used if so desired.

A slow influx of water-saturated air maintained a relative humidity of between 98% and 99.5% with variation of less than ±0.5% during a given test.

Electric potentials on the surface of the specimen were recorded by silver-silver chloride electrodes. Contact with the bone was made through a salt bridge and 0.75 mm diameter cotton wicks. *In vitro* experiments were made with a 0.9 saline bridge

TABLE XCVIII

PROGRAMS OF DEFORMATION
(Data from Cochran et al., 1968)

0-8 mm Series	*0-4 mm Series*	*Measured Rate (cm/sec)*
Normal Loading	*Normal Loading*	
0-1 (baseline)	0-1 (baseline)	25
0-2	0-0.05	20
0-3	0-1	25
0-4	0-2	34
0-5	0-1	25
0-6	0-3	35
0-7	0-1	25
0-8	0-4	40
0-1	0-1	25
Preloading	*Preloading*	
3-4	3-4	25
4-6	0-1	25
0-1		

and Ringer's solution in the *in vivo* experiments.

The test apparatus was screened. Bone potentials were recorded and amplified by a Offner Type R Dynograph Recorder with a differential input to an Offner 9808 A Electrometer Coupler. Frequency response was flat from d-c to 100 cycles. This response attenuated the absolute voltages recorded from the specimen by 10% to 20% but was adequate for comparable measurements if the pen deflections were in the same range to provide a nearly constant attenuation factor. Strain gauge and transducer recordings were also made.

All cortical specimens were tested in the same basic way. After taking the specimen from its storage place and putting it in the humidity chamber it was blotted free of excess moisture. Then 5 mm of the anatomically proximal end of the specimen was clamped in place with its periosteal surface upward. The electrode wicks were placed on opposite sides with electrode A on the inner surface opposite the plunger and 2.5 mm from the clamp. Electrode B was 2.5 mm from the plunger. Reproducibility of these positions was obtained via a lucite jig.

Prior to an experiment, potential differences between the electrode were measured and a pair of electrodes only used when the value was less than 200v.

When the plunger was fully retracted, its tip lightly touched the specimen to avoid impact loading. A predetermined amount of deformation of the specimen was produced by advancing the plunger. This constituted the first phase of the deformation cycle. Return of the specimen to its original condition by retraction of the plunger was the second phase. If the elastic limit of the specimen was not exceeded, its elasticity maintained its contact with the plunger.

Qualitative experiments to determine the voltage output with a constant rate and amount of deformation as well as quantitative experiments were performed. The latter experiments were divided into two series: (1) tests with standard specimens deformed up to 8 mm in one millimeter increments and (2) specimens deformed to 4 mm at faster rates of deformation. A specimen was only tested once at each amount of deformation.

The experiments were classified as: (1) normal loading and (2) preloading (Table XCVIII). Deformation rate was constant for each amount of loading. Deformation from the "resting position" (zero millimeters) in one continuous loading constituted "normal loading" while "preloading" was a slow deformation to a preset starting position, then one millimeter of deformation at a rapid rate. Voltage (V) produced by the first deformation cycle was measured in both types of deformation.

Reproducibility of the measurements was increased by a series of zero to one millimeter deformation cycles at a given rate. The zero to one millimeter deformations (baseline deformations) were repeated at two-minute intervals until the amplitude of the recorded potential was constant for at least five minutes. The test was then continued to the next five minutes and the "baseline" voltage rechecked periodically. Voltage data were normalized by giving recorded voltage as percentage of increase above the actual voltage produced by each zero to one millimeter "baseline" deformation.

In the *in vitro* experiments whole bones were tested like cantilever beams. In the *in vivo* experiments the bone was loaded like a simple beam.

Cochran et al. reported that the voltage wave forms in moist bone are qualitatively similar in bone from several species and persist without significant change, in spite of the variety of mechanical, physical and chemical treatment as long as the integrity of the bone is preserved.

In moist bone the voltage, secondary to charge displacement, was neutralized by charge leakage during deformation. Consequently, as the load was removed a second voltage of opposite polarity was generated. The amplitude of this second voltage was equivalent to the part of the first voltage that decayed before release of the initial deformation. This indicates the existence of a bi-directional current flow.

Forces similar to those produced by walking generated voltage in cat tibias. The voltages are qualitatively similar to those produced by a comparable preparation *in vitro* or in bending of cortical strips.

The amplitude of stress-generated voltages recorded from moist bone varied markedly with deformation rate unless it was very high. With a sufficiently high deformation rate the voltage amplitude generated by moist bone increases linearly with load through the regions of viscoelastic and plastic behavior until the bone breaks. If fatigue is present, the voltage amplitude decreases with load for a given deformation.

Voltage varies linearly with deformation in the elastic range but is nonlinear in the region of plastic deformation. The curve is almost the same as a load-deformation curve.

Cochran et al. believe that future attempts to understand the mechanism of how this electrical activity affects a biological system, the biphasic electrical signal that occurs during application, and release of a load on bone must be considered. Asymmetric wave forms are more apt to occur *in vivo* during unrestrained movements and are probably of greater significance with respect to effects on living cells.

SUMMARY

Strength and other mechanical properties of cancellous (vertebrae) and cortical bone are markedly decreased by immobilization for a few weeks.

Mechanical properties of cortical bone from purebred Beagle dogs are not significantly changed by injection of bone-seeking radioactive isotopes into the animal.

Piezoelectrical phenomena have been reported for dry and wet bone. However, it is a controversial subject and some of the investigators in the field are beginning to question its significance and reality.

CHAPTER 13

EFFECTS OF MICROSCOPIC STRUCTURE

I N ADDITION to the variables already discussed one must consider the structure of bone as a factor which also influences its mechanical properties. Since the present volume deals with bone as a material, only its microscopic structure will be discussed.

OSTEONS, LAMELLAE, CEMENT LINES AND SPACES

Rauber (1876) appears to be the first investigator to comment on the relation of the microscopic structure of compact bone to its mechanical properties. He noted that "the cell-containing bone substance is given an arrangement of particular importance for the strength of bone by the usual development into lamellae." He pointed out that the haversian canals are predominantly directed parallel to the longitudinal axis of a long bone. The outer and the inner circumferential lamellae are, according to Rauber, "particularly suited and needed to absorb bending stresses and to counteract a displacement and dislocation of haversian systems." No quantitative data were given in support of his arguments.

The relation between porosity and breaking load (under bending) in specimens of compact bone from the various quadrants of metacarpal and metatarsal bones of oxen and the anterior and the posterior aspect of the femur of a 79-year-old man was investigated by Maj (1938b). Five bony rings, 2 cm thick, were sawed at distances of 7, 12, 17, 22, and 27 cm from the proximal end of a metatarsal of a six-year-old ox. Another five rings of similar thickness were sawed at distances of 5, 8, 10, 15, and 20 cm from the proximal end of a metacarpal of the same animal. Test specimens 1.2 mm thick, 3 mm wide, and 10 to 20 mm long oriented in the long axis of the bone, were cut from the various quadrants of each ring and loaded to failure under bending. Porosity was determined by computing the volume of the cavities of the specimens.

In specimens from the anterior and the posterior aspects of the human femur the breaking load decreased and the porosity increased from the middle of the shaft toward the extremities of the bone. This was particularly true for the specimens from the posterior aspect of the bone. However, the decrease in the breaking load was not directly proportional to the porosity increase.

Maj, therefore, concluded that the degree of porosity was not responsible for variations in the breaking load except in the distal metacarpal rings in which the porosity was approximately 50%. According to Maj, regional differences in the strength characteristics of compact bone in a single skeletal segment are probably a function of the orientation and density of the collagen fibers.

Variations in the breaking strength and histological structure of specimens of compact bone from the anterior and the posterior half of metacarpal bones from two breeds of domestic cows, one from Holland and the other from Poland, were investigated by Toajari (1939). Test specimens, 1.2 mm thick and 3 mm wide, were tested like a simple beam with a span of 7 mm.

The average breaking load was greater in the posterior half of all metacarpals in both breeds of cows, but some overlapping was noted in the breaking load of individual specimens. The porosity of the bone, in terms of the percentage area of cavities (haversian canals and Volkmann's canals), was also greater in the posterior than in the anterior half of the metacarpals. Thus, the stronger half of the bone had the highest percentage (volume) of spaces. This suggests that the bone in the posterior half of the metacarpals is stronger than that in the anterior half, although the unit strength of the specimens was not determined.

The average breaking load in both halves of the metacarpal bones of the Polish cows was greater than that of the Dutch cows. On the other hand, the percentage volume of the cavities, i.e. the porosity of both halves of the metatarsals in the first and third Dutch cows, was greater than the corresponding porosity from the metacarpals in the first and third Polish cows. Thus, the degree of porosity and the breaking load seem to be parallel, the reverse of what was found in the anterior and posterior halves of the individual metacarpals in the two breeds of cattle.

The relations of osteons, osteon fragments (remnants), interstitial lamellae, and spaces of some of the mechanical properties of human cortical bone is being investigated in this laboratory.

In the first publication on this subject, Evans (1958) investigated the influence of the aforementioned histological elements on the tensile strength of standardized specimens of femoral, tibial, and fibular bone. In this and our subsequent studies the histological structure of the specimens was analyzed by a photographic-weight method.

Photomicrographs were taken of cross sections, from as near the fracture site as possible, of standardized specimens of cortical bone whose mechanical properties had been determined. Prints of the photomicrographs, enlarged to a standardized size, were then made on paper of a known weight. Knowing the weight (g) of a given area (mm²) of the paper, a conversion factor was obtained by means of which paper weight could be converted into area.

The enlarged print of the cross section was then carefully cut out, weighed and its area determined. This was called the *original break area* and corresponds to the break area measured at the time the strength and other mechanical properties of the specimen were determined. However, this break area did not allow for irregularities in the margins of or spaces within the specimen. Therefore, the spaces (representing haversian canals, Volkmann's canals, resorption spaces, and blood vessels) in the enlarged print of the cross section of the specimen were cut out, weighed and their area determined. The area of the spaces was then subtracted from the original break area to obtain the *corrected* (net) *break area* which was considered to represent the actual area, except for the lacunae and canaliculi, of bone subjected to stress during a test. Excluding the latter probably has little, if any, effect on the results of a test because, according to Frost (1960), the lacunae and the canaliculi represent an average of only 0.80% and 1.48%, respectively, of vascular-free cortical volume in human long bones.

It was found that the ultimate tensile strength, based on the corrected break area, was considerably higher than that originally calculated at the time of the test. This was to be expected because the original break area was measured with calipers and hence no allowance was made for irregularities in the margins of the specimen nor for spaces within it. Consequently, corrected break area was smaller than the original break area, which in turn means that the strength (force per unit area) based on the corrected break area, was greater than that originally computed at the time of the test.

The study also revealed that the tensile strength of the fibular specimens, which were characterized by having relatively few large osteons and fragments, was significantly greater than that of the femoral specimens which had many small osteons and fragments. Furthermore, a definite tendency was noted for fractures to follow the cement lines indicating that they represent areas of weakness where failure is most apt to occur. Consequently, the more cement lines per unit area the weaker the bone in tension. Therefore, it was concluded that many small osteons and their fragments reduce the tensile strength of bone because they provide for a greater abundance of cement lines per unit area.

Photomicrographs, taken under polarized light, showed that the fibular cross sections were darker in appearance than the femoral ones (Fig. 143). This indicated that the predominant direction of the collagen fiber bundles was more nearly parallel to the long axis of the specimen in the fibular than in the femoral specimens. Thus, the collagen fibers in the fibular specimens were in a better orientation to resist tensile stress and strain than they were in the femoral specimens.

Variations in the tensile strength of specimens of ox femoral bone of different histological types was investigated by Currey (1959) who also found a strong negative correlation between the amount of reconstruction that occurred in a piece of bone, and hence the number of osteons and tensile strength. Currey gave two complementary explanations for his results: (1) immature osteons have large central cavities thus reducing the actual amount of bone substance per unit volume, and (2) newly formed osteons are not fully mineralized and, therefore, are presumably weaker than the surrounding bony tissue.

The compressive and impact bending

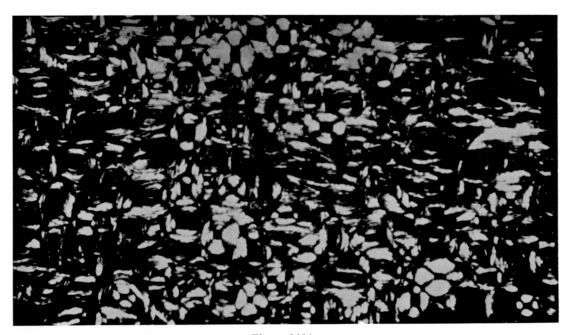

Figure 143A

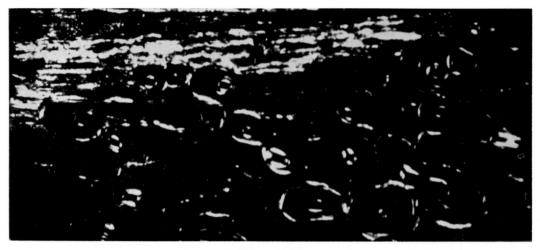

Figure 143B

Figure 143. Photomicrographs, taken under polarized light, of cross sections of a specimen from the embalmed femur of a 36-year-old Caucasian man *(A)* and the embalmed femur of a 33-year-old Caucasian woman *(B).* (From Evans: *Acta Anat,* 1958)

strength plus microhardness of primary and of haversian cortical bone from the long bones of cattle, a turtle *(Testudo graeca),* a rabbit, and man were investigated by Heřt et al. (1965). Cylinders of bone, 5 mm in diameter and 5 mm in length, with the long axis of the specimen in the longitudinal, the tangential, or the radial axis of the diaphysis of the intact bone were tested. The specimens obtained from the middle of the shaft were fixed in formaldehyde and preserved in ethyl alcohol.

The ultimate compressive strength (stress) of the specimens was determined by loading them to failure, at a rate of 5 mm/min, in a Schopper universal testing machine. Compressive stress-strain curves were obtained for a few specimens. A Charpy impact tester was used to determine the impact bending strength of unnotched cylinders. Microhardness of cross sections of the specimens was measured with a Poldi-Vickers' hardness tester and Meopta and Hanneman's microhardness apparatus (Zeiss).

TABLE XCIX

COMPRESSIVE STRENGTH OF PRIMARY AND HAVERSIAN BEEF BONE *(Bos taurus).*
LOADING SPEED = 5MM/MIN (Data from Heřt et al., 1965)

Bone Tissue	n	Dispersion kg/mm²	M ± σ kg/mm²	% Coefficient of Variation	σ M kg/mm²	σ d kg/mm²
Axial Pressure						
Primary	37	14.6-26.8	19.89 ± 2.81	14.13	0.468	0.536
Haversian	26	18.0-22.6	20.08 ± 1.30	6.47	0.262	
Radial Pressure						
Primary	4		19.37 ± 2.26			
Haversian	4		18.93 ± 1.56			
Tangential Pressure						
Primary	4		16.26 ± 1.12			
Haversian	4		15.44 ± 0.46			

TABLE C

AXIAL COMPRESSIVE STRENGTH OF PRIMARY AND
HAVERSIAN BONE. LOADING SPEED = 5 MM/MIN
(Data from Heřt et al., 1965)

Bone Tissue	Species	n	M kg/mm^2
Primary	*Testudo graeca*	5	23.77
	Oryctolagus cuniculus	5	17.72
Haversian	*Homo sapiens*	8	22.84

Data obtained in their tests showed that the average compressive strength of beef bone, in the axial direction, was slightly higher in haversian than in the primary bone but the difference was not statistically significant. Primary bone had a considerably greater dispersion than haversian bone (Table XCIX).

The compressive strength in the axial direction was greater than that in the tangential or the radial direction, a condition similar to that reported by Dempster and Liddicoat (1952) for human compact bone. Primary bone was also stronger in these directions than haversian bone. However, the number of specimens tested was not large enough for statistical evaluation. Stress-strain curves for both primary and haversian bone showed very small deformations, indicating that compact bone is a very brittle material. Comparison of the axial compressive strength of a small number of specimens from a turtle, a rabbit, and man (Table C) revealed no essential differences. The low strength values for the rabbit specimens may have been due to imperfect test specimens.

In discussing the results of their impact bending tests (Fig. 144) it is difficult to understand just what the authors mean. They state, "The values of impact bending strength keep constantly the same level. The variability of results, however, is extraordinarily striking, from 0.7 to 2.0 kg-cm, especially if compared with the values of the compressive strength." Perhaps they meant that the magnitude of the impact

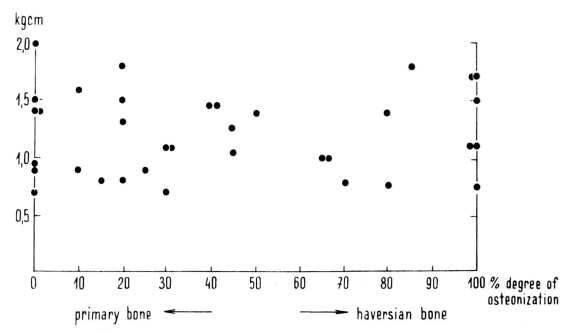

Figure 144. Impact bending strength of a cylindrical specimen of cortical beef bone tested with a Charpy impact tester. (From Heřt, Kučera, Vávra, and Voleník: *Acta Anat,* 1965)

TABLE CI

VICKERS' MICROHARDNESS (MACROMODIFICATION) OF PRIMARY AND HAVERSIAN BONE (Data from Heřt et al., 1965)

Species	Bone Tissue	No. of Samples	No. of Imprints	$M + \sigma$	Coefficient of Variation	T-test
Bos taurus	primary young	1	15	46.4 ± 3.84	8.29	
	primary old	1	18	62.7 ± 5.17	8.24	9.96
	haversian	1	13	47.2 ± 8.18	8.87	8.79
Homo sapiens	haversian	1	11	50.2 ± 6.14	6.14	

applied to the specimens was constant although the energy for failure varied.

The authors believe that this variability was the result of the low sensibility of the impact tester at low values or differences in the orientation of the specimen, because it was impossible to determine whether or not the specimens were subjected to tangential or to radial impact stress.

Histological examination of the fracture area revealed that most of the specimens had larger or smaller areas of haversian bone or haversian canals in primary bone. Separation of the two types of bone was very difficult and only approximate ratios of primary and haversian bone were obtained.

Microhardness tests of primary and haversian beef and human bone revealed no significant differences between young primary bone and haversian bone in either species (Table CI). However, microhardness of older bovine specimens was significantly greater than that of the other specimens.

The microhardness tests of individual osteons and primary lamellae, made with a Hanneman's microhardness apparatus under a 30 g load, showed that the older bovine sample (IA) consisting partly of primary (tested area) and partly of haversian bone was the hardest (Table CII). The authors believe that the high microhardness value (85 kg/mm²) of the older bone is due to greater mineralization than

in younger primary bone in which the microhardness was only 69.0 kg/mm². According to them, the coefficients of variation suggested that microhardness distribution was analogous in primary and in secondary bone.

It is the authors' belief that the mechanical properties of bone change in a typical way during growth. Young primary bone is relatively weak but its strength increases with increasing mineralization. A marked decrease in strength occurs with the onset of remodeling and only after the resorption cavities have been filled with new bone does bone strength increase and gradually stabilize with a progressive reduction in the modeling process. However, the strength of haversian bone never becomes as great as that of fully mineralized primary bone.

Recently Evans and Bang (1966) investigated the relations among several mechanical properties (ultimate tensile strength, single shearing strength, modulus of elasticity, hardness, density, and ratio between tensile and shearing strength) and the microscopic structure of forty-five femoral and thirty-two fibular specimens of embalmed adult human compact bone. The tensile strength was tested in the long axis of the specimen while the shearing strength was determined transverse to the long axis.

An analysis of variance of the mechanical properties revealed that the tensile

TABLE CII

VICKERS' MICROHARDNESS (MICROMODIFICATION) OF PRIMARY AND HAVERSIAN BEEF BONE
(Data from Heřt et al., 1965)

Species	Bone Tissue	Sample	Imprints	$M \pm \sigma$	Coefficient of Variation
Bos taurus	primary	I B	138	69.0 ± 8.7	12.6
	primary	I A	118	85.9 ± 15.2	17.7
	haversian	H 20	112	73.3 ± 10.4	14.2
	haversian	H 15	105	71.9 ± 13.6	18.9

strength and the modulus of elasticity of the fibular specimens were greater at the 0.01 significance level than the corresponding mechanical properties of the femoral specimens.

The single shearing strength of the fibular specimens was greater than that of the femoral specimens at the 0.05 significance level. No significant differences were found among the other mechanical properties of the two kinds of specimens.

A similar analysis of the various histological components showed that the number of osteons/mm², the percentage of the corrected break area formed by osteons, and the percentage of the original break area formed by spaces were greater, at the 0.01 significance level, in the femoral than in the fibular sections. However, the fibular specimens had a greater percentage, significant at the 0.01 level, of the corrected break area formed by interstitial lamellae.

A strong positive correlation, significant at the 0.01 and 0.02 levels for the fibular and femoral sections, respectively, was found between tensile strain and the percentage of the corrected break area formed by osteons. The fibular specimens also exhibited a strong positive correlation, at the 0.01 significance level, between tensile strain and the number of osteons/mm².

Strong negative correlations, at the 0.01 significance level, were found between the percentage of the original break area

formed by spaces and the modulus of elasticity, the ultimate tensile strength, and the hardness of the femoral specimens. The fibular specimens showed a strong negative correlation (at the 0.01 significance level) between tensile strain and the percentage of the corrected break area formed by interstitial lamellae, between tensile strain and the percentage of the original break area formed by spaces (at the 0.02 significance level), and between the single shearing strength and the cross-sectional area/osteon fragment (at the 0.01 significance level).

Evans and Bang (1967) extended their studies to include some specimens from embalmed adult human tibias. An analysis of variance showed that, at the 0.01 significance level, the tibial specimens had a higher tensile and shearing strength, tensile strain, modulus of elasticity, and density than the femoral specimens. Tibial specimens were significantly denser, at the 0.01 level, than fibular specimens. Tensile and shearing strength as well as the modulus of elasticity were all higher, at the 0.01 significance level, in the fibular than in the femoral specimens.

An analysis of variance of the histological components of cross sections from fifty-six femoral, seventy-nine tibial, and thirty-seven fibular specimens (Fig. 145) revealed the following differences at the 0.01 significance level: (1) femoral sections had larger osteons and osteon remnants (μ^2), which formed a greater percentage of the corrected break area than tibial sections; (2) the percentage of the corrected break area formed by interstitial lamellae was larger in the tibial than in the femoral sections; (3) femoral sections had more osteons/mm^2 and a greater percentage of the break area formed by osteons than fibular sections; (4) fibular sections had a larger percentage of the corrected break area formed by interstitial lamellae than femoral sections; (5) the number of osteons/mm^2 and the percentage of the break area formed by osteons was greater in the tibial than in fibular sections; and (6) fibular sections had larger osteons and osteon remnants than tibial sections.

Coefficients of correlation between me-chanical properties, and histological components were also computed (Table CIII). A strong positive correlation was found between the ultimate tensile strength of the specimens and the percentage of interstitial lamellae in the corrected break area. Hardness showed a strong positive correlation with the number of osteons/mm^2 and the percentage of the corrected break area formed by osteons. Strong negative correlations were found between the ultimate tensile strength and the percentage of the corrected break area formed by osteons; between the single shearing strength and the average area/osteon remnant; and between hardness and the percentage of spaces in the original break area. A negative correlation was found between mod-

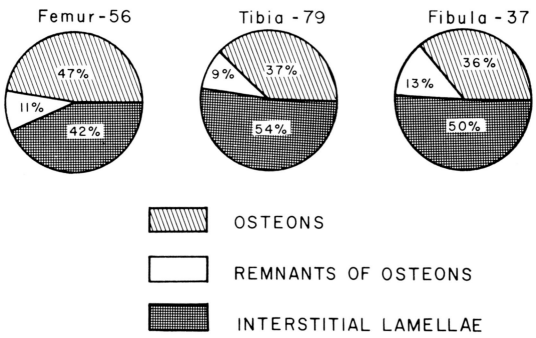

Figure 145. See text for definition of corrected break area. (From Evans and Bang: *Am J Anat*, 1967)

ulus of elasticity and the average area/osteon, and between modulus of elasticity and the percentage of the original break area formed by spaces. Single shearing strength showed a negative correlation with area/osteon.

These correlations strongly suggest that osteons and their fragments tend to decrease the tensile strength and modulus of elasticity of bone while interstitial lamellae tend to increase them. The presence of the cement lines surrounding the osteons and their fragments may account for the reduced strength of bone. The cement lines appeared to be the weakest material in the sections as evidenced by the marked tendency for fracture lines to follow the cement lines between osteons. This was true for fractures resulting from intrinsic tensile stresses and strains created by accidental drying of a section as well as by extrinsic tensile forces applied in the plane of a section. Thus, in areas of the bone with an abundance of osteons and their fragments there are more cement lines where failure can occur.

The tendency for fractures to follow cement lines between osteons was previously noted by Maj and Toajari (1937), who believed it was more frequent in decalcified than in undecalcified bone, and by Dempster and Coleman (1960). The latter investigators, on the basis of photomicrographs of wet and dry tested undecalcified specimens, concluded that the "weaker structural elements are the cement lines surrounding osteons and the planes between the lamellae of haversian systems." McElhaney (1966) also found that fractures produced at high strain rates of loading seemed to follow the cement lines bounding osteons.

Bird et al. (1968) investigated directional differences in compressive properties of fresh cortical bone from beef femurs tested at different stress rates of loading. The specimens were cylinders cut so that their long axis was longitudinal, radial, or circumferential with respect to the long axis of the shaft of the femur. At both low (1×10^2 psi/sec) and high (5×10^5 psi/sec) stress rates of loading the longitudinal specimens had the highest stress and modulus but the lowest strain to failure, while the radial specimens showed the lowest stress and the highest strain to failure. The circumferential specimens were intermediate but had the most uniform values for their mechanical properties. At the high loading rate the magnitude of the failure stress, strain, and the elastic and

TABLE CIII

CORRELATION BETWEEN PHYSICAL PROPERTIES AND HISTOLOGICAL ELEMENTS OF EMBALMED HUMAN CORTICAL BONE
(FEMUR, TIBIA, AND FIBULA) (Data from Evans and Bang, 1967)

Variables	Adjusted Number	Correlation Coefficient (R)	T-test (T)	Significance Level
E vs avg. area/osteon	115	−0.195	−2.109	> 0.05
E vs % OBA-spaces	115	−0.242	−2.648	> 0.01
UTS vs % CBA-osteons	119	−0.236	−2.628	> 0.01
UTS vs % CBA-interstitial lamellae	119	0.233	2.592	> 0.02
SSS vs avg. area/osteon	118	−0.188	−2.060	> 0.05
SSS vs avg. area/osteon remnant	118	−0.230	−2.541	> 0.02
Hardness vs no. osteons/mm²	113	0.259	2.827	> 0.01
Hardness vs % CBA-osteons	113	0.246	2.675	> 0.01
Hardness vs % OBA-spaces	113	−0.367	−4.158	> 0.001

E = tangent modulus of elasticity; OBA = original break area; UTS = ultimate tensile strength (stress); CBA = corrected break area; SSS = single shearing strength (stress); No. = number of specimens.

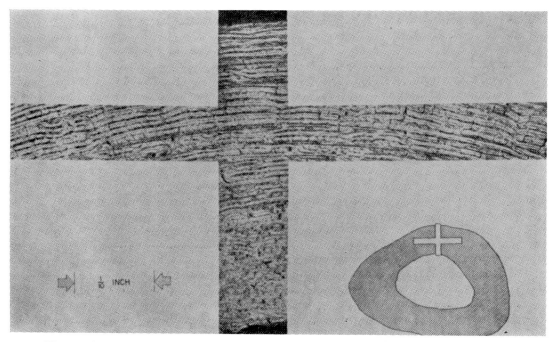

Figure 146. Photomicrograph mosaic showing details of differences in microscopic structure of bone. (From Bird, Becker, Healer, and Messer: *Aerosp Med,* 1968)

secant moduli were significantly greater than at the low loading rate.

As Bird et al. point out, osteons and collagen fibers are primarily oriented in a longitudinal direction with respect to the long axis of the bone. Therefore, one would assume that the mechanical properties in a direction perpendicular to the longitudinal axis of the bone would be the same regardless of whether the direction was radial or circumferential. The fact that this was found not to be true, Bird et al. believe, is due to structural differences in bone in the radial and circumferential directions (Fig. 146).

Photomicrographs of the surface of the samples used in the impact tests were made before and after testing in order to determine and classify damage caused by the test. Results of the tests were classified as (1) survival, (2) microcracking, and (3) gross failure. Survival was no evidence of macrocracks when examined at a 100× magnification. Gross failure was the breaking of the specimen into two or more pieces. Microcracks were found in all three categories and in many cases seemed to follow the contours of the osteons. This relation of microcracks to osteons is similar to that reported by other investigators and tends to support the contention of Evans (1958), Dempster and Coleman (1960) and Evans and Bang (1966, 1967) that cement lines are the weakest areas in bone.

COLLAGEN FIBERS AND CRYSTALS

The relationship of the predominant direction of the collagen fibers to the breaking load of twelve little parallelepipeds of cortical bone cut parallel, radial, and tangential to the long axis of ox tibias was investigated by Maj and Toajari (1937). The specimens were loaded to failure like a free simple beam and the fracture load in kilograms was determined for a span of 7 mm.

Results of the tests showed that the fracture load for specimens cut longitudinally to the long axis of the bone was three times greater than that for specimens cut tangentially and six times greater than that for specimens cut radially to the long axis of the bone. The tangentially cut specimens were about twice as strong as the radially cut ones.

Maj and Toajari explained the differences in the magnitude of fracture load on the basis of the predominant direction of the collagen fibers as revealed by polarized light in the individual specimens. In the strongest (longitudinal) specimens the collagen fibers were predominantly parallel to the long axis of the specimens, while in the weakest (radial) specimens only a few of the collagen fibers had a longitudinal orientation.

From their study Maj and Toajari concluded that (1) the resistance of compact bone to bending failure is directly proportional to the number of collagen fibers in the plane of the section of the bone; (2) the cohesiveness of the interfibrillar calcified substance is at least six times less than that of the collagen fibers; (3) the characteristic mechanical anisotropism of bone is a result of the distribution and the direction of the collagen fibers; and (4) the interfibrillar substance very probably confers homogeneity and isotropic properties to compact bone.

Olivo (1937) studied the relations between mechanical behavior and varying microscopic structures of specimens taken from various regions of metacarpal and metatarsal bones of the ox, the horse, the dog and, especially, the chamois. The regions of bone showing the highest resistance to fracture and a high modulus of elasticity had a predominance of osteons with vertically or steeply spiraling collagen fibers while areas with the least resistance to fracture had more circularly or obliquely oriented collagen fibers. Unfortunately, the actual values for the breaking load of the specimens were not reported.

The breaking strength, the modulus of elasticity, and the histological structure of cortical bone were investigated by Toajari (1938) in bones which, because of their position and function, were considered to be subjected continuously to a particular kind of mechanical stress. Test specimens, 1.2 mm thick and 3 mm wide, were cut, parallel to the long axis of the bone, from rings of bones taken from the radius, the ulna, and the olecranon process of oxen and from metacarpals and metatarsals of horses, oxen, and mules. The specimens were tested like a simple beam and progressively loaded to failure. The breaking load was computed in kilograms and the deformation, over a span of 7 mm, in 0.01 mm for 5 kg of load. Test specimens were obtained from the external, the middle, and the internal zones of the diaphysis of the bones—the external zone being nearest to the periosteum and the internal being closest to the medullary cavity.

From 271 observations Toajari concluded that, in general, the modulus of elasticity of bone increased with the increase in its breaking strength. This parallel behavior he felt was justified on the basis that the mechanical properties of bone were dependent upon the quality and orientation of the collagen fibers.

In a detailed analysis many differences, as far as its breaking strength was concerned, were found in the histological structure of the same skeletal segment. This was especially true in a large percentage of the metatarsals and the olecranon process in which the areas or zones of bone usually subjected to tension had a much higher elastic modulus and resistance to fracture than the areas of bones subjected to compression.

In a further attempt to verify his conclusions, Toajari examined splinters from fractured specimens under polarized light. He found that in longitudinal sections the luminosity of a specimen was significantly greater than in transverse sections because the collagen fibers usually ran longitudinally with respect to the major axis of the bone. A comparison of transverse sections from the strongest and the weakest specimens showed more pronounced luminosity in the latter. In the longitudinal sections the luminosity of the specimens with the greatest fracture strength (15 kg) was greater than that in the weakest specimens (9 kg).

Toajari (1939), in addition to porosity, studied differences in collagen fibers and breaking strength of compact bone from Dutch and Polish cows. He found that the higher breaking load of specimens from the Polish cows might be correlated with the greater percentage of the break area occupied by collagen fibers as well as the larger average cross-sectional area of the fibers (Table CIV). However, the specimens from the Dutch cattle had more collagen fibers/mm².

As suggested by Evans (1958) the significantly greater tensile strength of human fibular bone as compared with that of femoral bone may be partially explained by the predominantly longitudinal orientation of the collagen fibers in fibular bone in contrast to the more oblique direction of collagen fibers in femoral bone. This suggestion has recently been confirmed by Ascenzi and Bonucci (1964, 1965, 1967) and by Ascenzi et al. (1966) who dissected out and determined the tensile properties of single osteons from ox and human femurs. These investigators found that osteons with a markedly longitudinal spiral arrangement of their collagen fiber bundles had a higher tensile strength and modulus of elasticity than osteons with collagen fiber bundles whose direction alternately changed through an angle of about 90° in successive lamellae. As mentioned previously Maj and Toajari (1937) noted that their strongest specimens were the longitudinal ones whose collagen fibers were predominantly parallel with the long axis of the specimen.

Ascenzi and his associates also investigated the effects of the degree of calcification and of dehydration on the tensile properties of their osteons. They reported that drying increased the tensile strength and

TABLE CIV

Number and Size of Collagen Fibers in Metacarpal Bones of Two Breeds of Cattle
(Data from Toajari, 1939)

	Per Cent of the Area of Bony Tissue Occupied by Collagen Fibers	No. of Collagen Fibers/mm² of Bone	Average Area of Section of Collagen Fiber in Sq. Micra
Dutch Cows			
I	6.7	180,411	0.374
II	9.0	247,024	0.360
III	14.1	272,004	0.511
IV	11.2	266,902	0.410
Polish Cows			
I	30.6	147,104	2.046
II	24.6	102,695	2.338
III	15.7	152,695	1.517
IV	20.1	99,920	1.988

modulus of elasticity of the osteons but reduced the percent elongation. This confirms a similar finding reported by Evans and Lebow (1951) for larger specimens of cortical bone from adult human femurs. In wet osteons the relative degree of calcification produced significant changes in the shape of the stress-strain curves indicating an increase in the modulus of elasticity with increasing degree of calcification. The organic matrix of decalcified osteons has a modulus of elasticity similar to that of collagen. Age of the subject from whom the osteons were obtained appears to have little influence on their tensile properties. From a comparison of the tensile properties of single osteons and those of macroscopic bone specimens Ascenzi and his associates suggested "that the osteon is actually the mechanical unit of compact bone."

In a later publication, Ascenzi and Bonucci (1968) reported the results of an investigation on the compressive properties of single osteons from the shaft of adult human femurs. The method of dissecting out the individual osteons was the same as that employed in their earlier studies. In these experiments the osteon was subjected to longitudinal compressive instead of tensile stress.

On the basis of their appearance in polarized light, osteons were classified (1) light, (2) intermediate, and (3) dark. In the light (Type 1) osteons the collagen fiber bundles had a markedly transverse spiral course in successive lamellae. Intermediate (Type 2) osteons had fiber bundles in one lamella at nearly a 90° angle with those in the next lamella. Dark (Type 3) osteons had fiber bundles with a markedly longitudinal spiral course in successive lamellae. Each type of osteon in the complete and the initial stage of calcification was tested wet. Special apparatus was fabricated to test the specimens. Compressive

strain or shortening of the specimens during a test was measured with a microwave micrometer developed for that purpose.

Ascenzi and Bonucci found that ultimate compressive strength was greatest in the light (Type 1) osteons, lowest in the dark (Type 3) osteons, and intermediate in the intermediate (Type 2) osteons. In all three types of osteons the stress-strain curves for fully calcified osteons was markedly different from those of slightly calcified osteons which had a much lower modulus of elasticity. Comparison of the compressive properties of single osteons with those of macroscopic specimens supported their earlier opinion on the mechanical significance of the osteon.

Fractures of the osteons began with microscopic fissures induced by shearing. Regardless of the type of osteon the fissures were at a 30° to 35° angle with the long axis of the osteon. Electron microscopy revealed bone crystal distortion and rupture of collagen fibers at the edge of the fissures. Age had no measurable effects on the compressive properties of the osteons.

In an attempt to determine whether or not the results found by Ascenzi and Bonucci on single osteons would also apply for larger specimens, Evans and Vincentelli (1969) investigated the relation of collagen fiber orientation to the tensile properties and single shearing strength of sixteen femoral, twenty-eight tibial, and nine fibular specimens of embalmed adult human cortical bone. The tensile specimens (Fig. 8) were tested and then the middle reduced region used for the single shear tests. For details of the testing procedures see Chapter 2.

Cross sections of the specimens were made as close as possible to the fracture site and photomicrographs taken of them in polarized light. On the basis of their appearance in polarized light, osteons were classified as light, intermediate, or dark as was done by Ascenzi and Bonucci (1968). Prints of the photomicrographs were then enlarged to a standardized size and the percentage of the corrected break area formed by each of the three types of osteons and their fragments (remnants) was determined with the photomicrographic-weight method used by Evans (1958) and by Evans and Bang (1966, 1967).

On the basis of the results reported by Ascenzi and Bonucci for single osteons, it was assumed that significant positive correlations would be found between the percentage of the corrected break area formed by dark osteons and the tensile properties of the specimens. Such was not the case. None of the three types of osteons (dark, intermediate, and light) had any significant correlation with ultimate tensile strength (Table CV). However, intermediate osteons had a significant positive correlation with tensile strain (% elongation) and a highly significant positive correlation with modulus of elasticity. Light osteons had a significant negative correlation with modulus. Dark osteons had no significant correlations with any of the tensile properties or modulus of elasticity of the specimens.

Combining the osteons with their fragments (remnants) increased the correlation of the light group with the modulus of elasticity from 0.05 for osteons alone to 0.02 for the osteons plus their fragments although the correlation was still negative. However, the positive correlation between the intermediate group and modulus was decreased from 0.02 when the osteons were alone to 0.05 when they were combined with their fragments. No other correlations were found between osteons and fragments combined and tensile properties or modulus of elasticity.

Light osteons had a very high negative correlation and dark osteons an equally high positive correlation with single shearing strength (Table CV). Intermediate osteons had a high positive correlation with shearing strength. Combining the osteons with their fragments did not influence the correlation of the light or the dark group with shearing strength but reduced the correlation of the intermediate group with shearing strength from a high (0.01) to a lower (0.05) significance level.

It is interesting to note that Evans and Vincentelli also found significant differences between the means for the percentage of the corrected break area formed by different types of osteons and the different kinds of bone from which their material was obtained. Thus, the means for groups of light and dark osteons and of osteon

TABLE CV

CORRELATION COEFFICIENTS BETWEEN THE PERCENTAGE OF THE CORRECTED BREAK AREA
FORMED BY DIFFERENT TYPES OF OSTEONS AND PHYSICAL PROPERTIES OF EMBALMED BONE
(Data from Evans and Vincentelli, 1969)

	Modulus of Elasticity	Ultimate Tensile Strength	Percent Elongation	Single Shearing Strength
Light osteons	−0.315§	−0.052	−0.085	−0.474*
Intermediate osteons	0.329‡	0.283	0.313§	0.408†
Dark osteons	0.262	0.004	−0.025	0.507*

* = 0.001
† = 0.01
‡ = 0.02
§ = 0.05

fragments of the femoral and tibial sections and the means for the dark osteons and fragments of the tibial and fibular sections were significantly different at the 0.01 level. The percentage of the corrected break area formed by light osteons and their fragments in the tibial and the fibular sections were also different at the same significance level. No other significant differences were found in the histological structure of their specimens.

In a second publication (Vincentelli and Evans, 1971) a similar investigation was made on relations among mechanical properties, collagen fibers, and calcification of adult human cortical bone. This study was not directly comparable to their earlier one because it was based on unembalmed material from tibias of four white men ranging from 23 to 74 years of age. It was necessary to use unembalmed material because calcification was one of the variables involved and it might have been influenced by embalming. Collagen fiber orientation was studied by polarized light and calcification by microradiography. Osteons and their fragments were classified as before on the basis of their appearance in polarized light. Calcification of the osteons and their fragments was classified as slightly radiolucent, intermediately radiolucent, and markedly radiolucent on the basis of their appearance in the microradiographs.

The percentage of the corrected break area formed by the various types of osteons was analyzed as in their previous study.

Vincentelli and Evans found that ultimate tensile strength had a highly significant negative correlation with light osteons and an equally high positive correlation with dark osteons (Table CVI). This differed from their results with unembalmed bone for which they found no correlations between tensile strength and any of the three types of osteons. These results also varied from those reported for embalmed material in the absence of any correlations between the various types of osteons (light, intermediate, and dark) and modulus of elasticity. Light osteons had a very highly significant negative correlation and dark osteons an equally high positive correlation with tensile strain (% elongation). No correlation was found between intermediate osteons and tensile strain. Thus, the correlation between tensile strain and the various types of osteons was different than those reported for their embalmed material (*cf.* Tables CV and CVI).

Combining the different types of osteons with their fragments did not produce any significant correlations with modulus of elasticity. However, the light group (osteons plus fragments) had a very high negative correlation, significant at the 0.001 level, with ultimate tensile strength and

TABLE CVI

Correlation Coefficients Between Some Mechanical Properties of Wet, Unembalmed Cortical Bone from Tibias of Adult Men and Different Types of Osteons. See Text for Explanation of Osteon Types
(Data from Vincentelli and Evans, 1971)

	Modulus of Elasticity	Ultimate Tensile Strength	Percent Elongation
Light osteons	−0.228	−0.487†	−0.738*
Intermediate osteons	−0.010	−0.291	−0.031
Dark osteons	0.297	0.443†	0.530*

* = 0.001
† = 0.01

TABLE CVII

CORRELATION COEFFICIENTS BETWEEN SOME MECHANICAL PROPERTIES OF WET,
UNEMBALMED CORTICAL BONE FROM TIBIAS OF ADULT MEN AND DIFFERENT
RADIOLUCENT AREAS. SEE TEXT FOR EXPLANATION OF RADIOLUCENT AREAS
(Data from Vincentelli and Evans, 1971)

	Modulus of Elasticity	Ultimate Tensile Strength	Percent Elongation
Slight radiolucency	0.003	0.030	0.268
Intermediate radiolucency	−0.229	−0.409*	−0.055
Marked radiolucency	−0.153	0.008	−0.385*

* 0.05

strain. A negative correlation at the 0.05 significance level occurred between the intermediate group and tensile strength. The dark group had a positive correlation, at the 0.05 level with tensile strain.

Similar analysis of the microradiographs also revealed some significant correlations between the degree of radiolucency and mechanical properties (Table CVII). However, the number of correlations as well as the degree of significance between the various radiolucent osteons and mechanical properties was not as high as for osteons exhibiting various collagen fiber orientation (*cf.* Tables CVI and CVII). Thus, the only correlations found were a negative one between intermediate radiolucent osteons and ultimate tensile strength and between markedly radiolucent osteons and tensile strain (% elongation). Both were only significant at the 0.05 level.

The way in which various degrees of calcification would effect correlations between collagen fiber orientation and mechanical properties was investigated by partialing out the intermediate radiolucent group (which had the highest correlation with mechanical properties). Partial correlation coefficients were then computed between different osteon types, on the basis of their collagen fiber orientation, and tensile strength and strain. Interstitial lamellae, which also form a part of the corrected break area, were likewise partialed out. The results showed that the correlations found between histological components and mechanical properties still persisted although in some cases the significance level of some of the correlations was lower.

In order to estimate how accurately bone mechanical properties can be predicted from collagen fiber orientation and degree of mineralization, multiple correlations using tensile strength or percent elongation as the dependent variables, and all the histological and microradiographic components as the independent variables were computed. It was found that ultimate tensile strength and strain (% elongation) each had positive correlations, at the 0.001 significance level, with the percentage of the corrected and the original break areas formed by the various independent variables (Table CVIII). However, the magnitude of the correlation between tensile strength and the histological and microradiographic variables was greater with the original than with the corrected break area.

Two of the main constituents of bone are the collagen fibers and the hydroxyapatite crystals. As a consequence of this, several investigators have considered bone as a two-phase material, consisting of two different substances with contrasting mechanical properties which when combined is stronger than either substance alone.

TABLE CVIII

Multiple Correlation Coefficients Between Either the Ultimate Tensile Strength (UTS) or the Percent Elongation of Wet, Unembalmed Cortical Bone from Tibias of Adult Men and All Histologic and Microradiographic Variables Before (R) and After ($\overline{R}_c$) Correcting for Sample Size
(Data from Vincentelli and Evans, 1971)

Dependent Variable	Independent Variables				Break Area	R	$\overline{R}_c$	Error of $\overline{R}_c$
UTS	LF,	DF,	LO,	IO,				
	DO,	SR,	IR,	MR	CBA	0.688	0.564*	0.131
UTS	LF,	IF,	DF,	LO,				
	IO,	DO,	IL,	SP,				
	SR,	IR,	MR		OBA	0.845	0.764*	0.085
% Elongation	LF,	DF,	LO,	IO,				
	DO,	SR,	IR,	MR	CBA	0.824	0.765*	0.079
% Elongation	LF,	IF,	DF,	LO,				
	IO,	DO,	SP,	SR,				
	IR,	MR			OBA	0.838	0.764*	0.083

* 0.001.
CBA = corrected break area; OBA = original break area.
LF = light fragments, DF = dark fragments, IF = intermediate fragments, LO = light osteons, IO = intermediate osteons, DO = dark osteons, SR = slight radiolucency, IR = intermediate radiolucency, MR = marked radiolucency, SP = spaces, IL = interstitial lamellae.

The biphasic nature has been discussed by Knese (1958) who considers bone as a compound structure consisting of tension-resisting elements (the collagen fibers) and compression-resisting elements (the apatite crystals). He also assumes that bone is pre-stressed to prevent the collagen fibers from buckling under a compressive load. In support of his hypothesis of prestressed bone, Knese offers the following points: (1) the collagen fibers in bone are straight or gently curved rather than wavy or undulating as in other tissues which, he believes, indicates that the collagen fibers are under tension; (2) the course of collagen fibers in osteons is that of a catenary, e.g. a chain or a heavy rope hanging freely between two points of support, which indicates that they are stressed along their length even though no external force is acting; (3) the differences between the tensile and compressive strength of bone is not as great as would be expected for such a brittle material, but prestressing tends to produce such a similarity.

Knese gives an extensive review of the literature on the microscopic structure of bone with special emphasis on the orientation of the collagen fibers. He also discusses the mechanical significance of bone structure but gives no actual values for various mechanical properties of bone.

Currey (1964) considers bone as a two-phase material, such as fiberglass, consisting of a matrix with a low modulus of elasticity, in which are embedded hydroxyapatite crystals, with a high modulus of elasticity. He does not agree with Knese's argument that collagen fibers are straight or gently curved in bone while they undulate in other tissues or that they are in the form of a catenary in the walls of osteons. However, he thinks that Knese's argument that the difference between the tensile and compressive strength is less than would be expected for a brittle material like bone is a stronger one.

If the amount of prestressing is known, then the stresses in collagen and apatite, when bone is at the ultimate tensile or compressive stress, can be calculated for various prestress values (Table CIX). In calculating the values for the table, Currey assumed that the volumes of collagen and of apatite were equal and that each acts as it would in a compound bar, i.e. they have the same characteristics as they would if acting in bulk except for the restraining effect of the other component.

It is seen in Table CIX that the tensile stresses on the collagen must be about 20,000 lbf/in² (14.06 kgf/mm²) in order for the maximum tensile stress on the apatite to be small—5,000 to 10,000 lbf/in² (3.52 to 7.03 kgf/mm²). The amount of prestressing necessary to produce this low tensile stress in the apatite will range from 15,000 to 20,000 lbf/in² (10.6 to 14.1 kgf/mm²). With prestressing of this magnitude the apatite will be subjected to a stress of 65,000 lbf/in² (45.7 kgf/mm²) before bone failure at a compressive stress of 25,000 lbf/in² (17.6 kgf/mm²). Consequently, if prestressing occurs, it is unlikely that it could increase the apparent tensile stress of the apatite usefully without subjecting it to so much initial compression that it could not support the compressive loads acting on it near the ultimate stress. Currey cannot conceive how

such a large initial prestress could be applied. Furthermore, he does not think that the hypothesis of prestressing in bone provides any answers to problems arising from the peculiar properties of bone.

Mack (1964) has also treated bone as a two-phase material. Standardized specimens of cortical bone from the tibias of steers were treated selectively to remove the mineral, the protein, and the mucopolysaccharide components. The ultimate tensile and compressive strength and the modulus of elasticity of the specimens were then determined and compared with the same physical properties of the control specimens. The specimens were divided into five groups.

In Group 1, the organic material of twenty-eight specimens was removed by ethylenediamine in a Soxhlet's extraction apparatus at a boiling point of 117.5 to 118.5° C for forty hours and washing in running water for ten hours.

In the second group, twenty specimens were treated with Worthington collagenase prepared with bacteria in an attempt to disrupt the molecular structure. The total enzyme solution was made with 150 mg of collagenase dissolved in 1,500 cc of 0.067 molar dibasic sodium phosphate buffer so-

TABLE CIX

THE RELATION BETWEEN THE ULTIMATE STRESS IN BONE AND THE STRESS BORNE BY EACH OF THE TWO COMPONENTS WITH DIFFERENT AMOUNTS OF PRESTRESSING. IT IS ASSUMED THAT THE TWO COMPONENTS ACT AS IN A COMPOUND BAR. ALL STRESSES ARE GIVEN IN LBF/IN². E FOR APATITE ASSUMED AS 2.5×10^6 LBF/IN². + = COMPRESSION; − = TENSION. LOADING SPEED NOT GIVEN. (Data from Currey, 1964)

	Stress on Bone lbf/in²	kgf/mm²	Amount of Prestress lbf/in²	kgf/mm²	Stress in Apatite lbf/in²	kgf/mm²	Stress in Collagen lbf/in²	kgf/mm²
Compression	25,000	17.58	0	0	+46,640	+32.79	+3,360	+2.63
			5,000	3.52	+51,640	+36.20	−1,640	−1.15
			10,000	7.03	+56,640	+39.82	−6,640	−4.67
			15,000	10.55	+61,640	+43.33	−11,640	−8.18
			20,000	14.06	+66,640	+46.85	−16,640	−11.70
Tension	15,000	10.55	0	0	−27,980	−19.67	−2,020	−1.42
			5,000	5,000	−22,980	−16.15	−7,020	−4.94
			10,000	10,000	−17,980	−12.64	−12,020	−8.45
			15,000	15,000	−12,980	−9.12	−17,020	−11.97
			20,000	20,000	−7,980	−5.61	−22,020	−15.48

lution. The bones were treated with 500 cc of this solution for twenty-four hours each, under toluene, at 37° C. They were then washed for six hours in running tap water (Group II-A) and ten of them for another twenty-four hours in 500 cc of the solution and washed again (Group II-B).

The mineral content of twenty specimens (Group III) was removed by treating them in a vacuum with 9% nitric acid. Tensile specimens were treated for twenty-four hours and compression specimens for thirty-six hours. The presence of calcium was determined by staining sections of the specimens with chloraniliac acid. Roentgenograms were then taken for rapid determination of the demineralization.

Group IV specimens were treated with Versene for six months at constant agitation, in an attempt to remove minerals. However, after eight months of treatment the specimens were still incompletely demineralized, so the method was abandoned as being impractical.

The mucopolysaccharides were removed from the specimens in Group V by treatment with hyaluronidase for twenty-four hours and collagenase for twenty-four hours (Group V-A) or treatment with hyaluronidase for forty-eight hours and collagenase for forty-eight hours (Group V-B).

Mack found that the mineral component of bone was responsible for 30% of its compressive and 5% of its tensile strength whereas the protein (mainly collagen) component accounted for less than 0.1% of the compressive and 7% of the tensile strength (Table CX).

The modulus of elasticity of the mineral component of bone is 63% and 74% that of intact bone in compression and tension, respectively. Comparable values for the modulus of the protein component, in compression and tension, are less than 0.01% and 1%, respectively.

Removal of the mucopolysaccharides had no significant effect on the strength characteristics or the modulus of elasticity of bone. Treatment with collagenase alone or treatment first with hyaluronidase and then collagenase did not disturb the collagen fibers or change the ultimate strength or modulus of elasticity of intact cortical bone.

Bone consists of two main components: (1) mineral with a relatively high strength and modulus of elasticity and (2) protein (chiefly collagen) with a relatively low strength and modulus. According to Mack, mineral constitutes 70% of bone by weight and is present as finely divided units distributed in and around the collagen fibers. Protein, on the other hand, forms only 20% by weight of bone and is in the form of fine fibers. Because the ultimate strength of normal intact bone is greater than the combined strength of its components (mineral and protein) when tested separately, Mack considers bone as a two-phase material.

The two-phase nature of bone has likewise been investigated by Sweeney et al. (1965) who point out that in extracting one constituent for study it is necessary to leave the other as intact as possible.

Collagen properties were studied in specimens decalcified in *Decal* as much as possible after the specimens had been machined and before they were tested. Specimens, 0.029 inch in diameter, decalcified after nineteen hours in the solvent, maintained their shape well. After being washed in water, the specimens were translucent and as flexible as rubber.

The results obtained by Sweeney et al. were based on dense cortical bone from which the calcium was removed rather than on collagen fibrils (fibers) or on the collagen in a single osteon. Thus, the properties they found were a function not only of the strength of the collagen fibril but

TABLE CX

STRENGTH AND MODULUS OF ELASTICITY OF THE COLLAGEN AND MINERAL COMPONENTS OF BONE. LOADING SPEED IN GROUPS I, II, AND V IS 0.02 CM/MIN IN COMPRESSION; GROUP III = 0.2 CM/MIN IN COMPRESSION
(Data from Mack, 1964)

| | No. and type of specimens | Ultimate Strength (lbf/in²) | | No. of specimens | Modulus of Elasticity (× 10⁶ lbf/in²) | |
		Average	Range		Average	Range
Control Specimens						
Compression	28	21,400	14,700-30,800	28	1.48	1.14-2.00
Tension	17	14,300	11,400-17,800	12*	3.25	2.70-3.76
Group I						
Compression	10 (treated)	6,820	3,810-12,300		0.97	0.50-1.63
	8 (control)	22,600	17,800-30,800		1.54	1.07-1.93
Tension	4 (treated)	845	675-1,030		2.49	1.98-2.73
	2 (control)	16,900	16,000-17,800		3.36	2.97-3.76
Group II-A						
Compression	5 (treated)	21,900	20,100-23,900		1.61	1.47-1.78
	5 (control)	25,000	22,200-28,500		1.65	1.50-2.00
Tension	5 (treated)	14,200	12,700-17,100		0.40	0.18-1.19*
	5 (control)	14,400	11,400-16,500		0.29	0.16-0.68*
Group II-B						
Compression	5 (treated)	21,000	17,300-25,100		1.61	1.28-1.69
	5 (control)	22,700	15,100-26,400		1.40	1.27-1.60
Group III						
Compression	10 (treated)	16.9	9.2-39.2 (buckling failure)		0.000037	0.000025-0.000057
	10 (control*)	23,900	— (compression failure)		1.52	—
Tension	5 (treated)	1,010	654-1,790		0.0307	0.0253-0.0361
	17 (control)	14,300	—		3.25	—
Group V-A						
Compression	5 (treated)	18,300	16,400-22,600		1.46	1.05-1.64
	5 (control)	17,900	14,700-21,900		1.46	1.38-1.66
Tension	5 (treated)	14,500	12,300-18,200		3.28	2.78-3.85
	5 (control)	14,000	12,000-15,800		3.24	2.70-3.55
Group V-B						
Compression	5 (treated)	16,900	12,900-20,300		1.37	1.06-1.76
	5 (control)	17,800	15,300-22,300		1.32	1.14-1.54
Tension	5 (treated)	16,700	13,100-17,200		3.38	2.66-3.94
	5 (control)	13,600	12,100-14,200		3.22	2.78-3.41

Group I: Organic material removed by ethylenediamine.
Group II: Collagen disrupted by collagenase.
Group III: Minerals removed by nitric acid.
Group IV: Not used by Mack.
Group V: Mucopolysaccharides removed by hyaluronidase.
* Because of slipping of grips in testing of five specimens, their values are omitted here.

also the interrelations between fibrils, fibers, and their arrangement.

The collagen was extracted by putting the specimens in a modified Soxhlet extractor and allowing ethylenediamine, kept at a temperature of 118° C, to circulate as a continuously distilled solvent. The time required for extraction was thirty-two hours, and was performed in eight-hour periods. The specimens were then rinsed several times at room temperature in distilled water to remove all organic particles. The remaining mineral phase appeared to be unchanged. The specimens, which were white as chalk and easily scraped, were stored in alcohol and water until tested.

Because the mineral phase was very weak in tension, great care was necessary when putting the specimens into the testing apparatus. Many specimens were lost prematurely. Only five were successfully tested and their loads were so small that the reported strains (elongations) were probably inaccurate. Therefore, only the mean ultimate stress is given in Table CXI.

Compression tests of apatite were more reliable than those for tension for two reasons: (1) the compressive specimens were easily put into the testing jig and (2) apatite had a much greater compressive than tensile strength, although its compressive strength was far less than that of whole bone. The modulus of elasticity of apatite (Table CXI) is approximately 50% less while that of collagen is almost one hundred times less than in whole bone. It is interesting to note that apatite and collagen are both anisotropic, each of them having a greater strength and modulus in the longitudinal than in the transverse direction. As the authors state, "It is surprising that two constituents that are so weak by themselves combine to give strengths that compare with those of metals."

Stress-strain curves for tensile tests of collagen (Fig. 147A) showed that they underwent large strains before failure, accompanied by a noticeable reduction in the cross-sectional area of the specimens. The calculated stresses were based on their original cross-sectional areas. Three specimens (D, H, and J) which contained small amounts of calcium, had a noticeably higher tensile strength and modulus of elasticity than the other specimens. The authors presume that the roughly longitudinal orientation of the collagen fibers increases their strength in that direction.

Collagen in longitudinal tension followed Hooke's Law for a large part of the stress-strain curve (Fig. 147A). At the ultimate stress indicated in Figure 147A the specimens underwent partial failure so that the curve deviated from a straight line to final complete failure. Stress-strain curves for apatite in compression also deviated from a straight line when the specimen starts to fail (dotted line, Fig. 147B).

TABLE CXI

MECHANICAL PROPERTIES OF COLLAGEN AND APATITE ISOLATED FROM BEEF BONE.
LOADING SPEED NOT GIVEN (Data from Sweeney, Byers, and Kroon, 1965)

	Mean		Range		Mean		Range	
	lbf/in²	*kgf/cm²*	*lbf/in²*	*kgf/cm²*	*lbf/in²*	*kgf/cm²*	*×10⁶ lbf/in²*	*kgf/cm²*
Collagen	*Tensile Stress*				*Tensile Modulus of Elasticity*			
Longitudinal direction	2,403	169			30,400	2,137		
Transverse direction	848	60			16,700	1,124		
Apatite								
Longitudinal direction	983	69						
Transverse direction	452	32						
	Compressive Stress				*Compressive Modulus of Elasticity*			
Longitudinal direction	5,348	376	4,310-5,580	303-392	1,110,000	78,033	1,000,000-1,140,000	70,300-80,142
Transverse direction	2,818	698	2,460-3,820	173-269	480,000	33,744	455,000-496,000	31,987-34,869

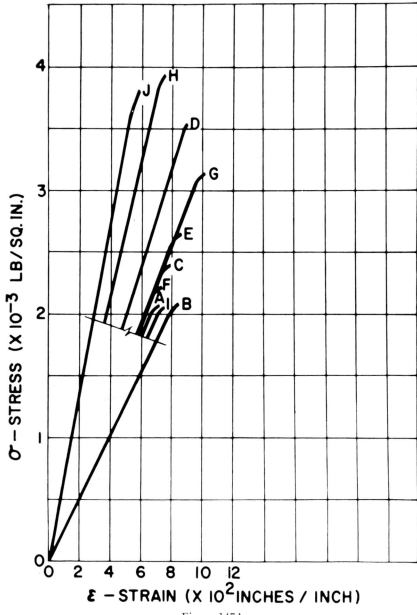

Figure 147A

In the region of the dotted line, the apatite started failing but the crushing allowed the stress to increase stepwise. Consequently, the dotted line does not represent simple plastic deformation. Generally, in both longitudinal and transverse specimens, failure occurred parallel to the axis of the specimens and often produced long thin plates. It is emphasized by the authors that their results are for a mineral structure produced by extracting the collagen from the bone. Consequently, the behavior they found is not that of individual mineral crystals, but that of a porous struc-

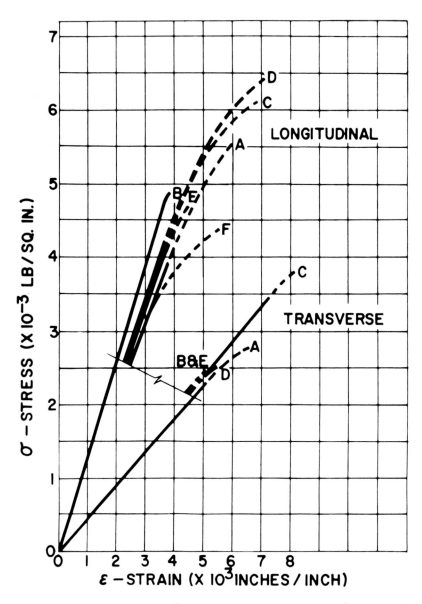

Compression tests on mineral matrix

B

Figure 147. *A*—Tensile stress-strain curves for collagen. (From Sweeney, Byers, and Kroon: ASME publ. 65-WA/HUF-7, 1965)

tural material. As they point out it would be very interesting to determine the strength characteristics of individual apatite crystals, but that is a very difficult problem.

When evaluating the data obtained by Sweeney et al. one must remember that their data are for dense cortical bone from which the collagen was removed. Consequently, their values are not those for collagen fibers alone nor for the collagen in one osteon, but those of collagen fibril strength combined with the interrelations and arrangement of the fibers.

The displacement of osteon lamellae, with special reference to the collagen fibers, under tensile and compressive stresses due to bending was investigated by Tischendorf (1951). Small L-shaped specimens of cortical bone from fresh adult human tibias were prepared so that the long arm and the short arm of the L represented the long and the horizontal axis, respectively, of the bone. The short horizontal arm was held in place while a bending force was applied to the free end of the long vertical arm, in a direction perpendicular to its long axis, by means of a thumb screw which pushed against the long arm. During bending the surface of the long arm facing the screw was subjected to tensile stresses while the opposite surface was undergoing compressive stresses.

Areas subjected to tensile and compressive stresses, in the longitudinal section of the specimen, were observed separately and at a sufficient distance from the neutral axis and the point of application of the force in order not to be affected. To investigate the effect of the bending on the cross-sectional area of the specimen the apparatus was tilted through 90°.

Specimens were tested in three steps by applying loads corresponding to one fifth, two fifths, and three fifths of the "empirically determined fracture load." Comparisons were made between the loaded and the unloaded condition. Drying was prevented by continuously wetting the specimens with Ringer's solution.

The observations were made in direct light with a Leitz-Ultropak equipped with a special condenser. The specimens were stained with supravital trypan blue so the lamellae and the collagen fibers could be visualized. Eighty photographs of the results of sixteen loadings were compared in

TABLE CXII

Summary of Hole Radius Estimates from Bone Models (Data from Stech, 1967)

Source or Model	Radius (non-dimensional)
Density	0.404-0.461
Shear Tests	0.390
Compression, column buckling failure	0.460
Compression, shear plane failure	3.375
Tensile	0.460

the loaded and the unloaded conditions. Investigations of a longitudinal section in a distinct outward shift in the lamellae on the loaded and the unloaded states showed both sides of the haversian canal. The magnitude of the shift was not the same on both sides and it was not always possible to verify identical lamellae on both sides of the haversian canal. Furthermore, the osteon is usually asymmetrical because of the strong eccentric arrangement of the blood vessels. Minute shifts were also observed in cross sections of the specimens in the loaded and unloaded conditions. The largest shifts seen were about 0.7μ and the smallest about 0.2μ.

Tischendorf concluded that (1) the collagen fibers were not calcified and, in concerted action with the ground substance, represented the mechanically effective principle; (2) minute interlamellar deflections, considerably less than one micron, were produced in the osteons by bending; and (3) minute deflections of the osteon lamellae were a stimulant for the bone cells. Thus, they probably caused and controlled a steady change in the functionally strained lamellar bone tissue.

Tischendorf's photographs clearly show the displacements of the lamellae referred to in the text of his paper. However, the actual magnitude of the force responsible for the displacements and the "empirically determined fracture load" of the specimens are not given.

TABLE CXIII

MECHANICAL PROPERTIES OF BONE BASED ON A
GEOMETRICAL MODEL (Data from Stech, 1967)

Mechanical Property	Matrix
Tensile strength	20 to 37 $\times$ 10^8 dynes/cm^2
Compressive strength	47 to 85 $\times$ 10^8 dynes/cm^2
Shear strength	23 $\times$ 10^8 dynes/cm^2
Tensile modulus of elasticity	5.95 $\times$ 10^{11} dynes/cm^2
Compressive modulus of elasticity	7.10 $\times$ 10^{11} dynes/cm^2
Density	3.0 to 3.5 gm/cm^3

An attempt to explain the anisotropy of lamellar bone, with its highly oriented collagen fibers, by a simple geometrical model was made by Stech (1967). The model was a cube with a series of holes running through it. The relationship of the holes or filler to matrix in the X and Y planes was dealt with separately for each type (compression and shear) of loading condition. Most of the model characteristics were a function of the hole radius which was a nondimensional measure of bone anisotropy (Table CXII).

Ultimate shear stress, parallel to and across the grain, was directly related to the model geometry. Cross-grain compression produced shear plane failures but compression, parallel to the axes of the collagen fibers, caused column buckling effects. Tensile strength data were more difficult to interpret in terms of the models, possibly because of crack-propagation effects.

On the basis of the model, equations were developed in connection with estimates of density and the strength characteristics of bone. The easiest and quickest application of the model was for density measurements as the author placed greater confidence in the density measurements, based on hole-size estimates, than in the strength calculations. Estimates of mechanical characteristics of bone matrix material are seen in Table CXIII.

VASCULAR PATTERN EFFECTS

Smith and Walmsley (1959), in their study of factors affecting the elasticity of bone, noted a vascular gradient effect on the modulus of elasticity of standardized specimens of cortical bone from the human tibia, the horse radius, the sheep metacarpal, and the dog femur. They determined the modulus of their specimens under pure tension and in bending produced by cantilever loading. The specimens were tested in a fluid medium and at different temperatures.

In some regions of their specimens the number and caliber of the vascular canals was found to be fairly uniform but in other regions there was a noticeable increase in the vascular field from the periosteal to the endosteal side of the specimen. On the basis of examination of cross sections of very narrow strips parallel to the periosteum of the specimen, they made a diagram (Fig. 148) showing the relative proportions of solid bone and vascular area. When the proportion of solid bone to vascular area was uniform throughout the specimen the line AB separating the two regions was perpendicular to the periosteal and endosteal surfaces of the specimen.

When the proportions of the two regions were not uniform there was a vascular gradient between the two surfaces which was expressed numerically as tan $<$ P. The AB was seldom straight but usually more like the situation found in a tibial specimen from a 72-year-old subject (Fig. 149). However, the situation seen in Figure 148 was used in their analysis.

When a vascular gradient was present the value for the modulus of elasticity varied progressively from the periosteal to the endosteal surface. If the modulus for

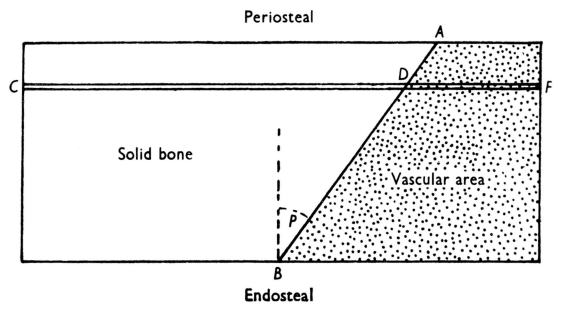

Figure 148. Diagrammatic representation of varying proportions of solid bone and vascular area in a bony rod. (From Smith and Walmsley: *J Anat*, 1959)

solid bone is assumed to be E_s then that for the elementary lamina CDF in Figure 148 will be E_s (CD/CF). Although Smith and Walmsley admit that this may be an over-simplification they are certain that the value for the elementary lamina is a function of CD, and that the suggested relationship is adequate for a qualitative analysis. In five representative cross sections, each 25×10 units in area, with a vascular gradient from zero in (a) to two in (e), the ratio of the modulus in tension (E_T) to that in bending (E_B) gave the curve seen in Figure 150 when plotted against the vascular gradient. This curve shows that the tensile modulus of elasticity (E_T) in specimens with a high vascular gradient (between 1 and 2) will be significantly greater than the bending modulus (E_B). Thus, bone with a high vascular gradient is always more flexible than is indicated by its tensile strain.

Smith and Walmsley also noted a partial lamination in some of their specimens as layers of predominantly solid bone alternated with layers of relatively porous bone. In its early stages of development bone has an extensive vascular labyrinth which is preferentially oriented in some regions so that thin layers of intervening bone, lying parallel to the bone surface, have a few radial interconnections. Primary osteons later form within the vascular labyrinth so that their longitudinal vascular canals occupy the site of the original vascular spaces. As a consequence of this, the vascular canals in cross sections of the bone appear as rows separated by solid bone. In some regions, e.g. the posterior aspect of the radius of the horse, this arrangement persists, but in other regions the vascular canals of the primary osteons enlarge into erosion spaces which are later occupied by secondary osteons. The canals of the secondary osteons usually are not aligned in the original vascular plane because the erosion phase of the reconstruction process typically progresses eccentrically from the primary osteon canals. This process results in the division of the bone

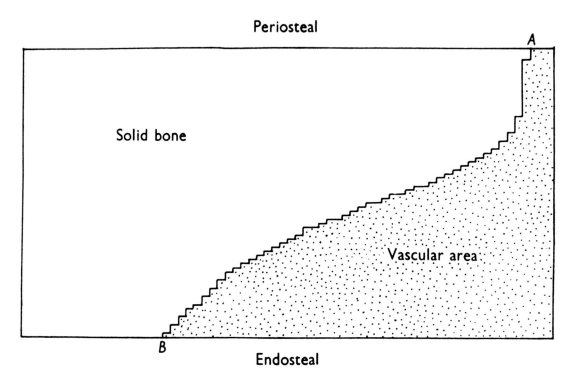

Figure 149. Variation, from the periosteal to the endosteal surface, in the proportion of solid bone to vascular area in a tibial specimen from a 72-year-old man. (From Smith and Walmsley: *J Anat,* 1959)

into vascular and nonvascular laminae which progressively become less distinct and are no longer evident in some adult mammalian bones.

Although Smith and Walmsley state that "It has not been possible to make any quantitative assessment of the physical results of such lamination . . ." they infer its effects on strain and flexibility from theoretical considerations of the effects of complete lamination. This was accomplished by comparing the theoretical effect of subjecting a solid rod and one consisting of four equal lamellae to a pure tensile stress and a bending stress produced by cantilever loading. It was found that lamination had no effect on the value for the tensile modulus of elasticity, but flexibility was increased if bending occurred at right angles to the plane of lamination. If bend-

ing occurred in the plane of lamination, flexibility was unaffected.

Smith and Walmsley also found that the elasticity of their specimens varied with the duration of stress as well as with the moisture content and temperature of the specimens. Under prolonged tensile or bending stress, immediate deformation occurred with application of the stress. This was followed by deformation that increased asymptotically with a constant stress. Cessation of stress promoted an incomplete recoil (the elastic aftereffect) followed by a similar but more prolonged asymptotic approach to zero. As a result of the elastic aftereffect the deformation of the bone occurred at a stress below the elastic limit. Deformation was a function of the duration of the stress and the difference between the immediate and ultimate deformation may be 10%. Modulus of elasticity has a similar relation to stress duration because it is computed from an observed deformation.

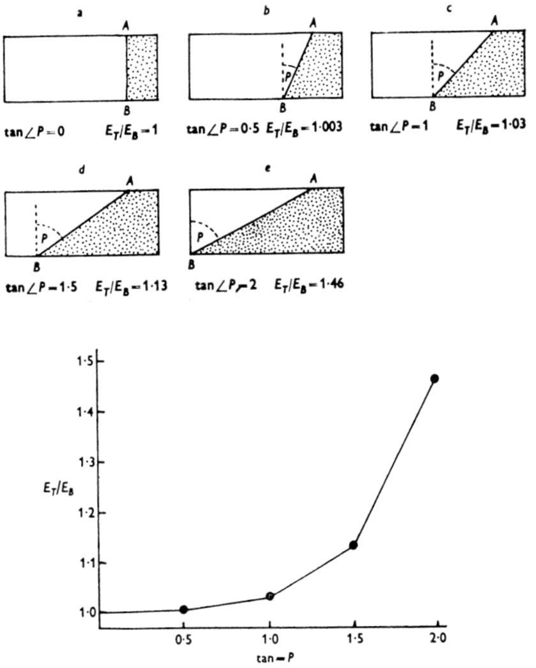

It was also reported by Smith and Walmsley that the rate of weight loss in their specimens due to evaporation progressively decreased with time, being 2.7% after five hours and 3.3% after twenty-four hours. Weight loss then continued until equilibrium with the atmosphere was established. Although weight loss varied with specimen size and atmospheric humidity it was practically complete within a week.

Tests to determine the effect of water content of a specimen on its tensile modulus of elasticity were also performed. For this purpose a tensile test was made with the specimen in a fluid. An hour later, when it was assumed that fluid loss due to evaporation had been corrected, a load was applied and the extension (tensile strain) occurring after two minutes was measured. The fluid circulation was then stopped and the specimen allowed to dry after which its contraction was observed for five hours with the extension produced by the same loading being measured at hourly intervals. After allowing for the contraction due to evaporation the strain was 7% greater at

Figure 150. Diagrammatic representation of vascular gradient and E_T/E_B ratio in 5 bone specimens. See text for explanation of the ratio. (From Smith and Walmsley: *J Anat*, 1959)

the start of the experiment than after one hour. The strain then remained constant. This experiment demonstrated that the modulus was inversely proportional to the tensile strain and that its value increased 7% during the first hour after which it remained unchanged.

SUMMARY

The mechanical properties of cortical bone are influenced by its microscopic structure. Osteons and their fragments tend to reduce the tensile strength and modulus of elasticity of bone while interstitial lamellae tend to increase them. Cement substance appears to be the weakest material in bone and fractures have a marked tendency to follow cement lines. Thus, the more osteons and their fragments in a given area of bone, the greater is the amount of cementing substance and

the lower the tensile strength and modulus of elasticity.

Microhardness is greater in older (secondary) than in younger (primary) beef bone apparently because the former is more mineralized.

The predominant orientation of collagen fibers, as revealed by polarized light, also influences mechanical properties of cortical bone. In beef bone, specimens with a predominantly longitudinal orientation of their collagen fibers have a greater breaking load in bending than do specimens with few such oriented fibers.

In individual osteons, tensile strength is greatest in those (dark in polarized light) whose collagen fibers have a steeply spiraling course around the long axis of the osteon, and least in those (light in polarized light) whose fibers have a low angle of spiral. Compressive strength is least in the former and greatest in the latter type of osteon. Osteons with fibers having an intermediate orientation (intermediate in polarized light) are intermediate in their strength characteristics.

The greater the percentage of the break area of a bone specimen formed by dark osteons the higher is its tensile strength and strain (% elongation). Light osteons have the opposite effect. The percentage of the break area occupied by intermediate osteons has no influence on tensile strain. Modulus of elasticity shows no significant correlations with the percentage of the break area formed by any of the three types of osteons.

The degree of mineralization of osteons, as revealed by microradiography, does not influence mechanical properties as much as collagen fiber orientation.

Bone, which consists chiefly of (1) mineral with a relatively high strength and modulus of elasticity, and (2) protein (collagen) with a relatively low strength and modulus, has often been considered as a two-phase material.

Mechanical properties of bone are also influenced by the amount of its vascularization. Thus, bone with a high vascular gradient is always more flexible than is indicated by its tensile strain.

Attempts have been made to explain the mechanical behavior of bone by geometrical or mathematical models.

BIBLIOGRAPHY

Aeby, K.: Ueber vergleichende Untersuchungen der Knochen. *Centralbl f d med Wissensch (Berlin)*, 10:98-102; 1872.

American Society for Testing and Materials. Terms relating to methods of mechanical testing. *Book of ASTM Standards*. ASTM Designation E 6-66. ASTM, Philadelphia, 1966.

Amprino, R.: Investigation on some physical properties of bone tissue. *Acta Anat*, 34 (3) : 161-186; 1958.

Amprino, R.: Microhardness testing as a means of analysis of bone tissue biophysical properties. In Evans, F. G. (Ed.).: *Biomechanical Studies of the Musculo-Skeletal System*. Springfield, Thomas, 1961, pp. 20-48.

Amtmann, E.: The distribution of breaking strength in the human femur shaft. *J Biomech*, 1 (4) :271-277; 1968.

Amtmann, E. and Schmitt, H. P.: Über die Verteilungder Corticalisdichte im menschlichen Femurschaft und ihre Bedeutung für die Bestimmung der Knochenfestigkeit. *Z Anat Entwicklungsgesch*, 127:25-41; 1968.

Armstrong, R. W., Arkayin, B. and Haddad, G.: Fracture of bone materials in compression at temperatures between −200° C and +200° C. *Nature*, 232 (5312) :576-577; 1971.

Arnold, J.: Quantitation of mineralization of bone as an organ and tissue in osteoporosis. *Clin Orthop*, 17:167-175; 1960.

Ascenzi, A. and Bonucci, E.: The ultimate tensile strength of single osteons. *Acta Anat*, 58:160-183; 1964.

Ascenzi, A. and Bonucci, E.: The measurements of the tensile strength of isolated osteons as an approach to the problem of intimate bone texture. *Calcif Tissue Res*, 31:325-335; 1965.

Ascenzi, A. and Bonucci, E.: The tensile proper-perties of single osteons. *Anat Rec*, 158 (4) : 375-386; 1967.

Ascenzi, A. and Bonucci, E.: The compressive properties of single osteons. *Anat Rec*, 161 (3) : 377-391; 1968.

Ascenzi, A., Bonucci, E. and Checcucci, A.: The tensile properties of single osteons studied using a microwave extensimeter. In Evans, F. G. (Ed.): *Studies on the Anatomy and Function of Bone and Joints*. Heidelberg, Springer-Verlag, 1966, pp. 121-141.

Bartley, M. H., Arnold, J. S., Haslam, R. K. and Jee, W. S. S.: The relationship of bone strength and bone quality in health, disease, and aging. *J Gerontol*, 21 (4) :517-521; 1966.

Bassett, C. A. L.: Electrical effects in bone. *Sci Am*, 213 (4) :18-25; 1965.

Bassett, C. A. L.: Electromechanical factors regulating bone architecture. In Fleich, H., Blackwood, H. J. J. and Owen, M. (Eds.) : *Third European Symposium on Calcified Tissues*. Heidelberg, Springer-Verlag, 1966, pp. 78-89.

Bassett, C. A. L. and Becker, R. O.: Generation of electric potentials by bone in response to mechanical stress. *Science*, 137:1063-1064; 1962.

Bassett, C. A. L., Pawluk, R. J. and Becker, R. O.: Effects of electric currents on bone *in vivo*. *Nature*, 204:652-654; 1964.

Baumeister, T. (Ed.) : *Marks' Standard Handbook for Mechanical Engineers*, 7th ed. New York, McGraw-Hill, 1967.

Becker, R. O.: Electron paramagnetic resonance in nonirradiated bone. *Nature*, 199:1304-1305; 1963.

Becker, R. O., Bassett, C. A. L. and Bachman, C. H.: Bioelectrical factors controlling bone structure. In Frost, H. (Ed.): *Bone Biodynamics*. Boston, Little, Brown and Co., 1964, pp. 209-232.

Bird, F., Becker, H., Healer, J. and Messer, M.: Experimental determinations of the mechanical properties of bone. *Aerosp Med*, 39 (1) :44-48; 1968.

Blanton, P. L. and Biggs, N. L.: Density of fresh and embalmed human compact and cancellous bone. *Am J Phys Anthropol*, 29 (1) :39-44, 1968.

Bonfield, W. and Li, C. H.: Deformation and fracture of bone. *J Appl Physics*, 37 (2):869-875; 1966.

Bonfield, W. and Li, C. H.: Anisotropy of non-elastic flow in bone. *J Appl Physics*, 38 (6) : 2450-2455; 1967.

Bonfield, W. and Li, C. H.: The temperature dependence of the deformation of bone. *J Biomech,* 1 (4):323-329; 1968.

Calabrisi, P. and Smith, F. C.: The effects of embalming on the compressive strength of a few specimens of compact human bone. Naval Medical Research Institute, Project NM 001 056.02, 1951.

Carlström, D.: Microhardness measurements on single Haversian systems in bone. *Experientia,* 10:171-172; 1954.

Carothers, C. O., Smith, F. C. and Calabrisi, P.: The elasticity and strength of some long bones of the human body. Naval Medical Research Institute, Project NM 001 056.02.13, 1949.

Chalmers, J. and Weaver, J. K.: Cancellous bone: Its strength and changes with aging and an evaluation of some methods for measuring its mineral content. I. Age changes in cancellous bone. *J Bone Joint Surg,* 48-A (2) :289-298; 1966.

Cochran, G. V. B., Pawluk, R. J. and Bassett, C. A. L.: Electromechanical characteristics of bone under physiologic moisture conditions. *Clin Orthop,* 58:249-270; 1968.

Coolbaugh, C. C.: Effects of reduced blood supply on bone. *Am J Physiol,* 169:26-33; 1952.

Currey, J. D.: Differences in the tensile strength of bone of different histological types. *J Anat,* 93 (1) :87-95; 1959.

Currey, J. D.: Strength of bone. *Nature,* 195 (4840) :513-514; 1962.

Currey, J. D.: Three analogies to explain the mechanical properties of bone. *Biorheology,* 2: 1-10; 1964.

Currey, J. D.: Anelasticity in bone and echinoderm skeletons. *J Exp Biol,* 43:279-292; 1965.

Davis, E., Troxell, G. E. and Wiskocil, C. T.: *The Testing and Inspection of Engineering Materials,* 3rd ed. New York, McGraw-Hill, 1964.

Dees, B. C.: *Fundamentals of Physics and Their Applications in Modern Life.* Philadelphia, The Blakiston Co., 1945.

Dempster, W. T. and Coleman, R. F.: Tensile strength of bone along and across the grain. *J Appl Physiol,* 16 (2) :355-360; 1960.

Dempster, W. T. and Liddicoat, R. T.: Compact bone as a non-isotropic material. *Am J Anat,* 91 (3):331-362; 1952.

Eichler, J.: Inaktivitätsosteoporose. *Aktuelle Orthopadie,* 3:1-80; 1970.

Evans, F. G.: Studies in human biomechanics. *Ann N Y Acad Sci,* 63 (4) :586-615; 1955.

Evans, F. G.: Relations between the microscopic structure and tensile strength of human bone. *Acta Anat,* 35:285-301; 1958.

Evans, F. G.: Regional differences in the compressive stress, strain and modulus of elasticity of human compact bone from unembalmed adult human tibias. *Anat Rec,* 139:226 (abstract) ; 1961a.

Evans, F. G.: Relation of the physical properties of bone to fractures. Instructional Course Lectures, *Am Acad Orthop Surg,* 28:110-121; 1961b.

Evans, F. G.: Significant differences in the tensile strength of adult human compact bone. In Blackwood, H. J. J. (Ed.): *Proceedings of the First European Bone and Tooth Symposium.* Oxford, Pergamon, 1964, pp. 319-331.

Evans, F. G.: Bibliography of the physical properties of the skeletal system. *Artif Limbs,* 11 (2) :48-66; 1967.

Evans, F. G.: The mechanical properties of bone. *Artif Limbs,* 13 (1):37-48; 1969.

Evans, F. G. and Lebow, M.: Regional differences in some physical properties of the human femur. *J Appl Physiol,* 3:563-572; 1951.

Evans, F. G. and Lebow, M.: The strength of human compact bone as revealed by engineering technics. *Am J Surg,* 83 (3) :326-331; 1952.

Evans, F. G. and Lebow, M.: Strength of human compact bone under repetitive loading. *J Appl Physiol,* 10:127-130; 1957.

Evans, F. G. and Lissner, H. R.: Tensile and compressive strength of human parietal bone. *J Appl Physiol,* 10 (3) :493-497; 1957.

Evans, F. G. and King, A. I.: Regional differences in some physical properties of human spongy bone. In Evans, F. G. (Ed.) : *Biomechanical Studies of the Musculoskeletal System.* Springfield, Charles C Thomas, 1961, pp. 49-67.

Evans, F. G. and Bang, S.: Physical and histological differences between human fibular and femoral compact bone. In Evans, F. G. (Ed.) : *Studies on the Anatomy and Function of Bone and Joints.* Heidelberg, Springer-Verlag, 1966, pp. 142-155.

Evans, F. G. and Bang, S.: Differences and relationships between the physical properties and the microscopic structure of human femoral, tibial and fibular cortical bone. *Am J Anat* 120 (1):79-88; 1967.

Evans, F. G. and Riolo, M. L.: Relations between the fatigue life and histology of adult human cortical bone. *J Bone Joint Surg,* 52-A (8) : 1579-1586; 1970.

Evans, F. G. and Vincentelli, R.: Relation of collagen fiber orientation to some mechanical properties of human cortical bone. *J Biomech*, 2 (1) :63-71; 1969.

Evans, F. G., Coolbaugh, C. C. and Lebow, M.: An apparatus for determining bone density by means of radioactive strontium (Sr^{90}) . *Science*, 114:182-185; 1951a.

Evans, F. G., Pedersen, H. E. and Lissner, H. R.: The role of tensile stress in the mechanism of femoral fractures. *J Bone Joint Surg*, 33-A (2) :485-501; 1951b.

Evans, F. G., Lissner, H. R. and Lebow, M.: The relation of energy, velocity and acceleration to skull deformation and fracture. *Surg Gynecol Obstet*, 107:593-601; 1958.

Friedenberg, Z. B. and Brighton, C. T.: Bioelectric potentials in bone. *J Bone Joint Surg*, 48-A (5):915-923; 1966.

Frost, H.: Measurement of osteocytes per unit volume and volume components of osteocytes and canaliculae in man. *Henry Ford Hosp Med Bull*, 8:208-211; 1960.

Frost, H. M., Roth, H. and Villaneuva, A. R.: Physical characteristics of bone. Part IV: Microscopic prefailure and failure patterns. *Henry Ford Hosp Med Bull*, 9 (1, pt.2) :163-170; 1961.

Fukada, E. and Yasuda, I.: On the piezo-electric effect of bone. *J Physical Soc Jap*, 12 (10) :1158-1162; 1957.

Fukada, E. and Yasuda, I.: Piezoelectric effects in collagen. *Jap J Appl Physics*, 3:117-121; 1964.

Galante, J., Rostoker, W. and Ray, R. D.: Physical properties of trabecular bone. *Calcif Tissue Res*, 5:236-246; 1970.

Garn, S. M.: An annotated bibliography on bone densitometry. *Am J Clin Nutr*, 10 (1) :59-67; 1962.

Gillespie, J. A.: The nature of the bone changes associated with nerve injuries and disease. *J Bone Joint Surg*, 36-B:464-473; 1954.

Göcke, C.: Beiträge zur Druckfestigkeit des spongiösen Knochens. *Bruns Beitr Klin Chir*, 143: 539-566; 1928.

Greenberg, S. W., Gonzalez, D., Gurdjian, E. S. and Thomas, L. M.: Changes in physical properties of bone between the *in vivo*, freshly dead and embalmed conditions. *Proceedings of Twelfth Stapp Car Crash Conference*. Society of Automotive Engineers, Inc., New York, pp. 271-279, 1968.

Gurdjian, E. S. and Lissner, H. R.: Deformation of the skull in head injury. A study with the "stresscoat" technique. *Surg Gynecol Obstet*, 81:679-687; 1945.

Hardinge, M. G.: Determination of the strength of the cancellous bone in the head and neck of the femur. *Surg Gynecol Obstet*, 89 (4) : 439-441; 1949.

Harris, C. O.: *Strength of Materials*. Chicago, American Technical Society, 1963.

Hazama, H.: Study on the torsional strength of the compact substance of human beings (Japanese text with English summary). *J Kyoto Pref Med Univ*, 60 (1) : 167-184; 1956.

Heřt, J., Kučera, P., Vávra, M. and Voleník, V.: Comparison of the mechanical properties of both the primary and Haversian bone tissue. *Acta Anat*, 61:412-423; 1965.

Hirsch, C. and Evans, F. G.: Studies on some physical properties of infant compact bone. *Acta Orthop Scand*, 35:300-313; 1965.

Hirsch, C. and da Silva, O.: The effect of orientation on some mechanical properties of femoral cortical specimens. *Acta Orthop Scand*, 38 (1) :45-56; 1967.

Hollingshaus, H. and Mays, C. W.: Changes in mechanical strength of bone due to internally deposited radioelements. Annual Progress Report (C00-215), Radiobiology Laboratory, College of Medicine, University of Utah, Salt Lake City, Utah, 1958.

Hubbard, R. P.: Flexure of layered cranial bone. *J Biomech*, 4 (4) :251-263; 1971.

Hülsen, K. K.: Specific gravity, resilience and strength of bone. (Russian text with German summary.) *Bull Biol Lab (St. Petersburg)*, 1: 7-35; 1896.

Ibuki, S.: Study on the shearing strength of human and animal compact bones. (Japanese text with English summary.) *J Kyoto Pref Med Univ*, 73 (6) :495-512; 1964.

Iida, H.: Study on dynamic and electric calluses of bone *in vitro*. *J Jap Orthop Surg Soc*, 31: 663-664; 1957.

Iida, H., Koh, S., Miyashita, Y., Sawada, T., Maeda, M., Nagayama, H., Kawai, A. and Kitamura, S.: On electric callus produced by an alternating current (Japanese text) . *J Kyoto Pref Med Univ*, 60:561-564; 1956.

Kazarian, L. E. and Von Gierke, H. E.: Bone loss as a result of immobilization and chelation: preliminary results in Macaca Mulatta. *Clin Orthop*, 65:67-75; 1969.

Kenedi, R. M.: Iatromathematics to biomechanics. *Proceedings,* 181 (1) :1-16. The Institution of Mechanical Engineers, London, 1966-67.

Kimura, H.: On the mechanical properties of the compact bone of a horse. *J Kyoto Pref Med Univ,* 51 (4):447-473; 1952.

King, A. I. and Evans, F. G.: Analysis of fatigue strength of human compact bone by the Weibull method. In Jacobson, B. (Ed.) : *Digest of the Seventh International Conference on Medical and Biological Engineering.* Stockholm, The Organizing Committee of the Conference, 1967, p. 514.

Knese, K. H.: Knochenstruktur als Verbundbau, Versuch einer technischen Deutung der Materialstruktur des Knochens. In Bargmann, W. and Doerr, W. (Eds.): *Zwangslose Abhandlungen aus dem Gebiet der Normalen und Pathologischen Anatomie.* Stuttgart, Georg Thieme, 1958, No. 4.

Ko, R.: The tension test upon the compact substance of the long bones of human extremities. (Japanese text with English summary.) *J Kyoto Pref Med Univ,* 53 (4):503-525; 1953.

Krause, W. and Fischer, L.: Neue Bestimmungen des specifischen Gewichts von Organen und Geweben des menschlichen Körpers. *Z Rationelle Medicin,* 26:306-334; 1866.

Lease, G. O'D. and Evans, F. G.: Strength of human metatarsal bones under repetitive loading. *J Appl Physiol,* 14 (1) :49-51; 1959.

Lexer, E. W.: Untersuchungen über die Knochenhärte des Humerus. *Z Konstitutionslehre,* 14: 227-243; 1928.

Lindahl, O. and Lindgren, A. G. H.: Cortical bone in man. I. Variation of the amount and density with age and sex. *Acta Orthop Scand,* 38: 133-140; 1967a.

Lindahl, O. and Lindgren, A. G. H.: Cortical bone in man. II. Variation in tensile strength with age and sex. *Acta Orthop Scand,* 38:141-147; 1967b.

Lindahl, O. and Lindgren, A. G. H.: Cortical bone in man. III. Variation of compressive strength with age and sex. *Acta Orthop Scand,* 39:129-135; 1968.

Lissner, H. R. and Evans, F. G.: Engineering aspects of fractures. *Clin Orthop,* 8:310-322; 1956.

Lissner, H. R. and Roberts, V. L.: Evaluation of skeletal impacts of human cadavers. In Evans, F. G. (Ed.): *Studies on the Anatomy and Function of Bone and Joints.* Heidelberg, Springer-Verlag, 1966, pp. 113-120.

Mack, R. W.: Bone—a natural two-phase material. Technical Memorandum, Biomechanics Lab., University of Calif., San Francisco-Berkeley, 1964.

Maj, G.: Resistenza meccanica del tessuto osseo a diversi livelli di uno stesso osso. *Boll Soc Ital Biol Sper,* 13 (6) :413-415, 1938a.

Maj, G.: Osservazioni sulle differenze topografiche della resistenze meccanica del tessuto osseo di uno stesso segmento scheletrico. *Monit Zool Ital,* 49:139-149; 1938b.

Maj, G.: Studio sulle variazioni indivualie topografiche della resistenze meccanica del tessuto osseo diafisario umano in diverse età. *Arch Ital Anat Embriol,* 67:612-633; 1942.

Maj, G. and Toajari, E.: Osservazioni sperimentali sul meccanismo di resistenza del tessuto osseo lamellare compatto alle azioni meccaniche. *Chir Organi Mov,* 22:541-557; 1937.

Marino, A. A., Becker, R. O. and Bachman, C. H.: Dielectric determination of bound water of bone. *Phys Med Biol,* 12 (3) :367-378; 1967.

Melick, R. A. and Miller, D. R.: Variations of tensile strength of human cortical bone with age. *Clin Sci,* 30:243-248; 1966.

Melvin, J. W., Robbins, D. H. and Roberts, V. L.: The mechanical behavior of the diploë layer of the human skull in compression. *Proceedings of the Eleventh Midwestern Mechanics Conference.* 1969a, vol. 5, pp. 811-816.

Melvin, J. W., Fuller, P. M., Daniel, R. P. and Pavliscak, G. M.: Human head and knee tolerance to localized impacts. Publ. Society of Automotive Engineers, #690477, 1969b.

Messerer, O.: *Uber Elasticitat und Festigkeit der Menschlichen Knochen.* Verlag der J. G. Cotta'schen Buchhandlung, Stuttgart, 1880.

Mueller, K. H., Tries, A. and Ray, R. D.: Bone density and composition. *J Bone Joint Surg,* 48-A (1) :140-148; 1966.

McElhaney, J. H.: Dynamic response of bone and muscle tissue. *J Appl Physiol,* 21 (4) :1231-1236; 1966.

McElhaney, J. H.: The charge distribution of the human femur due to load. *J Bone Joint Surg,* 49-A (8) :1561-1571; 1967.

McElhaney, J. H. and Byars, E. F.: Dynamic response of biological materials. ASME publ. 65-WA/HUF-9:1-8; 1965.

McElhaney, J., Fogle, J., Byars, E. and Weaver, G.: Effect of embalming on the mechanical properties of beef bone. *J Appl Physiol,* 19 (6) : 1234-1236; 1964.

McElhaney, J. H., Stalnaker, R. and Bullard, R.: Electric fields and bone loss of disuse. *J Biomech*, 1 (1):47-52; 1968.

McElhaney, J. H., Fogle, J. L., Melvin, J. W., Haynes, R. R., Roberts, V. L. and Alem, N. M.: Mechanical properties of cranial bone. *J Biomech*, 3 (5) :495-512; 1970a.

McElhaney, J. H., Alem, N. M. and Roberts, V. L.: A porous block model for cancellous bone. American Society of Mechanical Engineers, Publ. #70-WA/BHF-2, New York, 1970b.

Neuman, W. F. and Neuman, N. W.: Emerging concepts of the structure and metabolic functions of bone. *Am J Med*, 22 (1) :123-131; 1957.

Noguchi, K.: Study on dynamic callus and electric callus. *J Jap Orthop Surg Soc*, 31:641-642; 1957.

Oda, M.: The influence of the environment upon the strength of compact bone. (Japanese text with English summary.) *J Kyoto Pref Med Univ*, 57 (1) :1-24; 1955a.

Oda, M.: The strength of buried human bones. (Japanese text with English summary.) *J Kyoto Pref Med Univ*, 57 (1) :25-27; 1955b.

Olivo, O. M.: Rispondenza della funzione meccanica varia degli osteoni con la loro diversa minuta architettura. *Boll Soc Ital Biol Sper*, 12 (8):400-401; 1937.

Olivo, O. M., Maj, G. and Toajari, E.: Sul significato della minuta struttura del tessuto osseo compatto. *Bull Sci Med (Bologna)*, 109:369-394; 1937.

Policard, A. and Roche, J.: La formation de la substance osseuse. *Ann Physiol Phys Biol*, 13 (4) :663-668; 1937.

Rafel, S. S.: Temperature changes during high-speed drilling on bone. *J Oral Surg*, 20:475-477; 1962.

Rauber, A. A.: *Elasticität und Festigkeit der Knochen*. Leipzig, Wilhelm Engelmann, 1876.

Reiner, M.: The flow of matter. *Sci Am*, 201:122-138; 1959.

Reiner, M.: *Deformation, Strain and Flow*, 2nd ed. London, H. K. Lewis and Co., Ltd., 1960.

Roberts, V. L. and Melvin, J. W.: The measurement of the dynamic mechanical properties of human skull bone. *Applied Polymer Symposia*, 12:235-247; 1969.

Robinson, R. A. and Elliott, S. R.: The water content of bone. I. The mass of water, inorganic crystals, organic matrix, and "CO_2 space" components in a unit volume of dog bone. *J Bone Joint Surg*, 39-A (1) :167-188; 1957.

Rockoff, S. D., Sweet, E. and Bluestein, J.: The relative contribution of trabecular and cortical bone to the strength of human lumbar vertebrae. *Calcif Tissue Res*, 3:63-175; 1969.

Rosate, A.: Distribuzione della microdurezza del tessuto osseo nella compatta di ossa lunghe in accrescimento. *Monit Zool Ital*, Supplement 67:428-435; 1958.

Rosate, A.: Variazioni della microdurezza nell'osso primario di bovini di varia eta. *Arch Putti Chir Organi Mov*, 28:391-417; 1963.

Roth, H., Frost, H. M. and Villanueva, A. R.: Physical characteristics of bone. Part I. The existence of plastic flow *in vitro*. *Henry Ford Hosp Med Bull*, 9 (1, part 2) :149-152; 1961a.

Roth, H., Frost, H. M. and Villanueva, A. R.: Physical characteristics of bone. Part II. Biphasic elastic behavior of fresh human bone. *Henry Ford Hosp Med Bull*, 9 (1, part 2) :153-156; 1961b.

Salvadori, M. and Heller, R.: *Structure in Architecture*, 2nd ed. New Jersey, Prentice-Hall, 1963.

Sedlin, E. D.: A rheological model for cortical bone. *Acta Orthop Scand*, Supplement 83, 1965.

Seireg, A. and Kempke, W.: Behavior of *in vivo* bone under cyclic loading. *J Biomech*, 2 (4) : 455-461; 1969.

Shamos, M. H., and Lavine, L. S.: Peizoelectricity as a fundamental property of biological tissues. *Clin Orthop*, 35:177-188; 1964.

Shamos, M., and Lavine, L.: Peizoelectricity as a fundamental property of biological tissues. *Nature*, 213:267-269; 1967.

Shamos, M. H., Lavine, L. S. and Shamos, M. J.: Piezoelectric effect in bone. *Nature*, 197 (4862) :81; 1963.

Singer, F. L.: *Strength of Materials*. New York, Harper and Bros., 1951.

Smith, R. W. and Keiper, D. A.: Dynamic measurement of viscoelastic properties of bone. *Am J Med Electronics*, Oct.-Dec.:156-160; 1965.

Smith, J. W. and Walmsley, R.: Factors affecting the elasticity of bone. *J Anat*, 93 (4) :503-523; 1959.

Sonoda, T.: Studies on the strength for compression, tension and torsion of the human vertebral column. (Japanese text with English summary.) *J Kyoto Pref Med Univ*, 71 (9):659-702; 1962.

Sorenson, J. A. and Cameron, J. R.: A reliable *in vivo* measurement of bone mineral content. *J Bone Joint Surg,* 49-A (3) :481-497; 1967.

Stech, E. L.: A descriptive model of lamellar bone anisotropy. In Byars, E. F., Contini, R. and Roberts, V. L. (Eds.) : *Biomechanics Monograph.* New York, The American Society of Mechanical Engineers, 1967, pp. 236-245.

Steinberg, M. E., Bosch, A., Schwan, A. and Glazer, R.: Electrical potentials in stressed bone. *Clin Orthop,* 61:294-299; 1968.

Stevens, J. and Ray, R. D.: An experimental comparison of living and dead bone in rats. 1. Physical properties. *J Bone Joint Surg,* 44-B: 412-423; 1962.

Swanson, S. A. V., Freeman, M. A. R. and Day, W. H.: The fatigue properties of human cortical bone. *Med Biol Eng,* 9:23-32; 1971.

Sweeney, A. W., Byers, R. K. and Kroon, R. P.: Mechanical characteristics of bone and its constituents. American Society of Mechanical Engineers publication #65-WA/HUF-7:1-17; 1965.

Takezono, K., Yasuda, H. and Maeda, M.: The impact snapping strength of human and animal compact bone. (Japanese text with English summary.) *J Kyoto Pref Med Univ,* 73: 72-74; 1964.

Taysum, D. H., Evans, F. G., Hammer, W. M., Jee, W. S. S., Rehfield, C. E. and Blake, L. W.: Radionuclides and bone strength. In Doughtery, T. F., Jee, W. S. S., Mays, C. W. and Stover, B. J. (Eds.) : *Some Aspects of Internal Radiation.* Oxford, Pergamon Press, 1962, pp. 145-162.

Thompson, H. C.: Effect of drilling into bone. *J Oral Surg,* 16 (1) :22-30; 1958.

Timoshenko, S. and Young, D. H.: *Elements of Strength of Materials,* 4th ed. Princeton, D. Van Nostrand Co., 1962.

Tischendorf, F.: Das Verhalten der Haversschen Systeme bei Belastung I. Mitteilung. Untersuchungen über das Knochengewebe. *Roux' Arch Entwicklungmech,* 145:318-332; 1951.

Toajari, E.: Resistenza meccanica ed elasticita del tessuto osseo studiata in rapporto alla minuta struttura. *Monit Zool Ital,* 48:148-154; 1938.

Toajari, E.: Differenze nella struttura e resistanza meccanica del tessuto osseo in due razze *Bos taurus. Arch Sci Biol,* 25:544-557; 1939.

Tsuda, K.: Studies on the bending test and the impulsive bending test on human compact bone. (Japanese text with English summary.) *J Kyoto Pref Med Univ,* 61 (6):1001-1025; 1957.

Uehira, T.: On the relation between the chemical components and the strength of the compact bone. (Japanese text with English summary.) *J Kyoto Pref Med Univ,* 68 (4) :923-940; 1960.

Valentin, G. G.: *Lehrbuch der Physiologie des Menschen,* 2nd ed. Braunschweig, Druck und Verlag von Friedrich Vieweg und Sohn, 1847.

Vincentelli, R. and Evans, F. G.: Relations among mechanical properties, collagen fibers, and calcification in adult human cortical bone. *J Biomech,* 4 (3) :193-201; 1971.

Weaver, J. K.: The microscopic hardness of bone. *J Bone Joint Surg,* 48-A (2):273-288; 1966.

Wertheim, M. G.: Mémoire sur l'élasticite et la cohésion des principaux tissus du corps humain. *Ann Chim Phys,* 21:385-414; 1847.

Wistar, C.: In Horner, W. E., Carey, H. C. and Lea, I. (Eds.) : *A System of Anatomy,* 3rd ed. Philadelphia, 1825, Vol. I, p. 2.

Wood, J. L.: Dynamic response of human cranial bone. *J Biomech,* 4 (1) :1-12; 1971.

Woodard, H. Q.: The elementary composition of human cortical bone. *Health Phys,* 8:513-517; 1962.

Yamada, H.: Die mechanischen Eigenschaften der Knochen, besonders beim Zugversuch. (Japanese text with German summary.) *J Kyoto Pref Med Univ,* 33 (1):263-323; 1941.

Yamada, H.: In Evans, F. G. (Ed.) : *Strength of Biological Materials.* Baltimore, Williams and Wilkins Co., 1970.

Yasuda, I., Noguchi, K. and Sata, T.: On the piezoelectric activity of bone. (Japanese text.) *J Jap Orthop Surg Soc,* 28:267-268; 1954.

Yasuda, I., Noguchi, K. and Sata, T.: Dynamic callus and electric callus. *J Bone Joint Surg,* 37-A:1292-1293; 1955.

Yokoo, S.: Compression test of the cancellous bone. (Japanese text with English summary.) *J Kyoto Pref Med Univ,* 51 (3):273-276; 1952a.

Yokoo, S.: The compression test upon the diaphysis and the compact substance of the long bone of human extremities. (Japanese text with English summary.) *J Kyoto Pref Med Univ,* 51 (3) :291-313; 1952b.

Zarek, J. M.: Biomechanics—Its application to surgery. In Gillis, L. (Ed.) : *Modern Trends in Surgical Materials.* London, Butterworths and Co., Ltd., 1958, pp. 106-123.

AUTHOR INDEX

SUBJECT INDEX